Essentials of Perioperative Nursing

Third Edition

CYNTHIA SPRY, RN, MA, MSN, CNOR
International Clinical Consultant
Advanced Sterilization Products
Johnson and Johnson

JONES AND BARTLETT PUBLISHERS
Sudbury, Massachusetts
BOSTON   TORONTO   LONDON   SINGAPORE

World Headquarters
Jones and Bartlett Publishers
40 Tall Pine Drive
Sudbury, MA 01776
978-443-5000
info@jbpub.com
www.jbpub.com

Jones and Bartlett Publishers Canada
2406 Nikanna Road
Mississauga, ON L5C 2W6
CANADA

Jones and Bartlett Publishers International
Barb House, Barb Mews
London W6 7PA
UK

Library of Congress Cataloging-in-Publication Data

Spry, Cynthia.
  Essentials of perioperative nursing / Cynthia Spry.— 3rd ed.
    p. ; cm.
  Includes bibliographical references and index.
  ISBN 0-7637-4835-8 (casebound : alk. paper)
  1. Operating room nursing—Programmed instruction.   I. Title.
  [DNLM: 1. Perioperative Nursing—Programmed Instruction. WY 18.2 S771e 2005]
RD32.3.S65 2005
617'.0231—dc22

                                2004021985

Production Credits
Acquistions Editor: Kevin Sullivan
Production Director: Amy Rose
Associate Production Editor: Renée Sekerak
Associate Editor: Amy Sibley
Marketing Manager: Ed McKenna
Associate Marketing Manager: Emily Ekle
Manufacturing and Inventory Coordinator: Amy Bacus
Composition: Auburn Associates, Inc.
Cover Design: Timothy Dziewit
Printing and Binding: Malloy, Inc.
Cover Printing: Malloy, Inc.

Printed in the United States of America
09 08 07 06 05   10 9 8 7 6 5 4 3 2 1

Introduction

Nursing shortages, insufficient staff, inexperienced staff, and budget constraints have not reduced the pressure upon operating room managers to turn over rooms quickly and to work at full capacity. The number of surgical procedures escalates each year, and managers and educators are faced with the responsibility of orienting nurses with no operating room experience as quickly as possible. Nursing curriculums rarely include a course in perioperative nursing, and a morning observing surgery may be the extent of the nurse's operating room experience. Coupled with this reality is the fact that many operating rooms do not have an educator on staff. As a result, the nurse new to the operating room may be assigned to work with a senior nurse or preceptor who demonstrates excellence in practice, but who probably has not been schooled as an educator.

Essentials of Perioperative Nursing is intended as an educational tool that can be used independently by the inexperienced orientee or may serve as a supplement to the education provided by the educator or preceptor. The text can also be used by experienced perioperative nurses in preparation for the certification exam or by perioperative nurses who simply want to review basic concepts of perioperative nursing and/or test their knowledge. Finally, the educator will find the text helpful in preparing inservice programs for the entire perioperative nursing staff.

The text covers the basics of perioperative nursing and provides information the perioperative nurse must retain and skills that require early mastery to be able to function independently at an entry level. It is an introductory perioperative nursing text only and does not cover all aspects of perioperative nursing, surgical specialties, or specific procedures.

Each chapter contains learning objectives, an outline, content, references, suggested readings, section questions and answers, a test of chapter content, and a competency check-off list. There is a final comprehensive exam available on CD-ROM.

The learner may progress independently through the text and refer to the competency checklist to identify the competencies that must be achieved to complete learning related to chapter content. The educator can use the competency checklist to assess the orientee's mastery of the lesson content. Section questions throughout the text include a reference that directs the user to the information necessary to answer the question correctly. Questions are designed to test the learner's retention of information, comprehension of the material, and ability to synthesize the information.

The perioperative educator may find it most appropriate to use the learning objectives and chapter outline to prepare a lesson, and the chapter content and references to supplement other instructional materials. The test following each chapter can be used to evaluate learning. The tests can also be used as a learning needs assessment tool for the nurse with limited operating room experience or as a starting point for ongoing inservice presentations.

Objectives

Upon completion of this text, the learner will be able to:

- describe essential elements of perioperative nursing practice
- list nursing diagnoses commonly applicable to the surgical patient
- identify desired patient outcomes relative to surgical intervention
- discuss the responsibility of the perioperative nurse in achieving desired patient outcomes
- demonstrate understanding of basic principles and concepts of perioperative nursing by attaining a passing score on all tests contained in the text
- identify behavioral skills necessary to demonstrate competency in essential perioperative practice

Assumptions about the Learner

The learner:

- is a registered nurse
- may have no experience or may have varied clinical experience
- is self-motivated
- does not function at the expert level
- views knowledge of perioperative nursing practice as desirable and useful
- desires immediate feedback to identify additional learning needs
- demonstrates competence in using the nursing process

The first edition of *Essentials of Perioperative Nursing* was published in 1987 and the second in 1997. Although basic principles have not changed markedly since the last edition, practice has changed as the body of knowledge related to desired patient outcomes has grown. Evidence-based practice is a key phrase in the current literature. Essentially it means that practice should be based on evidence that what is being done has been shown to contribute to desired patient outcomes. As a result, this third edition has been significantly revised and reflects current literature and the most recent AORN Standards and Recommended Practices. One new chapter on staff safety has been added. Patient safety is the focus of much of today's research and is imperative, thus it is covered throughout the text. Staff safety, however, is equally important. Perioperative nurses work in a very high-tech, equipment-filled, oxygen-enriched environment, and on a daily basis are at risk for exposure to bloodborne pathogens, which have the potential to cause life-threatening illness. Lifting and moving patients and lifting and moving heavy equipment present significant risk for back or other musculoskeletal injury. Fire is not uncommon and in an oxygen-enriched environment can become deadly in a matter of seconds. These topics are addressed in Chapter 12.

One other addition to this third edition of *Essentials of Perioperative Nursing* is a CD-ROM with a test covering all of the material in the book. This allows the learner to work independently on a home computer.

Over the past 15 years since the first edition of *Essentials of Perioperative Nursing* was published, I have been honored by many perioperative nurses who have seen me at an AORN Congress or other meetings and have taken the time to tell me how much they appreciate my book. The nurse new to the educator role has found it a valuable teaching aid, and many nurses have used it to prepare for the certification exam. "I use your book all the time" is something I have often heard, and because of that I decided to write this latest edition. For me, it is a labor of love and a gift I can bring to the perioperative nursing community that has given so much to me and has enriched my life. I am close to retirement and consider this part of my legacy to perioperative nursing. My hope is that the book will serve as a guide to teach those nurses who will take the place of the many perioperative nurses who are also nearing retirement. At no other time in history have so many perioperative nurses been just a few years short of retirement. A shortage of nurses with perioperative experience is a threat to the profession. There are purse-string holders who believe the work of perioperative nursing can be accomplished with lesser qualified individuals who are paid lower wages than nurses. Every perioperative nurse knows that replacing nurses with ancillary personnel is not cost effective and not in the best interests of patient safety. Every surgical patient deserves a perioperative nurse. Hopefully, this book will contribute to filling the ranks of perioperative nurses with competent practitioners.

ACKNOWLEDGMENTS

I would like to thank the following people for their contributions to this third edition of *Essentials of Perioperative Nursing*:

Vangie Dennis, RN
Advanced Technology Coordinator
Gwinnett Health Systems
Lawrenceville, Georgia

Dorothy Fogg, RN
AORN Center for Nursing Practice
Denver, Colorado

Dianna Heikkila, RN
Certified Registered Nurse Anesthetist
Boise, Idaho

Cecil King, RN
Perioperative Clinical Nurse Specialist, UWMC
Clinical Instructor SON, Biobehavioral Nursing & Health Systems
University of Washington Medical Center
Seattle, Washington

Marsha Miller, RN—Author of Chapter 12, "Workplace Safety"
Manager of Professional Education
Advanced Sterilization Products
Irvine, California

Table of Contents

Introduction   iii

Chapter 1   **Introduction to Perioperative Nursing**   1
Phases of the Surgical Experience   2
   Preoperative   2
   Intraoperative   2
   Postoperative   2
Nursing Process throughout the Perioperative Period   2
   Assessment   3
   Nursing Diagnoses   3
   Planning   3
   Intervention   3
   Evaluation   3
Patient Outcomes: Standards of Perioperative Care   4
Roles of the Perioperative Nurse   4
Expanded and Advanced Practice Roles   5
Practice Settings   5
Members and Responsibilities of the Surgical Team   5

Chapter 2   **Preparing the Patient for Surgery**   11
Nursing Diagnoses   12
Desired Patient Outcomes   12
Preoperative Preparation   12
Preoperative Assessment and Interventions   14
   Overview   14
   Sources of Patient Information   14
   Assessment Parameters   14
      Physiologic   14
      Psychosocial   14
Nursing Diagnoses and Interventions   17
   Preoperative Period   17
   Intraoperative Period   18
Prevention of Wrong Site Surgery   18
Patient-Family Teaching   19
Communication of Relevant Patient Data   20

Chapter 3   **Prevention of Infection—Preparation of Instruments and Items Used in Surgery: Sterilization and Disinfection**   27
Definitions   29
Desired Patient Outcomes   29
Sterilization and Disinfection   31
   Critical, Semicritical, and Noncritical Items   31
      Critical Items—Examples   31
      Semicritical Items—Examples   31
      Noncritical Items—Examples   31
   Sterility Assurance Level (SAL)   31
   Disinfection   31

Methods of Sterilization   32
   Overview   32
   Thermal Sterilization—Steam under Pressure: Moist Heat   33
      Advantages   33
      Disadvantages   33
   Steam Sterilizers—Autoclaves   34
      Overview   34
      Gravity Displacement   35
      Prevacuum Sterilizer (Dynamic Air Removal)   37
         Bowie-Dick Test   38
      Steam-Flush-Pressure-Pulse Sterilizer   38
Flash Sterilization   38
   Overview   38
Chemical Sterilization—Ethylene Oxide Gas (EO)   40
   Description   40
      Advantages   41
      Disadvantages   41
Low–Temperature Hydrogen Peroxide Gas Plasma Sterilization   41
   Description   41
      Advantages   42
      Disadvantages   42
Chemical Sterilization—Liquid Peracetic Acid   42
   Description   42
      Advantages   43
      Disadvantages   43
Other Emerging Sterilization Technologies   43
Sterilization—Quality Control   45
   Overview   45
   Mechanical Process Indicators   45
   Chemical Indicators   47
   Biological Monitors   48
   Rapid Readout Biological Monitors   48
Record Keeping   49
Disinfection   50
   Overview   50
   Levels of Disinfectants—Application   50
      Glutaraldehyde   51
      Ortho-phthalaldehyde   51
Disinfection—Quality Control   52
Documentation   52

Chapter 4   **Prevention of Infection—Preparation of Instruments and Items Used in Surgery:
Cleaning, Packaging, and Storage**   **63**
Definitions   64
Nursing Diagnosis—Desired Patient Outcomes   65
Nursing Responsibilities   65
Preparation of Items and Instruments for Sterilization   65
   Cleaning   65
      Intraoperative Cleaning   65
      Postoperative Cleaning   66
      Manual Cleaning   66
      Mechanical Cleaning   66
      Special Protocols for Instruments Exposed to Prions   66
      Ultrasonic Cleaning   67

Lubrication   67
Inspection   68
Packaging Materials—Barriers   69
Selection Criteria   69
Types of Packaging   70
Overview   70
Woven Fabric   70
Nonwoven Materials   70
Plastic/Paper, Plastic/Tyvek®—Pouches   71
Rigid Containers   71
Principles of Packaging—Steam   72
Instruments   72
Other Items   73
Basins, Bowls, Cups   73
Rubber Goods, Tubing, Items with a Lumen, Wood Items   73
Reusable Textiles—Linen Packs   73
Packaging for Alternate Methods of Sterilization   73
Package Information and Identification   74
Chemical Indicators   74
Sealing   74
Labels   74
Shelf Life   74
Storage Considerations   74
Determining Factors   75
Reuse of Single-Use Devices   75

Chapter 5   **Prevention of Infection—Aseptic Practices: Attire, Scrubbing, Gowning, Gloving, Draping, Prepping, Creating and Maintaining a Sterile Field, and Sanitation   83**
Nursing Diagnosis—Desired Patient Outcomes   85
Overview   85
Nursing Responsibilities   85
Pathogenic Microorganisms   86
Sources of Infection (Endogenous)   86
Patients   86
Sources of Infection (Exogenous)   87
Personnel   87
Environment   87
Equipment   87
Standard and Transmission-Based Precautions   87
Control of Sources of Infection   90
Control of Patient Sources of Infection—Skin Prep   90
Control of Personnel Sources of Infection   96
Attire   96
Scrubbing, Gowning, and Gloving   97
Definitions   97
Traditional Surgical Hand Antisepsis (Traditional Scrub Procedure)   99
Use of Alcohol-Based Hand Rubs   99
Gowning and Gloving Procedure   100
Assisting Others to Gown and Glove   103
Creating a Sterile Field   106
Draping   106
Draping Guidelines   107
Standard Drapes   108
Maintaining a Sterile Field   108

Control of Environmental Sources of Infection   114
Traffic Patterns   114
Operating Room Environment   115
Operating Room Sanitation   115
Additional Considerations—Cleaning and Scheduling   117

Chapter 6   Prevention of Injury—Positioning the Patient for Surgery   131
Overview   132
Desired Patient Outcomes   132
Impact of Surgical Positioning   133
Overview of Injuries   133
Respiratory and Circulatory System Compromise   133
Neuromuscular—Injury   133
Facial Nerves   134
Brachial Plexus   134
Lower Extremity Nerves   134
Integumentary System Injury   135
Responsibilities of the Perioperative Nurse   139
Patient Advocate   139
Nursing Considerations   139
Patient Assessment   139
Planning Care   139
Additional Considerations for Positioning   140
Surgical Procedure   140
Anesthesia   140
Patient Dignity   141
Positioning Devices   141
Implementation of Patient Care   142
Transportation and Transfer   142
Initial Position Techniques   143
Basic Surgical Positions   144
Supine (Dorsal Recumbent)   144
Trendelenburg   145
Reverse Trendelenburg   146
Lithotomy   146
Sitting (Semi-sitting; Semi-Fowler's; Lawnchair)   147
Prone   148
Jackknife (Kraske's)   149
Lateral   150
Evaluating Implementation of Positioning   154
Postoperative Transfer   154
Documentation of Nursing Actions   154

Chapter 7   Prevention of Injury—Counts in Surgery   167
Description   168
Nursing Diagnosis—Desired Patient Outcome   168
Overview   168
Nursing Responsibilities   168
Count Procedures   170
Sponge Counts   170
Sharps Counts   172
Instrument Counts   172
Documentation   173

Chapter 8   **Prevention of Injury—Hemostasis, Tourniquet, and Electrosurgical Equipment**   183
Hemostasis   184
    Natural Methods of Hemostasis   185
    Artificial Methods of Hemostasis   185
        Chemical Hemostasis   185
            Thrombin   185
            Absorbable Gelatin   185
            Oxidized Cellulose   185
            Microfibrillar Collagen   185
            Styptic   186
        Mechanical Hemostasis   186
            Instruments, Ties, Suture Ligatures, Ligating Clips   186
            Bonewax   186
            Pressure   186
    Tourniquet   187
        Overview   187
        Nursing Diagnosis—Desired Patient Outcome   187
        Nursing Interventions   187
    Electrical Hemostasis—Electrosurgery   190
        Overview   190
        Electrosurgical Components   190
            The Generator   190
            The Active Electrode   191
            The Dispersive Electrode   192
        Application   193
        Nursing Diagnosis—Desired Patient Outcomes   194
            Desired Patient Outcome/Criteria   196
        Nursing Interventions—Patient and Staff Safety   196
            Electrosurgical Use During Endoscopic Surgery—Special Precautions   197
Ultrasonic Energy Devices   198
    Overview   198
    System Components   198
    Tissue Effects   198
    Technology Characteristics   199
    Applications   199
Argon Beam–Enhanced Electrosurgery   199
    Overview   199
    System Components   199
    Application/Characteristics   199
Chapter 9   **Prevention of Injury—Use and Care of Basic Surgical Instrumentation**   213
Nursing Diagnosis—Desired Patient Outcome   214
Overview   214
    Evolution of Surgical Instruments   214
    Proper Care and Handling—Departmental Impact   215
    Manufacture of Surgical Instruments   215
Nursing Responsibilities Related to Surgical Instrumentation   216
Categories of Instruments   216
    Cutting and Dissecting Instruments   216
    Clamps   218
        Hemostatic Clamps   218
        Noncrushing Vascular Clamps   218

Occluding Clamps   218
Grasping/Holding Clamps   218
Grasping Forceps   219
Retractors   219
Suction   221
Other   222
Care and Handling   225
Cleaning   225
General Guidelines for Care and Cleaning   225
Inspection   226

Chapter 10   **Prevention of Injury—Wound Management   235**
Nursing Diagnoses—Desired Patient Outcomes   236
Potential Injury   236
Desired Patient Outcomes/Criteria   236
Surgical Wounds   236
Surgical Wound Classification   236
Wound Healing   237
Primary, Secondary, and Tertiary Intention or Delayed Primary Closure   237
Process of Wound Healing   237
Suture Material   238
Classification of Suture Material   240
Monofilament and Multifilament   240
Absorbable Suture   240
Nonabsorbable Suture   241
Suture Diameter   242
Suture Selection—Considerations   242
Suture Package Information   244
Surgical Needles   245
Needle Characteristics   245
Needle Attachment   245
Other Wound Closure Devices   248
Stapling Devices   248
Skin Tapes, Skin Adhesives   248
Drains   249
Dressings   249
Nursing Responsibilities Related to Wound Management   250

Chapter 11   **Prevention of Injury—Anesthesia   259**
Potential Injury—Desired Patient Outcomes   260
Nursing Diagnoses   261
Desired Patient Outcomes   261
Outcome Criteria   261
Overview of Nursing Responsibilities   261
Preanesthesia   265
Assessment Data   265
American Society of Anesthesiologists Classification   265
Patient Teaching   266
Patient Instructions   266
Selection of Anesthetic Agents and Technique   266
Anesthesia Techniques—Overview   267
Premedication   267
Goals   267
Medications/Protocols   267
Monitoring   268
Practice Recommendations and Standards   269

Monitoring Devices 269
    Precordial or Esophageal Stethoscope 269
    Electrocardiogram (ECG) 270
    Pulse Oximetry 270
    Blood Pressure 270
    Temperature 270
    Capnography 271
General Anesthesia 273
  Inhalation Agents 273
  Anesthesia Machine 275
  Intravenous Agents 276
    Barbiturate Induction Agents 276
    Nonbarbiturate Induction Agents 276
    Dissociative Induction Agent 276
    Narcotics 276
    Tranquilizers—Benzodiazepines 276
    Neuromuscular Blockers (Muscle Relaxants) 276
  Stages of Anesthesia 280
  Preparation for Anesthesia—Nursing Responsibilities 281
  Sequence for General Anesthesia—Nursing Responsibilities 281
Malignant Hyperthermia 284
  Overview 284
  Treatment 285
  Nursing Responsibilities 286
Moderate Sedation/Analgesia 287
  Overview 287
  Nursing Responsibilities 288
Regional Anesthesia 289
  Overview 289
  Spinal 289
  Epidural and Caudal 290
  Intravenous Block (Bier Block) 290
  Nerve Block 291
  Local Infiltration 291
  Topical 291
  Regional Anesthesia—Nursing Responsibilities 292

Chapter 12   **Workplace Safety 307**
Regulations 308
Standards and Recommendations 308
Job Safety Analysis 309
Physical Hazards 310
  Fire 310
  Electricity 315
  Radiation 315
  Lifting and Moving 317
  Slips, Trips, and Falls 319
Chemical Hazards 320
  Formaldehyde 320
  Methyl Methacrylate 320
  Waste Anesthetic Gases 321
  Latex Considerations 321

Glossary 329
Index 337

Introduction to Perioperative Nursing

LEARNER OBJECTIVES

After reading and completing "Introduction to Perioperative Nursing," the learner will:

- define the three phases of the surgical experience
- describe the scope of perioperative nursing practice
- identify members of the surgical team
- discuss the outcomes a patient can be expected to achieve during surgical intervention
- describe the roles of surgical team members
- describe the responsibilities of the perioperative nurse in the circulating role

• • • • • • • • • • • • •

Lesson Outline

I. PHASES OF THE SURGICAL EXPERIENCE
    A. Preoperative
    B. Intraoperative
    C. Postoperative
II. NURSING PROCESS THROUGHOUT THE PERIOPERATIVE PERIOD
    A. Assessment
    B. Nursing Diagnoses
    C. Planning
    D. Intervention
    E. Evaluation
III. PATIENT OUTCOMES: STANDARDS OF PERIOPERATIVE CARE
IV. ROLES OF THE PERIOPERATIVE NURSE
V. EXPANDED AND ADVANCED PRACTICE ROLES
VI. PRACTICE SETTINGS
VII. MEMBERS AND RESPONSIBILITIES OF THE SURGICAL TEAM

PHASES OF THE SURGICAL EXPERIENCE

1. The surgical experience can be segregated into three phases: (1) preoperative, (2) intraoperative, and (3) postoperative. The word *perioperative* encompasses and is used to describe all three. The perioperative nurse provides nursing care in all three phases.

Preoperative

2. The preoperative phase begins at the point in time when the patient, or someone acting on the patient's behalf, makes the decision to have surgery. This phase ends when the patient is transferred to the operating room bed.

3. The preoperative phase is the period that is used to physically and psychologically prepare the patient for surgery. The length of the preoperative period varies. For the patient whose surgery is elective, the period may be lengthy. For those patients whose surgery is emergent, the period is brief or the patient may have no awareness of this period.

4. Diagnostic studies and medical regimens are initiated in the preoperative period. Information obtained from preoperative assessment and interview in this period is used to prepare a plan of care for the patient.

5. Nursing activities in the preoperative phase are directed toward patient support, teaching, and preparation for the procedure.

Intraoperative

6. The intraoperative phase begins when the patient is transferred to the operating room bed and ends with transfer to the postanesthesia care unit or other area where immediate postsurgical recovery care is given.

7. During the intraoperative period the patient is monitored, anesthetized, prepped, and draped, and the operation is performed.

8. Nursing activities in the intraoperative period center on patient safety, facilitation of the procedure, prevention of infection, and satisfactory physiologic response to anesthesia and surgical intervention.

Postoperative

9. The postoperative phase begins with the patient's transfer to the recovery unit and ends with the resolution of surgical sequelae. The postoperative period may be brief or extensive and most commonly ends outside the facility where the surgery was performed. The perioperative nurse provides care for the patient in the postoperative period. For patients that will remain in the hospital for an extended stay, the perioperative nurse may not provide care beyond patient transfer to the recovery room or postanesthesia care unit. Care in the recovery unit is assumed by postanesthesia care nurses, and care at home, if required, is delivered by home health care nurses. Recently, however, in an effort to better utilize nursing resources, many perioperative nurses have been given training in postanesthesia care and are increasingly responsible for providing care in both the operating room and postanesthesia care units.

The majority of surgeries performed today are done on an ambulatory basis. For patients who undergo surgery in ambulatory or day surgery centers, where the expectation is that they will return home on the same day they have surgery, it is not uncommon for the perioperative nurse to provide the postoperative as well as the intraoperative care.

10. Perioperative nursing activities in the immediate postoperative phase center on support of the patient's physiologic systems. In the later stages of recovery much of the focus is on reinforcing patient education in preparation for discharge.

NURSING PROCESS THROUGHOUT THE PERIOPERATIVE PERIOD

11. The words *perioperative* and *perioperative nursing* are accepted and utilized in nursing and medical literature. Perioperative nursing was formerly referred to as *operating room nursing*. Operating room nursing generally referred to patient care provided in the intraoperative period and administered within the operating room itself. However, as the responsibilities of the nurse who specialized in this area expanded to include care in the pre- and postoperative periods as well as the intraoperative period, the term *perioperative* became more appropriate. In fact the organization that represents perioperative nurses, once known as the Association of Operating Room Nurses (AORN), changed its name in 1999 to the Association of Perioperative Registered Nurses (AORN).

12. The perioperative nurse is a nurse who specializes in perioperative practice and who provides nursing care to the surgical patient throughout the continuum of care. The AORN Perioperative Patient Focused Model identifies four specific domains: patient safety, physiologic response, behavioral responses, and the health system. These are the areas of concern for the perioperative

nurse. The domains of safety, physiologic responses, and behavioral responses of patients reflect the nature of the surgical experience for the patient and serve as a guide for providing care. The fourth domain represents other members of the health care team and the health care system. Perioperative nurses work collaboratively with other health care team members to formulate nursing diagnoses, identify desired outcomes, and provide care within the context of the health care system in order to achieve desirable patient outcomes (Association of Perioperative Registered Nurses [AORN], 2004a, p. 16).

13. Perioperative nurses provide patient care within the framework of the nursing process. They use the tools of patient assessment, care planning, intervention, and evaluation of patient outcomes to meet the needs of patients who are undergoing operative or other invasive procedures. Much of perioperative nursing is technical. Equipment, instrumentation, and surgical techniques are areas of major responsibility. The patient, however, is the focus of the perioperative nurse's activities. Technical skills and responsibilities are purposeful within the nursing process during the implementation phase. The goal of perioperative nursing is to provide care to patients and support to their families. The perioperative nurse utilizes the nursing process to assist patients and their families in making decisions to meet and support the needs of patients undergoing surgical or other invasive procedures. The overall desired outcome is that the patient will achieve a level of wellness after surgery that is equal to or greater than the level prior to surgery.

14. Perioperative nursing care is provided in a variety of settings including acute care facilities, ambulatory settings, physician-based office settings, and the patient's home. Perioperative nurses provide care to patients and their families and/or those who support the patient. Three major activities of perioperative nurses are providing direct care, coordinating comprehensive care, and educating patients and their families.

Assessment

15. Nursing assessment of the patient may take place in a number of settings and time frames. Assessment may be performed a week or more before surgery or just prior to the procedure. Assessment may occur in the patient's inpatient hospital unit, the surgeon's office, the preadmission testing unit of the surgical facility, or the same-day/ambulatory surgery unit. In some instances the assessment process is initiated in a phone conversation with the patient several days prior to surgery and completed on the day of surgery at the surgical facility. Often the initial nursing assessment is performed by a nurse who is not assigned to the operating room. Although the perioperative nurse may perform the initial nursing assessment, it is more likely that the perioperative nurse will perform an assessment just prior to patient entry into the operating room. Assessment at this time will include a brief interview, a quick inspection of the patient, and a review of the patient's record, including assessment data obtained previously by other caregivers.

Nursing Diagnoses

16. Assessment data provide information that the perioperative nurse uses to formulate nursing diagnoses and identify desired outcomes. Although there are several nursing diagnoses that are typical of the surgical patient, such as knowledge deficit and high risk for infection, assessment data form the foundation for patient-specific nursing diagnoses and individualized care tailored to meet individual and unique patient needs.

Planning

17. The perioperative nurse uses knowledge of the patient, the proposed procedure, patient needs, related nursing diagnoses, and desired outcomes to plan care for the patient.

18. Care planning usually begins before the patient is seen. The perioperative nurse begins the care planning prior to interviewing the patient by combining knowledge of the planned procedure, needed resources, and common nursing diagnoses related to surgical intervention. Knowledge of the individual patient obtained during the assessment stage is combined with this previous planning to prepare for the unique needs of the patient and to provide care that is individually tailored to each patient.

Intervention

19. In the intervention stage of the nursing process the perioperative nurse provides, coordinates, supervises, and documents care within the framework of accepted standards of nursing care, such as the standards of clinical practice and professional performance developed by AORN.

Evaluation

20. In the final evaluation stage of the nursing process, the perioperative nurse evaluates the results of nursing care in relation to how well expected patient outcomes have been met.

PATIENT OUTCOMES: STANDARDS OF PERIOPERATIVE CARE

21. Perioperative nursing is patient oriented, not task oriented. Perioperative nurses must use knowledge, judgment, and skill based on the principles of biological, physiological, behavioral, social, and nursing sciences to plan and implement care to achieve desired patient outcomes (AORN, 2004a, p. 17). The Association of Perioperative Registered Nurses (AORN, 2004b) has identified patient outcomes that describe the results a patient can expect to achieve during surgical interventions. These standards reflect the responsibilities of the perioperative nurse and may serve as a framework to evaluate patient response to perioperative nursing interventions. They are as follows:

- The patient is free from signs and symptoms of injury caused by extraneous objects.
- The patient is free from signs and symptoms of chemical injury.
- The patient is free from signs and symptoms of electrical injury.
- The patient is free of signs and symptoms of injury related to positioning.
- The patient is free from signs and symptoms of laser injury.
- The patient is free from signs and symptoms of radiation injury.
- The patient is free from signs and symptoms of injury related to transfer/transport.
- The patient receives appropriate medication(s) safely administered during the perioperative period.
- The patient is free from signs and symptoms of infection.
- The patient has wound/tissue perfusion consistent with or improved from baseline levels established preoperatively.
- The patient is at or returning to normothermia at the conclusion of the immediate postoperative period.
- The patient's fluid, electrolyte, and acid-base balances are consistent with or improved from baseline levels established preoperatively.
- The patient's respiratory function is consistent with or improved from baseline levels established preoperatively.
- The patient's cardiovascular function is consistent with or improved from baseline levels established preoperatively.

- The patient demonstrates and/or reports adequate pain control throughout the preoperative period.
- The patient's neurological function is consistent with or improved from baseline levels established preoperatively.
- The patient demonstrates knowledge of expected responses to the operative or invasive procedure.
- The patient demonstrates knowledge of nutritional requirements related to the operative or other invasive procedure.
- The patient demonstrates knowledge of medication management.
- The patient demonstrates knowledge of pain management.
- The patient participates in the rehabilitation process.
- The patient demonstrates knowledge of wound healing.
- The patient participates in decisions affecting his or her perioperative care.
- The patient's care is consistent with the perioperative plan of care.
- The patient's right to privacy is maintained.
- The patient is the recipient of competent and ethical care within legal standards of practice.
- The patient receives consistent and comparable care regardless of the setting.
- The patient's value system, lifestyle, ethnicity, and culture are considered, respected, and incorporated in the perioperative plan of care. (pp. 197–206)

Other desired patient outcomes not specifically listed in the AORN Outcome Standards may be identified by the perioperative nurse and included in the plan of care. New knowledge regarding patient response to surgery and the effect of nursing interventions will lead to new desired patient outcomes that have implications for perioperative nursing practice. The perioperative nurse who plans patient care should be guided by, but not limited by, established patient outcome standards. (See AORN's *Perioperative Nursing Data Set,* 2nd edition for more information.)

ROLES OF THE PERIOPERATIVE NURSE

22. Perioperative nurses function in various roles, including those of manager/director, clinical practitioner (e.g., scrub nurse, circulating nurse,

clinical nurse specialist), educator, and researcher. In these roles responsibilities include but are not limited:

- patient assessment before, during, and after surgery
- patient and family teaching
- patient and family support and reassurance
- patient advocacy
- performing as scrub or circulating nurse during surgery
- control of the environment
- efficient provision of resources
- coordination of activities related to patient care
- collaboration and consultation with other health care team members
- maintenance of asepsis
- ongoing monitoring of patient's physiological and psychological status
- supervision of ancillary personnel

Additional responsibilities that promote personal and professional growth and contribute to the profession of perioperative nursing include but are not limited to:

- participation in professional organization activities
- participation in research activities that support the profession of perioperative nursing
- exploration and validation of current and future practice
- participation in continuing education programs to enhance personal knowledge and development and to promote the profession of perioperative nursing
- functioning as a role model for nursing students and perioperative nursing colleagues
- mentoring other perioperative nurses

EXPANDED AND ADVANCED PRACTICE ROLES

23. The Registered Nurse First Assistant (RNFA) is an expanded role of perioperative nursing. The RNFA practices under the direction of the surgeon and assists the surgeon during the intraoperative phase of the perioperative experience. A more complete definition of the RNFA and the qualifications for this role are outlined in the Revised AORN Official Position Statement on RN First Assistants (AORN, 2004c, p. 163).

24. The perioperative nurse with an advanced/graduate degree may function in an advanced

role. Examples of advanced practice roles are Clinical Nurse Specialist, Nurse Practitioner, and RNFA. Responsibilities and job description may vary with employment setting.

PRACTICE SETTINGS

25. Technological advances have resulted in dramatic changes in surgical technique within the last 15 years. Many procedures that once involved utilizing a hospital-based operating room, that necessitated a large incision, and that required a hospital stay and an extended recovery can now be performed in same-day or ambulatory settings. Minimally invasive surgical techniques, in which surgery is performed through a small puncture hole with specialized instruments and equipment, facilitate rapid recovery and same-day discharge. Reimbursement guidelines also encourage same-day or ambulatory surgery and early discharge. As a result, surgery has moved into settings outside the acute-care hospital-based operating room. These settings include free-standing surgical centers, satellite surgery facilities, mobile surgical units, surgeon office–based operating rooms, and clinics. As long as reimbursement favors physician office–based surgery, the numbers of surgeries performed in the physician's offices will continue to increase.

26. Perioperative nursing, once practiced exclusively within the hospital, is now practiced in a variety of settings. However, the needs of the patient undergoing surgery transcend the setting, and in all settings the perioperative nurse brings specialized skills, technical competence, knowledge, and caring that is essential to a successful surgical experience.

MEMBERS AND RESPONSIBILITIES OF THE SURGICAL TEAM

27. Safe and effective care of the patient in surgery requires a team effort. Each member of the surgical team brings unique skills that must be coordinated to achieve the desired patient outcomes.

28. Team members may be categorized according to their responsibilities during the procedure. Sterile team members are those who scrub their hands and arms, don sterile attire, contact sterile instruments and supplies, and work in the sterile field, i.e., the area immediately surrounding the surgical site. They are referred to as the "scrubbed" members of the team.

29. Members of the sterile surgical team may include the primary surgeon; assistants to the

surgeon, i.e., other surgeons, residents, physician assistants, and RNFAs; and the scrub person, who may be a registered nurse, a licensed practical nurse, a surgical technologist, or a surgical technician.

30. Members of the nonsterile surgical team carry out their responsibilities outside the sterile field and do not wear sterile attire. Members of the nonsterile surgical team may include the anesthesiologist, the nurse anesthetist, the circulating nurse, and others.

31. The primary surgeon is responsible for the preoperative diagnosis, selection of the procedure to be performed, and the actual performance of surgery.

32. The assistants work under the direction of the primary surgeon and are responsible for providing assistance during surgery, such as exposing the site, suctioning, handling tissue, and suturing. The nature of the surgery, the state in which the surgery is performed, the medical board and the boards of nursing regulations, the surgeon's preference, and the hospital policies are factors that determine who may function as an assistant.

33. The scrub person works primarily with instruments and equipment. Responsibilities of the scrub person may include:

    - selecting instruments, equipment, and other supplies appropriate for the surgery
    - preparing the sterile field and setting up sterile table(s) with instruments and other sterile supplies needed for the procedure
    - scrubbing, donning gown and gloves
    - maintaining integrity and sterility of the sterile field throughout the procedure
    - having knowledge of the procedure and anticipating the surgeon's needs throughout
    - providing instruments, sutures, and supplies to the surgeon in an appropriate and timely manner
    - preparing sterile dressings
    - implementing procedures that contribute to patient safety, i.e., surgical counts for instruments, sponges, and sharps
    - cleaning and preparing instruments for terminal sterilization

34. Factors that determine the most appropriate scrub person include the nature of the surgery, the skills required for the procedure, the staffing skill mix, and hospital policy.

35. The anesthesiologist is responsible for assessing the patient prior to surgery and for administering anesthetic agents to facilitate surgery and provide pain relief. The certified registered nurse anesthetist (CRNA) administers anesthesia under the direct supervision of the anesthesiologist or, in some cases, the surgeon.

36. The perioperative nurse in the circulating role coordinates the care of the patient, is the patient's advocate throughout the intraoperative experience, and has responsibility for managing and implementing activities outside the sterile field. Activities are directed toward achieving desired patient outcomes. The nursing process is used as a framework for these activities. Examples of activities performed by the perioperative nurse in the circulating role include:

    - providing emotional support to the patient prior to the induction of anesthesia
    - performing ongoing patient assessment
    - formulating a nursing diagnosis
    - developing and implementing a plan of care
    - documenting patient care
    - evaluating patient outcomes
    - teaching patient and family
    - obtaining appropriate surgical supplies and equipment
    - creating and maintaining a safe environment
    - administering drugs
    - implementing and enforcing policies and procedures that contribute to patient safety, e.g., surgical counts for instruments, sponges, and sharps, as well as performing equipment checks
    - preparing and disposing of specimens
    - communicating relevant information to other team members and to the patient's family

37. Perioperative nurse managers assume a variety of roles. In a very small facility, the perioperative nurse may serve as manager and also scrub or circulate on cases as needed. In very large facilities it is common for there to be several managers within the department. In addition to administrative department manager(s), other leadership/management positions include team leaders, specialty managers, or specialty coordinators, who typically assume responsibility for a particular surgical specialty. Responsibilities may include assigning staff, ensuring availability of supplies and equipment needed for scheduled surgeries, managing and ensuring adequate inventory of specialty supplies, maintaining and updating surgeon preference cards that identify supplies needed for each case by each surgeon in the specialty, creating preference cards for sur-

geons new to the service, periodically reviewing contents of instrument trays for appropriateness, standardizing supplies and trays whenever possible, and promoting or providing education for other staff. They may also be responsible for ordering supplies. Scheduling coordinators who "run the desk" are personnel whose responsibilities typically may include assigning staff to procedures, surgeries to rooms, and generally moving the schedule along throughout the day. This position may or may not be held by a perioperative nurse. An unanticipated emergency often requires quickly altering the daily schedule. The scheduling coordinator must understand patient acuity, know the skill level of the staff, and be able to schedule accordingly. Perfusionists, radiology and laboratory technicians, perioperative educators, pathologists, nurse's aides, clerks, and personnel from materials management, environmental services, and central service are some of the other personnel that are necessary to achieve desired patient outcomes. All have a role in ensuring a safe surgical experience. It is the perioperative nurse who coordinates the contributions of each team member.

• • • References

Association of Perioperative Registered Nurses (AORN). (2004a). Perioperative patient focused model. In *Standards, recommended practices, and guidelines* (pp. 15–19). Denver, CO: Author.

AORN. (2004b). Perioperative patient outcomes. In *Standards, recommended practices, and guidelines* (pp. 197–206). Denver, CO: Author.

AORN. (2004c). Revised official statement on RN first assistants. In *Standards, recommended practices, and guidelines* (pp. 163–165). Denver, CO: Author.

Appendix 1-A

• •

Chapter 1 Post Test

Instructions: Fill in the blank(s), mark the correct answer(s), or answer the question as appropriate.

1. Explain why the term *perioperative nurse* is more appropriate than the term *operating-room nurse*. (Ref. 11)

   _____

   _____

2. The preoperative period may be as long as 3 weeks or as short as a half hour. (Ref. 2, 3)

   True   False

3. Although the perioperative nurse must be skilled in technology, responsibilities related to technical equipment are outside the scope of the nursing process. (Ref. 13)

   True   False

4. The perioperative nurse may begin planning care for the patient scheduled for surgery prior to performing a nursing assessment; however, the plan of care can only be individualized after the assessment. (Ref. 18)

   True   False

5. Desired outcomes related to surgical intervention are as follows (Ref. 21):

   a. The patient is free from signs and symptoms of chemical, electrical, laser, radiation, and position-related injury.

   b. The patient demonstrates knowledge of expected responses to the operative procedure.

   c. The patient is pain free.

6. The RNFA role is a(n) (Ref. 23, 24):

   a. expanded perioperative nursing practice role

   b. advanced perioperative nursing practice role

   c. expanded or advanced role depending upon the level of education achieved

7. The nurse providing care to a patient undergoing a surgical procedure in a physician's office-based procedure room is technically not a perioperative nurse. (Ref. 26)

   True   False

8. The following persons might ordinarily function as members of the nonsterile surgical team (Ref. 30, 37):

   a. scrub person

   b. circulating nurse

   c. anesthesiologist

   d. surgical resident

   e. nurse anesthestist

   f. perfusionist

9. Arrangement of instruments on the sterile back table prior to surgery is the responsibility of (Ref. 29, 33):

    a. the perioperative nurse in the scrub role

    b. the perioperative nurse in the circulating role

    c. the scrub person who is not a nurse

    d. all of the above

10. Responsibilities of the perioperative nurse in the circulating role would appropriately include (Ref. 36):

    a. communicating with the patient's family to provide a report of the patient during surgery

    b. sending specimens to the laboratory

    c. testing a tourniquet

    d. donning sterile attire to assist the surgeon

    e. informing the surgeon that his or her glove has become contaminated and needs to be changed

Chapter 1—Post Test Answers

1. Responsibilities of the perioperative nurse include providing care in the pre- and postoperative periods as well as the intraoperative period.
2. True
3. False
4. True
5. a, b
6. c
7. False
8. b, c, e, f
9. a, c
10. a, b, c, e

Preparing the Patient for Surgery

LEARNER OBJECTIVES

After reading and completing "Preparing the Patient for Surgery," the learner will:

- state desired patient outcomes related to the preoperative phase
- identify the critical factors included in a preoperative patient assessment
- recognize nursing diagnoses common to the surgical patient in the preoperative phase
- describe interventions in the preoperative phase to achieve desired patient outcomes
- list at least eight factors that may contribute to wrong site surgery
- describe the three components of the JCAHO protocol to prevent wrong site surgery
- discuss the content of preoperative patient teaching

. . . .

Lesson Outline

I. NURSING DIAGNOSES
II. DESIRED PATIENT OUTCOMES
III. PREOPERATIVE PREPARATION
IV. PREOPERATIVE ASSESSMENT AND INTERVENTIONS
   A. Overview
   B. Sources of Patient Information
   C. Assessment Parameters
      1. Physiologic
      2. Psychosocial
V. NURSING DIAGNOSES AND INTERVENTIONS
   A. Preoperative Period
   B. Intraoperative Period
VI. PREVENTION OF WRONG SITE SURGERY
VII. PATIENT-FAMILY TEACHING
VIII. COMMUNICATION OF RELEVANT PATIENT DATA

NURSING DIAGNOSES

1. The perioperative nurse combines unique knowledge of the surgical procedure with patient assessment data and formulates nursing diagnoses that serve as the basis for the patient's plan of care.

2. Over 150 nursing diagnoses and hundreds of nursing interventions have been identified through the North American Nursing Diagnosis Association (NANDA, 2003). These diagnoses and interventions are not mutually exclusive, and any one or more may be appropriate for an individual patient.

3. The plan of care is developed as the perioperative nurse identifies nursing actions to be taken based on the patient's nursing diagnoses. Some nursing diagnoses will require interventions in all three phases of the surgical experience. For other nursing diagnoses the interventions will be confined to a single period or to a period when the patient has left the operating and recovery room. (Exhibit 2-1)

4. Each plan of care must be individualized based on specific individual patient needs. There are, however, several nursing diagnoses that are common to the surgical patient and that require nursing intervention in the preoperative period.

DESIRED PATIENT OUTCOMES

5. A well-prepared patient will have an understanding of the events that can be anticipated to occur in the preoperative and immediate postoperative periods. The Association of Perioperative Nurses (AORN) Outcome Standard states, "The patient demonstrates knowledge of expected responses to the operative or invasive procedure" (AORN, 2004, p. 202). The patient should have knowledge of the procedure to be performed and should confirm consent. The patient should also be prepared for discharge and demonstrate some essential understanding of expected participation in his or her own recovery and rehabilitation. The patient should feel supported in the preoperative period and be encouraged to express feelings about the surgical experience. Finally, the patient's level of anxiety or fear should be reduced to a minimum.

PREOPERATIVE PREPARATION

6. Preparations for surgery are begun in the preoperative period as the patient is psychologically and physiologically prepared for surgery. Activities are directed toward treating or minimizing preexisting medical conditions and providing information and support to assist the patient through the surgical experience. Nursing activities are planned to achieve positive patient outcomes.

7. Preparations focus on a variety of nursing activities, including data collection through patient assessment, patient-family teaching, emotional support, planning care with the patient for the intra- and postoperative periods, and communicating patient information to health care team members.

8. Planning for the achievement of desired patient outcomes begins with a patient assessment. The desired outcome, that the patient demonstrates knowledge of expected responses to the operative or invasive procedure, can be achieved by providing appropriate information and support during the preoperative period. The content of that information and the patient's unique learning needs can only be ascertained through an assessment process.

9. Additional desired patient outcomes, such as freedom from infection, freedom from injury, maintenance of skin integrity, maintained electrolyte balance, and patient participation in the rehabilitation process, are planned or based on information obtained from the preoperative assessment. For example, assessment data that reveal a patient has limited range of motion in a shoulder will lead to planned positioning interventions that will prevent further shoulder injury.

10. The perioperative nurse may be responsible for antibiotic administration prior to surgery. Administration of prophylactic antibiotics prior to the incision in certain types of surgery has been shown to significantly reduce the rate of surgical infection (OR Manager, 2004, p. 13). Many health care facilities have preoperative prophylactic antibiotic protocols that identify the type of surgery, the type of antibiotic, and the time frame in which the antibiotic should be given. Prophylactic antibiotics should be given far enough in advance of the start of surgery so that the level of antibiotic in the patient's serum and tissue is sufficient to destroy microorganisms that may be encountered during surgery. The ideal time frame is typically one hour prior to incision. Traditionally, prophylactic antibiotics are given just prior to the patient's transport to the operating room. However, delays in transport and preparations for surgery often result in delay of the surgical incision by more than one hour, and the antibiotics are therefore not effective. A number of facilities have determined that compliance with the 60-minute time frame is best achieved when the perioperative nurse assumes responsibility for antibiotic administration.

Exhibit 2–1 Preop Visit Assessment Form

OR #: _____				PRE-OP VISIT	

PERSONAL PHYSICIAN	SURGEON	ANESTHESIOLOGIST	SEX □ M □ F	AGE	
DATE	TIME	PROCEDURE		NICKNAME	
ALLERGIES			ISOLATION PRECAUTIONS □ TB □ HIV □ HEPATITIS		

MEDICAL & SURGICAL HISTORY:

_____

_____

_____

_____

_____

_____

	SKIN ASSESSMENT	MENTAL/ EMOTIONAL	VISION	PRE-OP TUBES	LABORATORY INFORMATION	PRE-OP:
HT:	COLOR:	□ Oriented	□ Adequate	□ Foley		_____
WT:	□ Pale	□ Disoriented To:	□ Decreased	□ NG		TIME:
T:	□ Flushed	□ Time	□ Blind	□ Other:		_____
	□ Dusky	□ Place	□ Rt □ Lt			
P:	□ Cyanotic	□ Person	□ Glasses	**CHART REQUIREMENTS**		ROUTINE MEDS:
R:	□ Jaundice	□ Lethargic	□ Contacts	□ Permit		_____
	□ Normal	□ Comatose	**HEARING**	□ H & P		_____
BP RANGE:	□ Other:	□ Dementia/ Alzheimers	□ Adequate			_____
			□ Decreased			_____
PERIPHERAL PERFUSION:	CONDITION:	□ Protective Devices	□ Deaf	**DENTURES**	□ BLOOD GLUCOSE MONITORING	_____
	□ No Problem		□ Rt □ Lt	□ Upper	SHA / OR / PACU INSTRUCTIONS:	
PULSES:	□ Rash	□ Calm		□ Lower		
RR:	□ Boney Area	□ Apprehensive	□ Hearing Aide	□ Partial	X-RAYS:	
LR:	□ Redness	□ Emotional Disorders	COMMUNICATION BARRIERS:			
RP:	□ Decubiti					
LP:	□ Contusions/ Abrasions	UNITS OF BLOOD:			SCANS:	
SMOKES:	□ Edema	□ T & C	CONSULTING PHYSICIANS/ SPECIALTY:			
□ Yes	□ Other:	Number of Units on Hand:			EKG:	
□ No						
□ PPD _____						
□ Quit _____					FAMILY □ FWA □ ICU FWA □ HOME □ OTHER:	

COMMENTS:

_____

_____

_____

_____

IVs: □ Central □ Peripheral DATE OF INSERTION: _____	Fluids: _____ Support Meds: Type _____ Rate _____ TPN & Rate: _____	□ OR RN □ PACU RN Signature:

Source: Pilot DRAFT form courtesy of St. Luke's Medical Center, Milwaukee, Wisconsin.

PREOPERATIVE ASSESSMENT AND INTERVENTIONS

Overview

11. The perioperative nurse is the patient's advocate during surgery. The patient, whose protective reflexes are compromised by anesthesia or other requirements for surgery, is dependent on members of the health care team to be his or her advocate. Knowledge of the patient gained through assessment in the preoperative period provides the information that is necessary for advocacy responsibilities.

12. The perioperative nurse may have the opportunity to perform a complete and thorough assessment of the patient a day or more prior to surgery at the time of preoperative testing. This is most likely to occur only in a small surgical center where the perioperative nurse practices in the preoperative testing unit as well as the operating room and the recovery area. More commonly, preoperative testing is accomplished at another site by someone other than the perioperative nurse who will actually provide the intraoperative care. Typically, during the preoperative period the patient will interact with nurses other than the perioperative nurse. The perioperative nurse often will first encounter the patient in the holding area immediately prior to surgery. Under these conditions, there is insufficient opportunity to carry out a comprehensive history and assessment. The perioperative nurse must therefore focus on essential elements that are necessary for desired patient outcomes.

Sources of Patient Information

13. Assessment data may be obtained from a combination of chart review, patient-family interview, patient observation, and communication with other health care providers. The patient's chart may include an assessment and preoperative checklist that was completed prior to transport to the holding area. This document is a valuable resource when performing a patient assessment. (Exhibit 2-2)

14. With the exception of emergency surgery, where life may depend on immediate surgical intervention, a rapid but thorough chart review and patient-family interview can be sufficient to accomplish the essential assessment.

Assessment Parameters

Physiologic

15. Critical physiological assessment data include the following:

- medical diagnosis, chronic diseases, and treatment
- medications, especially antibiotics, herbal medications; anticoagulants, including aspirin; and diuretics that deplete potassium
- surgery to be performed and verification of surgical site
- previous surgeries and any complications, including anesthesia complications
- vital signs, diagnostic and laboratory data **as ordered**—abnormalities

  hemoglobin and hematocrit

  white blood count

  platelet count

  serum electrolytes

  urine analysis

  chest X-ray

  diagnostic X-rays pertinent to surgical procedure

  electrocardiogram

  blood type and cross match information and availability of replacement blood

  results of specific tests or studies specific to the planned procedure

- age—very young or very old
- substance abuse—smoking, alcohol, drugs
- skin condition—color, rashes, lesions
- allergies—medication and latex allergies are especially critical
- nutritional and nothing by mouth (NPO) status
- sensory impairments—presence of lenses, hearing aids, dentures
- mobility impairments
- presence of prosthetic devices—orthopedic implants, pacemaker, vascular prosthesis
- weight and height—extreme under- and overweight, height greater than length of the operating room table

Psychosocial

16. Critical psychosocial assessment data include the following:

- understanding and perception of the procedure to be performed
- coping ability
- ability to comprehend
- readiness to learn

Exhibit 2–2 Perioperative Nursing Diagnosis Flowsheet

PROBLEM	PAT	PRE-OP	INTRA-OP	PACU I	PACU II

DIAGNOSIS #1   DATE:
 Potential knowledge deficit R/T unknown;
 the environment and surgical procedures.
 1. Assess present knowledge level with patient quote
     on record.
 <u>DESIRED OUTCOME</u>
 1. Patient will demonstrate understanding of all
     phases of care by accurately verbalizing knowledge
     or return demonstration.
	——	——	——		

<u>INTERVENTIONS</u> 1. Explain your (nurse) role to patient.					
2. Provide information regarding perioperative nursing.					
3. Clarify previous physician explanations. Refer appropriate personnel for clarification.					
4. Provide written instructions/audiovisual aids.					

DIAGNOSIS #2   DATE:
 Potential alteration in family and individual coping
 mechanisms R/T anxiety, fear, and/or inadequate
 support systems.
 1. Assess support person's understanding of patient's
     perioperative experiences.
 <u>DESIRED OUTCOME</u>
 1. Patient/support person will demonstrate appropriate
     coping mechanisms.
	——	——	——		

<u>INTERVENTIONS</u> 1. Have patient identify support person.					
2. Communicate any specific support needs of family/patient to appropriate personnel.					
3. Keep support person informed.					
DIAGNOSIS #3 DATE: Potential for infection R/T surgical procedures, foreign environment. 1. Assess patient for history and current risk factors. <u>DESIRED OUTCOME</u> 1. Patient will remain free of nosocomial infection.	——	——	——		
<u>INTERVENTIONS</u> 1. Monitor for break in aseptic technique, and take corrective measures.					
2. Monitor and limit excessive travel into/from operating suite.					
3. Proper handwashing.					
4. Use universal precautions.					

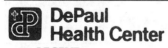

DePaul Health Center

<u>LEGEND</u>
O = Ongoing
O/N = Ongoing, No Intervention
R = Resolved
N/A = Not Applicable

PERIOPERATIVE NURSING DIAGNOSES

FORM NO. 2-417 (REV. 3/93) APPROVED BY MRC 1/93

(continues)

Exhibit 2–2 *continued*

PROBLEM	PAT	PRE-OP	INTRA-OP	PACU I	PACU II
DIAGNOSIS #4 DATE: Potential alterations in ventilation and cardiovascular function R/T anesthesia with surgical procedures. 1. Assess patient's current and review past history for potential risk factors. 2. Assess need for O_2 therapy. 3. Assess peripheral circulatory status. DESIRED OUTCOME 1. Patient will maintain or improve pulmonary functions. 2. Patient will maintain or improve cardiovascular functions.	____	____	____ *GEN.		
INTERVENTIONS 1. Respiratory a. Assist with anesthesia induction/assist with O_2 therapy.			*		
b. Observe respiratory function.					
c. Auscultate lung fields.					
d. Elevate HOB.					
e. Deep breathe/cough.					
f. Suction prn.					
g. Monitor ABG/SAO_2.					
2. Cardiovascular a. Monitor heart rhythm.					
b. Implement usage of thermal support.			*		
c. Monitor pulses.					
d. Apply and/or monitor TED/sequential stockings.			*		
3. Monitor skin color.					
4. Teach s/s of alterations expected at home, leg exercises/deep breathing.					
DIAGNOSIS #5 DATE: Potential alterations in fluid/electrolyte balance R/T surgical procedure, blood loss, & NPO status. 1. Assess patient fluid/electrolyte status during perioperative experience. DESIRED OUTCOME 1. Patient will maintain fluid balance.	____	____	____		
INTERVENTIONS 1. Maintain IV fluid therapy.					
2. Notify physician of abnormal lab values.					
3. Monitor blood/fluid loss.					
4. Assist with insertion of invasive hemodynamic monitors.					
5. Monitor for and notify physician of abnormal hemodynamic monitor values.					
6. Teaching of drainage output including amount, frequency, character/follow-up.					

NAME _____ MEDICAL RECORD NO. _____

Source: Courtesy of DePaul Health Center, Bridgeton, Missouri.

- anxiety related to surgical intervention or surgical outcome
- knowledge of perioperative routines
- cultural or spiritual beliefs relevant to surgical intervention

NURSING DIAGNOSES AND INTERVENTIONS

Preoperative Period

17. The most common nursing diagnoses requiring nursing intervention in the preoperative period are knowledge deficit and anxiety.

18. Knowledge deficit may be related to perioperative routines, surgical interventions, or outcome expectations. Knowledge deficit may be the result of impaired communication ability, a language barrier, a patient's insufficient mental capacity, or a lack of information regarding the surgical procedure. Nursing interventions must be appropriate to the etiology of the patient's knowledge deficit and to the patient's learning needs.

19. Anxiety can range from mild to severe and may have a variety of etiologies. A patient's level of anxiety may be more acute at some periods throughout the surgical experience than at others. For some patients, anxiety is at its height just prior to surgery. For others, it is most acute at the time the decision to have surgery is made. Patients who are anxious cannot always identify the exact cause of their anxiety. They may express an uneasiness or nervousness.

20. Anxiety is different from fear. An anxious patient may not be able to state the exact cause for his or her anxiety. An increased heart and respiratory rate and an elevated blood pressure can be signs of anxiety. The patient may feel nervous or tense and may not be able to concentrate or retain information. The fearful patient, however, can state the source of fear. Fear is marked by apprehension and dread and may be related to surgical intervention, surgical outcome, anesthesia, impact of surgery on lifestyle, loss of control, pain, death, and so forth. Although some patients will exhibit fear, an anxious state is more common.

21. Another likely nursing diagnosis in the preoperative period may be anticipatory grieving related to possible changes in body image.

22. Each patient is unique and nursing diagnoses are not the same for all surgical patients. Nursing diagnoses and nursing interventions must be determined through individual patient assessment and must be individualized for each patient.

23. The desired outcome related to knowledge deficit is that the patient will demonstrate knowledge of the physiological and psychological responses to surgery.

24. Nursing interventions that assess knowledge and address knowledge deficit should include:
- confirmation of the patient's identity
- verification of the surgical site and procedure
- verification of consent
- solicitation of the patient's perception of planned surgery
- solicitation of questions related to surgery
- identification of teaching needs, readiness, and ability to learn
- explanation of surgical routines
- explanation of procedures that need to be followed postoperatively upon discharge (especially critical for patients who are intended to be discharged on the day of their surgery, therefore limiting the time available for teaching)
- provision of appropriate information with consideration for the patient's level of understanding, ability to comprehend, desired information, culture, and religious beliefs, as well as medical concerns referred to the surgeon
- solicitation of feedback regarding perioperative procedures

25. The desired outcome related to anxiety is that anxiety and fear will be lessened through gained knowledge and expression of feelings about the surgical intervention. It is important to assess readiness to learn, because providing more information than the patient desires or can handle can exacerbate anxiety.

26. Nursing interventions that address anxiety and fear should include:
- attentive listening
- provision of information as needed and desired (Providing information the patient does not wish can increase the patient's anxiety.)
- solicitation of patient expressions of anxiety or fear
- provision of emotional support and reassurance

27. Criteria that may be used to evaluate the achievement of these outcomes are that the patient will (1) confirm the consent, (2) describe the expected sequence of events, (3) express feelings about the surgical experience, (4) indicate knowledge of expected surgical outcomes, and (5) confirm procedures to be followed upon discharge.

Intraoperative Period

28. The intraoperative period begins when the patient enters the actual operating room. During the intraoperative period, the patient is at high risk for injury. A variety of injuries may result from interventions such as positioning, transport and transfer, use of equipment such as electrocautery or tourniquet, application of chemical agents such as skin prep solutions, extraneous objects such as sponges inadvertently left in the wound, and use of X-ray or laser. The patient is also at high risk for infection injury as a result of surgical intervention. Other possible nursing diagnoses include but are not limited to: fluid deficit or excess and impaired gas exchange related to general anesthesia. (Nursing interventions to prevent these injuries are presented in other chapters.)

PREVENTION OF WRONG SITE SURGERY

29. In 1999 the Institute of Medicine issued a report, "To Err Is Human: Building a Safer Health System," that reported as many as 98,000 patients die in hospitals each year as a result of errors (Kohn, Corrigan, & Donaldson, 2000, p. 1). In response, health care facilities, professional organizations, and the Joint Commission on Accreditation of Healthcare Organizations (JCAHO) have focused intently on initiatives to improve patient safety. In 2003, in an effort to improve patient safety, the JCAHO established six National Patient Safety Goals for 2004. One goal is the elimination of wrong site, wrong patient, wrong procedure surgery (JCAHO, 2003).

30. Over 150 cases of wrong site surgery are listed in the Joint Commission's Sentinel Event database and five to eight new reports of wrong site surgery are received each month (JCAHO, 2001). Because reporting is voluntary, the actual number is not known. What is known is that the patient is at high risk for injury related to wrong site surgery and that wrong site surgery can have serious consequences for the patient.

31. Wrong site surgery may be surgery on the wrong patient, body part, side, level, or site, or it may be performance of the wrong procedure. Factors that contribute to wrong site surgery can include (AORN, 2003):

    - emergency surgery
    - unusual equipment or setup in the room
    - multiple surgeons involved in the procedure
    - multiple procedures on multiple body parts during a single surgical experience
    - physical deformity

- inadequate patient assessment
- miscommunication among members of the surgical team
- inadequate medical record review
- pressure to reduce preoperative preparation time
- unusual time pressures
- lack of institutional policies
- illegible handwriting
- use of abbreviations
- failure to include the patient and/or family members when identifying the correct site
- relying solely upon the surgeon to determine surgical site

32. As a patient advocate, the perioperative nurse has a responsibility to verify the patient's identity and to protect the patient from wrong site surgery. The surgeon is responsible for determining the patient's need for surgery, identifying the procedure, and delineating the surgical site. Verifying patient identification and the correct surgical site is the responsibility of all team members, including the perioperative nurse.

33. In the preoperative period, the nurse performing the patient assessment should verify the patient's identity and the procedure. This should be done verbally with the patient and by checking the name band. Chart review should begin by ascertaining that the patient, the chart, and the name band are all in the same name. If the patient is unable to communicate, verification should be with the family or authorized representative and through chart review. A patient should never be transferred into the operating room suite without an identification band that has been verified for accuracy. Often the perioperative nurse is the first to greet the patient upon arrival to the operating room. Verification of identity and surgical procedure must be a priority for the perioperative nurse.

34. JCAHO, AORN, and the American College of Surgeons are among the organizations that have guidelines regarding marking the surgical site. These guidelines specify what is marked, how it is marked, and by whom. They also provide guidelines for verifying the surgical site. Individual institutional policies and procedures may vary; however, as of July 2004, health care organizations must comply with a JCAHO (2003) Universal Protocol for preventing wrong site surgery. The Protocol includes:

    - a preoperative verification process—all documents and studies available prior to procedure, reviewed, consistent with each other and patient's expectations and with the team's understanding of the intended patient, procedure, site and, as applicable, any implants. Missing information or discrepancies must be addressed before starting the procedure.

- marking the operative site—to identify unambiguously the intended site of incision or insertion (all procedures involving right/left distinction, multiple structures such as fingers and levels such as the spine)
- a "time out" immediately before starting the procedure—to conduct final verification of the correct patient, procedure, site, and as applicable, implants (JCAHO, 2003, p. 1).

At this time all team members should verify the name of the patient, the procedure, and the site and should validate that the site is marked. Documentation should indicate that a "time out" was performed in accordance with health care facility policy, what was verified, and who participated in the "time out." Many facilities have developed forms specific for this purpose to streamline documentation requirements.

35. Most health care facilities have policies that identify how verification should occur, who is responsible for verification, and what documentation must be completed. Typically, the surgeon, the anesthesiologist, and the circulating nurse must all participate in verification.

PATIENT-FAMILY TEACHING

36. Patient teaching is ideally begun during a preadmission workup or in the physician's office or clinic where the prospect of surgery is discussed. When possible, the patient's family or support persons should be included in the teaching process. Patient teaching must be appropriate to the patient's and family's ability and readiness to understand and to learn.

37. The patient's age must be considered when patient teaching is implemented.

38. Elderly patients are no less intelligent than younger patients; however, short-term memory may be diminished and additional time and reinforcement may be necessary in order for them to learn, comprehend, and retain information. Additional time should be planned for instruction. Instructional materials and voice level should take possible sight and hearing deficits into consideration.

39. Pediatric patients have special needs. The school-age child may view the surgical experience as a threat to recently achieved independence and control. Children under 7 years of age may view illness as a punishment for wrongdoings, and surgery may invoke fear of body mutilation and death (Redman, 1993, pp. 90–91). Patient teaching for pediatric patients may include an opportunity for them to handle simple items that they will be faced with in surgery. The ability, for example, to touch and manipulate an anesthesia mask may provide the child with a needed feeling of control.

40. Patient teaching during a preadmission workup will be more extensive than teaching in the holding area just prior to surgery. Teaching during a preadmission process should include content that is directed toward preparation for surgery and participation in the postoperative rehabilitation process. An example of teaching content in preparation for colon surgery is instruction in bowel cleansing. An example of preoperative teaching directed toward patient participation in postoperative rehabilitation is crutch walking. Written instructions, pamphlets, and videos related to preparation for surgery and rehabilitation may be provided. Teaching in the preoperative holding area will be abbreviated and will reinforce previous teaching. Teaching directed toward discharge will be reinforced in the postoperative period prior to discharge.

41. Preoperative teaching content should include at least:

- the procedure, anticipated duration, and expected outcome
- specific instructions such as whether to bathe or shower, to hold or take medications, and whether to maintain NPO status from a designated time onward
- an explanation of preoperative events such as diagnostic tests, skin preparation, intravenous (IV) insertion, sedation, and transfer to holding area
- an explanation of intraoperative events such as function of the circulating nurse or case manager, application of monitoring equipment, administration of anesthesia, maintenance of privacy and dignity, staff communication with family members during the procedure, and transport to the postanesthesia care unit
- an explanation of postoperative events such as expected length of stay, coughing and deep breathing expectations, turning, presence of lines, drains, and indwelling catheters, pain control, and discharge to a step-down or other unit or to home

42. The nurse who performs an assessment of teaching needs in the holding area may identify that the patient is anxious and unable to recall information presented earlier in preparation for surgery. The anxious patient may have difficulty concentrating or retaining information. Information given earlier about surgical interventions may need to be repeated, and information pertaining to discharge and expected recovery will need to be reinforced with both the patient and the family in the postoperative period.

43. In addition to providing information to the patient, the perioperative nurse provides emotional support and reassurance. The perioperative nurse should solicit the patient's expression of feelings and concerns regarding surgery.

44. Anxiety and fear can be alleviated through attentive listening and reassurance as well as through information that is delivered calmly and candidly. An attentive, caring attitude, coupled with appropriate touch, can serve as a source of patient comfort and reassurance. It may be necessary to reduce anxiety and fear through these interventions in order to prepare the patient for teaching.

COMMUNICATION OF RELEVANT PATIENT DATA

45. Assessment information with relevance to intra- and postoperative care must be communicated to other members of the health care team. Continuity of care and appropriate therapeutic interventions cannot be assured without the communication of information. Documentation of findings and verbal communication of patient data and responses to interventions must be part of the surgical patient's ongoing care.

46. Forms for documenting patient assessment and care in the preoperative period may be stand-alone forms or may be part of an integrated form that includes patient assessment and care

throughout the pre-, intra-, and postoperative periods.

• • • References

Association of Perioperative Registered Nurses (AORN). (2004). Outcome standards. In *Standards, recommended practices, and guidelines* (pp. 197–206). Denver, CO: Author.

AORN. (2003). *AORN position statement on correct site surgery*. Retrieved January 27, 2004, from http://www.aorn.org/about/positions/correctsite.htm

Joint Commission on Accreditation of Healthcare Organizations (JCAHO). *2004 National patient safety goals*. Retrieved January 28, 2004, from http://www.jcaho.org/accredited+organizations/patient+safety/03+npsg/index.htm

JCAHO. (2001). *Sentinal event alert*. Retrieved January 28, 2004, from http://www.jcaho.org/about+us/news+letters/sentinel+event+alert/sea_24htm

JCAHO. (2003). Universal protocol for preventing wrong site, wrong procedure, wrong person surgery. Retrieved January 28, 2004, from http://www.jcaho/org/accredited+organizations/patient+safety/universal+protocol/universal+protocol.pdf

Kohn L., Corrigan J., & Donaldson, M. (Eds). (2000). *To err is human: Building a safer health system*. Committee on Quality of Healthcare in America, Institute of Medicine. Washington, DC: The National Academy Press.

NANDA International. (Feb. 2003). *NANDA Nursing diagnoses: Definitions and classification, 2003–2004*. Retrieved May 2003 from http://www.iom.edu/file.asp?id=4117

OR Manager. (Feb. 2004). Tightening up the process for use of prophylactic antibiotics. (pp. 13–15). Santa Fe, NM: Author.

Redman, B. (1993). *The process of patient education*. St. Louis, MO: Mosby Year Book.

Appendix 2-A

· ·

Chapter 2 Post Test

Instructions: Fill in the blank(s), mark the correct answer(s), or answer the question as appropriate.

1. Nursing diagnoses made by the perioperative nurse should not require interventions outside the operating room or postanesthesia care unit. (Ref. 3)

   True   False

2. List four nursing activities the perioperative nurse might perform in the preoperative period to prepare the patient for surgery. (Ref. 6, 7)

   _____

   _____

   _____

   _____

3. The perioperative nurse in the holding area may share responsibility for patient assessment with nurses outside the operating room. (Ref. 12, 13)

   True   False

4. Assessment of the patient's understanding and perception of the surgical procedure to be performed should always be included in the assessment process. (Ref. 16)

   True   False

5. Anxiety increases the patient's ability to concentrate. (Ref. 20)

   True   False

6. Before implementing patient teaching, the perioperative nurse must assess the patient's (Ref. 16, 20):

   a. knowledge of perioperative routines

   b. understanding of the procedure to be performed

   c. expected cost of services

   d. readiness to learn

   e. anxiety

7. Nursing diagnosis must be individualized and based on patient assessment; however, there are two nursing diagnoses that are typically appropriate for the surgical patient in the preoperative period. These two nursing diagnoses are (Ref. 17, 18, 19):

   _____

   _____

8. Asking the patient if he or she has any questions about the pending surgery is a nursing intervention appropriate to a patient with the nursing diagnosis of knowledge deficit. (Ref. 24)

   True   False

9. Soliciting feelings about the patient's pending surgery is a nursing intervention appropriate to a patient with the nursing diagnosis of anxiety. (Ref. 26)

   True   False

10. List three criteria to evaluate whether the desired outcome, that the patient will demonstrate knowledge of the physiological and psychological response to surgery, has been achieved. (Ref. 27)

    _____

    _____

    _____

11. List eight factors that may contribute to wrong site surgery. (Ref. 31)

    _____   _____

    _____   _____

    _____   _____

    _____   _____

12. The JCAHO Universal Protocol to prevent wrong site surgery identifies three steps that must be taken. One is a preoperative verification process. The other two are (Ref. 34):

    _____

    _____

13. Elderly patients may have diminished vision; therefore instructional materials should not be printed in very small letters that may be difficult to see. Instructional materials for the elderly should take into consideration the possibility of diminished vision. List two other considerations that should be taken when teaching elderly patients. (Ref. 38)

    _____

    _____

14. A 5-year-old child may believe that the pending surgery is a punishment for wrongdoings. (Ref. 39)

    True   False

15. Nursing interventions for the school-age child should be directed toward providing the child with a feeling of some control over the pending activities. This may be accomplished by permitting the child to handle items that he or she may come in contact with, such as a blood pressure cuff. (Ref. 39)

    True   False

Appendix 2-B

· ·

Competency Checklist: Preparing the Patient for Surgery

Under "Observer's Initials," enter initials upon successful achievement of competency.
Enter N/A if competency is not appropriate for institution.

NAME _____

	OBSERVER'S INITIALS	DATE

1. Patient is identified.   _____ _____

2. Surgical procedure and operative site are verified with the patient.   _____ _____

3. Operative consent is verified with the patient.   _____ _____

4. Patient is assessed (or chart reviewed) for:

   a. medical diagnosis   _____ _____

   b. medications (prescription, over-the-counter, herbal)   _____ _____

   c. laboratory data (tests ordered, lab results, blood type and cross)   _____ _____

   d. previous surgeries   _____ _____

   e. anesthesia complications   _____ _____

   f. substance abuse   _____ _____

   g. skin condition   _____ _____

   h. allergies   _____ _____

   i. nutritional and NPO status   _____ _____

   j. sensory impairments   _____ _____

   k. dentures   _____ _____

   l. mobility impairments   _____ _____

   m. presence of prosthesis   _____ _____

   n. weight and height   _____ _____

   o. vital signs

   p. age   _____ _____

   _____

5. Patient is assessed for:

   a. level of understanding   _____ _____

   b. ability to comprehend   _____ _____

   c. information desired   _____ _____

   d. cultural and religious beliefs   _____ _____

6. Patient is asked to verbalize understanding of the surgical experience.   _____ _____

7. Patient is encouraged to ask questions regarding the surgical procedure.   _____ _____

8. Patient is encouraged to verbalize concerns about the surgical experience.   _____ _____

9. Intraoperative routines that the patient should expect are explained.   _____ _____

10. Patient teaching takes patient's age and level of understanding into consideration.   _____ _____

11. Universal Protocol to prevent wrong site surgery is implemented.   _____ _____

12. Postoperative routines are explained to the patient.   _____ _____

13. The above information is communicated to the surgical team.   _____ _____

OBSERVER'S SIGNATURE   INITIALS   DATE

_____

ORIENTEE'S SIGNATURE

_____

Chapter 2—Post Test Answers

1. False
2. Patient assessment, patient/family teaching, emotional support, planning care, communicating information
3. True
4. True
5. False
6. a, b, d, e
7. Knowledge deficit, anxiety
8. True
9. True
10. Patient confirms consent, patient describes sequence of events, patient expresses feelings about the surgery, patient indicates knowledge of expected surgical outcomes, patient confirms procedures to be followed upon discharge
11. Emergency surgery, unusual equipment or setup in the room, multiple surgeons involved in the procedure, multiple procedures on multiple body parts during a single surgical experience, physical deformity, inadequate patient assessment, miscommunication among members of the surgical team, inadequate medical record review, pressure to reduce preoperative preparation time, unusual time pressures, lack of institutional policies, illegible handwriting, use of abbreviations, failure to include the patient and/or family members when identifying the correct site, relying solely upon the surgeon to determine surgical site
12. Marking the operative site, a "time out" immediately before starting the procedure to conduct final verification
13. Additional time may be needed, additional reinforcement may be needed, hearing deficit may be present requiring the nurse to speak more loudly, special instructional materials
14. True
15. True

Prevention of Infection—Preparation of Instruments and Items Used in Surgery: Sterilization and Disinfection

LEARNER OBJECTIVES

After reading and completing "Prevention of Infection—Preparation of Instruments and Items Used in Surgery: Sterilization and Disinfection," the learner will:

- discuss the relationship of sterilization and disinfection to the prevention of patient infection
- identify the critical factors that determine whether an item must be sterile or whether disinfection is sufficient
- describe at least four methods used to accomplish sterilization
- discuss critical factors that determine the selection of the sterilization method
- discuss advantages and disadvantages of sterilization methods
- compare and contrast gravity displacement and high-vacuum sterilization cycles
- discuss appropriate uses of flash sterilization
- discuss appropriate use of disinfectants
- list hazards associated with sterilization and disinfection processes
- identify methods for monitoring sterilization and disinfection processes

• • • • • • • • • • • • •
Lesson Outline

I.   DEFINITIONS
II.   DESIRED PATIENT OUTCOMES
III. STERILIZATION AND DISINFECTION
    A.   Critical, Semicritical, and Noncritical Items
        1. Critical Items—Examples
        2. Semicritical Items—Examples
        3. Noncritical Items—Examples
    B.   Sterility Assurance Level (SAL)
    C.   Disinfection
IV.   METHODS OF STERILIZATION
    A.   Overview
    B.   Thermal Sterilization—Steam under Pressure: Moist Heat
        1. Advantages
        2. Disadvantages
    C.   Steam Sterilizers—Autoclaves
        1. Overview
        2. Gravity Displacement
        3. Prevacuum Sterilizer (Dynamic Air Removal)
            a. Bowie-Dick Test
        4. Steam-Flush-Pressure-Pulse Sterilizer
V.   FLASH STERILIZATION
    A.   Overview
VI.   CHEMICAL STERILIZATION—ETHYLENE OXIDE GAS (EO)
    A.   Description
        1. Advantages
        2. Disadvantages
VII. LOW-TEMPERATURE HYDROGEN PEROXIDE GAS PLASMA STERILIZATION
    A.   Description
        1. Advantages
        2. Disadvantages
VIII. CHEMICAL STERILIZATION—LIQUID PERACETIC ACID
    A.   Description
        1. Advantages
        2. Disadvantages
IX.   OTHER EMERGING STERILIZATION TECHNOLOGIES
X.   STERILIZATION—QUALITY CONTROL
    A.   Overview
    B.   Mechanical Process Indicators
    C.   Chemical Indicators
    D.   Biological Monitors
    E.   Rapid Readout Biological Monitors
XI.   RECORD KEEPING
XII. DISINFECTION
    A.   Overview
    B.   Levels of Disinfectants—Application
        1. Glutaraldehyde
        2. *Ortho*-phthalaldehyde
XIII. DISINFECTION—QUALITY CONTROL
XIV. DOCUMENTATION

DEFINITIONS

1. **Autoclave:** A steam sterilizer
2. **Bioburden:** A population of viable microorganisms on a product
3. **Biological Indicator:** A sterilization monitor consisting of a known population of resistant spores that is used to test the sterilizer's ability to kill microorganisms
4. **Bowie-Dick Test:** An air removal test designed to test the ability of the autoclave to remove air and noncondensable gases from the chamber and of steam to penetrate into a specified pack
5. **Chemical Indicator:** A device used to monitor one or more process parameters in the sterilization cycle. The device responds with a chemical or physical change (usually a color change) to conditions within the sterilizer chamber.

   Chemical indicators are usually supplied as a paper strip, tape, or label that changes color when the parameter has been met.
6. **Disinfectant:** An antimicrobial agent used to destroy microorganisms on inanimate surfaces. The composition and concentration of the disinfectant and the amount of time an item is exposed to it determines the number and types of organisms that will be killed.
7. **Disinfection:** Process that kills all living microorganisms with the exception of high numbers of spores. Low-level disinfection kills vegetative forms of bacteria, lipid viruses, and some fungi. Intermediate-level disinfection kills vegetative bacteria, mycobacteria, viruses, and fungi but not spores. High-level disinfection kills vegetative bacteria, mycobacteria, viruses, fungi, and some spores.
8. **Flash Sterilization:** A steam sterilization process for sterilizing items that are needed immediately.
9. **Spore:** An inactive or dormant, but viable, state of a microorganism, that is difficult to kill. Sterilization methods are monitored by their ability to kill a known population of highly resistant spores.
10. **Sterile:** Free of all viable microorganisms, including spores.
11. **Sterility Assurance Level (SAL):** The probability of a viable microorganism being present on an item after sterilization
12. **Sterilization:** A process that kills all living microorganisms, including spores

DESIRED PATIENT OUTCOMES

13. Freedom from infection is a critical desired patient outcome.

14. Postoperative wound infection is a complication of surgery with potentially dire consequences for the patient. The result can be delayed recovery, increased patient suffering, and even death. Postoperative wound infection contributes to extended hospital stays and significantly increases the costs for care.

15. Skin is the body's first line of defense against infection, and surgical intervention interrupts skin integrity. Invasive drains, catheters, and monitors also alter skin integrity. These all put the patient at risk for infection by providing a portal of entry for pathogenic microorganisms.

16. Perioperative nursing activities are directed toward prevention of infection with the goal that the patient will be free from infection following the operative procedure.

17. Pathogenic microorganisms are capable of causing disease when they invade human tissue. Contaminated equipment has been reported as a source of hospital-acquired infection (US Dept. Health and Human Services, Centers for Disease Control, 1999, pp. 557–560). Every effort must be made to remove microorganisms from articles and instruments that contact human tissue during surgical intervention.

18. Sterilization and disinfection are two processes used to destroy microorganisms. These processes are the cornerstones of infection control. Prevention of infection requires the perioperative nurse to have an in-depth understanding of principles and practices of sterilization and disinfection.

19. Advances in surgical techniques have resulted in the proliferation and routine use of a wide variety of complex, sophisticated, and expensive surgical instrumentation. As an example, fiberoptic instruments costing many thousands of dollars are a standard component of many procedures. Cleaning, disinfection, and sterilization procedures can vary according to the composition and configuration of the instrumentation. The composition and configuration of the instrument, its compatibility with the disinfection and sterilization methods available within the health care facility, and the manufacturer's instructions for processing must be considered when purchasing and processing decisions are made.

20. Most instrument processing is performed by ancillary personnel; however, the perioperative nurse assumes varying degrees of responsibility for the care and preparation of instruments. Selecting the appropriate method of processing requires a broad knowledge of disinfection and sterilization principles and procedures.

21. Acceptance of just-in-time sterilization (sterilizing an item just prior to its use) has required the movement of some sterilization procedures from the sterile processing department to the point where the instrument is to be used. When disinfection and sterilization are accomplished within the operating room department, it is often the perioperative nurse who is responsible for the process.

. . . .

SECTION QUESTIONS

Q1. Disinfectants are used to kill microorganisms on instruments and on the patient's skin. (Ref. 6)

   True   False

Q2. Low-level disinfectants kill mycobacteria. (Ref. 7)

   True   False

Q3. Sterilization is a process that will kill all microorganisms except high numbers of spores. (Ref. 12)

   True   False

Q4. Complications of postoperative surgical wound infection affect the patient and impact the cost of health care. Describe two consequences to the patient. (Ref. 14)

   _____

   _____

Q5. Explain how a drain that was placed into the wound during surgery can put the patient at risk for infection. (Ref. 15)

   _____

Q6. Explain why the nursing diagnosis of high risk for infection is appropriate for patients undergoing surgery and other invasive procedures. (Ref. 14, 15, 17)

   _____

   _____

Q7. Sterilization procedures are carried out primarily by ancillary personnel; however, the perioperative nurse must have an in-depth knowledge of these procedures because (Ref. 16, 20, 21):

   a. responsibility for care and preparation of instrumentation is a shared responsibility

   b. the perioperative nurse is responsible for prevention of infection

   c. sterilization of surgical instrumentation usually takes place in the operating room

Q8. _____ and _____ are two processes used to destroy pathogenic microorganisms. (Ref. 18)

. . . .

STERILIZATION AND DISINFECTION

Critical, Semicritical, and Noncritical Items

22. How an instrument should be processed is dependent upon its intended use. The Spaulding classification of devices, developed in 1968 by Earle Spaulding, was adopted by the Centers for Disease Control. It categorizes devices as critical, semicritical, or noncritical (Favero & Bond, 2001, p. 883–884). This categorization is used today to determine whether an item must be sterilized or whether disinfection is sufficient.

Critical Items—Examples

23. Critical items come in contact with sterile tissue or the vascular system, i.e., devices introduced beneath a mucous membrane. Critical items *must* be sterile. Sterilization may be defined as a process that kills all living microorganisms, including spores.
24. Critical items contaminated with microorganisms present a high risk of infection.
25. Examples of critical items include surgical instruments, orthopedic implants, sutures, and cardiac catheters.

Semicritical Items—Examples

26. Items that contact unbroken mucous membranes but do not penetrate them are considered semicritical items. Semicritical items may be sterile but *must* at least be disinfected. High-level disinfection is appropriate for semicritical items.
27. Examples of semicritical items include thermometers, cystoscopes, and dental dams.

Noncritical Items—Examples

28. Noncritical items contact intact skin and require only low-level disinfection or cleaning.
29. Examples of noncritical items include crutches, blood pressure cuffs, and stethoscopes.

Sterility Assurance Level (SAL)

30. The process of sterilization provides the greatest assurance that items are sterile, i.e., free of known and unsuspected microorganisms.
31. Devices sterilized for use in surgery must be sterilized with a sterility assurance level (SAL)

of 10^{-6}. This mathematical expression means that there is equal to, or less than, one chance in a million that any viable microorganism remains on an item after sterilization. This is a very high level of sterility assurance. For example, in some industries a sterility assurance of 10^{-3} (one chance in a thousand) might be acceptable.

32. In addition to the requirement for such a high level of sterility assurance, manufacturers of sterilizers must demonstrate that the sterilizer kills one million spores in half the programmed exposure time. Therefore, if the exposure phase in the sterilization cycle (the time within the cycle when the parameters required for sterilization are achieved) is programmed for four minutes, the sterilizer manufacturer must demonstrate that the kill is achieved in two minutes. In other words, a sterilizer must be capable of killing one million spores in half the time for which the sterilizer is programmed for hospital use (Favero & Bond, 2001, pp. 885–886).
33. Certain pathogenic bacteria such as *Clostridium tetani*, which produces tetanus, and *Clostridium perfidens*, which results in gas gangrene, are capable of developing spore forms. The environmental conditions that make it possible for spore formation are unknown; however, spores can remain alive for many years. When conditions are favorable for growth, such as when the spore is permitted entry into the body, the spore will germinate to produce a vegetative cell.
34. Spores are resistant, to a greater degree than are other bacteria, to heat, drying, and chemicals. Spores can survive long exposures to these processes. Only the process of sterilization can render an item free of all microorganisms, including spores.

Disinfection

35. Disinfection, a process that kills all living microorganisms with the exception of high numbers of bacterial spores, does not provide the same margin of safety associated with sterilization. Disinfectants vary in their ability to destroy microorganisms and are classified according to their cidal activity (ability to kill microorganisms).

• •

SECTION QUESTIONS

Q9. An arthroscope (instrument used to examine the inside of a joint) is an example of a (Ref. 23):

a. critical item

b. semicritical item

c. noncritical item

Q10. According to the Spaulding Classification System, the following item(s) may be sterile but must be at least high-level disinfected (Ref. 25, 26, 27):

a. cardiac catheter

b sutures

c. bedpan

d. thermometer

Q11. An example of a semicritical item is a laryngoscope. Acceptable infection control practice mandates that this item be sterilized before use. (Ref. 26)

True   False

Q12. An SAL of 10^{-6} means there is equal to or less than one chance in a million that any viable microorganisms remain on a device after sterilization. (Ref. 31)

True   False

Q13. Once a pathogenic bacterium forms a spore, that bacterium is no longer capable of causing an infection. (Ref. 33)

True   False

Q14. Spores are _____ resistant to heat than are nonspore-forming bacteria. (Ref. 34)

a. more

b. less

Q15. _____ is the process that kills all living microorganisms except high numbers of bacterial spores. (Ref. 35)

• •

METHODS OF STERILIZATION

Overview

36. There are a number of methods of sterilization. The choice of method is dependent on the compatibility of the item to be sterilized with the sterilization process, configuration of the item, required equipment, cost, availability, safety factors, packaging of the item, and length of time of the sterilization process. Each method has both advantages and disadvantages.

37. Methods of in-house sterilization have traditionally been dominated by steam and ethylene oxide gas and more recently include liquid peracetic acid and hydrogen peroxide gas plasma. Steam is used for heat and moisture-stable items. Ethylene oxide and hydrogen peroxide gas plasma are appropriate for sterilization of items that cannot withstand moisture or the

high temperatures of steam sterilization. Liquid peracetic acid sterilization is a just-in-time process suitable for heat-sensitive items that can tolerate immersion.

38. Steam and ethylene oxide have been used in hospitals for more than 50 years. Liquid peracetic acid gained acceptance in the 1980s, and hydrogen peroxide gas plasma was introduced in the 1990s.

39. Two other accepted methods of sterilization are dry heat and ionizing radiation.

40. Dry heat is appropriate for powders, oils, and petroleum products that cannot be penetrated by steam or ethylene oxide or other sterilizing agents. Most of these products are supplied sterile from the manufacturer; therefore, dry heat sterilization is rarely used in hospitals today.

41. Because of equipment, safety, and cost considerations, ionizing radiation is confined to industrial settings and is used for bulk sterilization of commercially prepared items.

Thermal Sterilization—Steam under Pressure: Moist Heat

42. Moist heat in the form of saturated steam under pressure is an economical, safe, and effective method of sterilization used for the majority of surgical instruments. It is the most common sterilization method used within health care facilities. Sterilization by this method is accomplished in a steam sterilizer referred to as an autoclave.

43. For sterilization to be achieved, steam must penetrate every fiber of the packaging and contact every surface of the item; and the intended parameters of moisture, temperature, and time must be met.

44. Steam that is saturated (contains the greatest amount of water vapor possible) and is heated to a sufficient temperature is capable of destroying all living microorganisms, including spores, within a relatively short amount of time.

45. Saturated steam destroys microorganisms through a thermal process that causes denaturation and coagulation of protein or the enzyme protein system contained within the microorganism's cell.

46. Steam at atmospheric pressure has a temperature of 212°F (100°C). This temperature is inadequate for sterilization. The addition of pressure to raise the temperature of steam is necessary for the destruction of microorganisms.

47. An increase in pressure of 15 to 17 pounds per square inch will increase steam temperature to 250°F to 254°F (121°C to 123°C). Twenty-seven pounds of pressure per square inch will increase steam temperature to 270°F (132°C).

48. The minimum generally accepted temperature required for sterilization to occur is 250°F (121°C) (Perkins, 1969, p. 161). Typical temperatures for the operation of steam sterilizers are 270°F to 275°F (132°C to 135°C), although 250°F (121°C) is also used (Association for the Advancement of Medical Instrumentation [AAMI], 2002, p. 36).

49. Steam sterilization is a function of time and temperature. A temperature of 250°F (121°C) requires more time than a temperature of 270°F (132°C).

Advantages

50. Some of the many advantages to steam sterilization include:

- Steam is readily available (most often supplied from the health care facility boiler).
- Steam is economical.
- Steam is compatible with most in-house packaging materials.
- Steam leaves no toxic residue and is environmentally safe.
- Steam sterilization is suitable for a wide range of surgical instrumentation. (The majority of items used for surgery can withstand repeated steam sterilization without sustaining damage).
- Steam sterilization is fast. Destruction of most resistant spores occurs quickly.

Disadvantages

51. Disadvantages associated with steam sterilization include:

- A variety of instruments and devices used in surgery cannot withstand moist heat at temperatures of 250°F (121°C) or above.
- Steam sterilization is prone to operator error with regard to preparation and packaging of items, setting of parameters, and loading of the autoclave.
- Timing of the sterilization cycle must be adjusted for type of cycle, variances in materials, and size of the load.
- A temperature of 270°F cannot be used for all items. The temperature may need to be reduced from 270°F to 250°F to be compatible with a specific item being sterilized.

Efficacy depends on attention to detail. Improper preparation of items or improper placement within the autoclave can result in trapped air that can prevent steam contact with all surfaces and thus prevent sterilization. Items must be disassembled in order for steam to contact all surfaces.

Steam Sterilizers—Autoclaves

Overview

52. A steam sterilizer, referred to as an *autoclave*, generally consists of a rectangular metal chamber and a shell. Between the two is an enclosed space referred to as a *jacket*. When the autoclave is activated, steam and heat fill the jacket and are maintained at a constant pressure, keeping the autoclave in a heated, ready state. (Figure 3-1, 3-2)

53. Items are placed in the chamber, the door is shut tightly, and the sterilization cycle is initiated. Steam enters the chamber and displaces all the air from the contents of the load. As the pressure rises, steam penetrates the contents and contacts all surfaces. The steam forces the

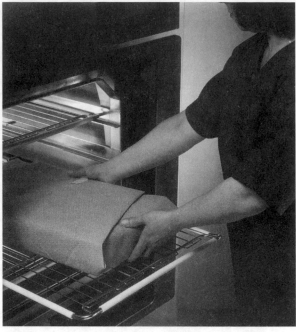

FIGURE 3-2   Loading the steam autoclave.
Source: Printed with permission from STERIS Corporation, Mentor, Ohio.

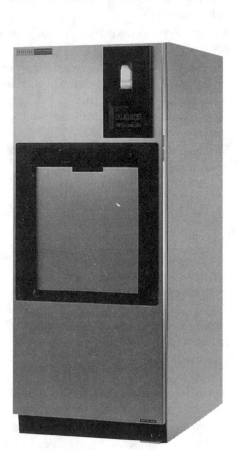

FIGURE 3-1   Steam Sterilizer.
Source: Printed with permission from STERIS Corporation, Mentor, Ohio.

air out through a discharge port outlet at the bottom front of the autoclave.

54. The discharge port outlet is the beginning of a filtered waste line. Beneath the filter is a thermometer. This is the coolest part of the autoclave.

55. The actual exposure or sterilization time does not begin until the temperature rises and the thermometer senses that the steam has reached the necessary preset temperature.

56. It is essential that all the air in the chamber is displaced by steam. Air that is trapped will act as an insulator and prevent heating and moisture contact with every surface of every item, and the sterilization process will be compromised. For this reason, loading of the autoclave is critical. Items must be placed so that steam can circulate freely throughout the chamber and can contact all surfaces.

57. If air is not trapped and parameters of time, moisture, and temperature have been met, microbial destruction will occur.

58. Items such as cups or basins must be placed within the sterilizer so that they do not become receptacles of water and compromise the sterilization process.

59. When the exposure time is complete, the steam is exhausted through the outlet port, and if de-

sired, a drying cycle follows. A drying cycle must be used for wrapped items.

60. Wrapped packages should be allowed to cool on the rack in the sterilizer while the door is open. They should not be touched during this time. Once removed from the autoclave they are allowed to continue cooling on wire mesh shelves that are covered with material that will absorb heat and condensation. A minimum of 30 minutes is recommended, although some instrument sets may require as much as 2 hours to adequately cool (AAMI, 2002, p. 36). Warm packages are not placed on cool surfaces because condensate will form, causing the package to become damp.

61. Microorganisms are capable of penetrating wet materials; therefore, moist packages that contact an unsterile surface must be considered contaminated.

62. There are three types of steam sterilizers or autoclaves: (1) gravity displacement, (2) pre-vacuum or high vacuum, and (3) steam-flush-pressure-pulse. These autoclaves differ in how air is removed from the chamber during the sterilization process.

63. Sterilizers vary in design and performance characteristics. Some sterilizers may be operated with either a gravity displacement or a high vacuum cycle and some offer only one type of cycle.

64. The nature of the items and the container in which they are sterilized determine the necessary time and temperature. There is no single setting that is appropriate for all items. Manufacturer's guidelines for the items and for the autoclave must be consulted to determine correct cycle settings.

Gravity Displacement

65. In a gravity-displacement cycle or autoclave the air in the chamber is displaced by gravity.

66. As steam enters from a port located near the top and rear of the chamber, it is deflected upward. Air is heavier than steam and, by the force of gravity, the air is forced to the bottom while the steam rides on top of the air. The steam rapidly displaces the air under it and forces the air out through the discharge outlet port. (Figure 3-3)

67. Most gravity displacement autoclaves are usually operated at temperatures between 250°F and 274°F (121°C to 134°C) with a 10- to 30-minute exposure time. For example, a wrapped instrument set requiring 30 minutes at 250°F (121°C) might require a 15-minute exposure at 270°F (134°C) (AAMI, 2002,

p. 36). (Certain powered equipment may require prolonged exposure times of as much as 55 minutes.)

68. A higher temperature requires less time than a lower temperature. A temperature of 270°F (132°C) will accomplish sterilization more rapidly than a temperature of 250°F (121°C).

69. The disadvantage of a gravity-displacement process is the length of time required for sterilization and the dependence on gravity to remove air. A high vacuum or steam-flush-pressure-pulse cycle offer a greater margin of safety with regard to air removal.

70. Gravity displacement cycles should not be used when a high vacuum or steam-flush-pressure-pulse cycle can be used.

71. Gravity displacement sterilizers are common in dentist and physician offices where sterilization is needed. Sterilizers that operate only with a gravity displacement cycle can still be found in health care facilities; however, most sterilizers sold today for hospitals and large ambulatory surgery centers run high vacuum cycles but may offer gravity displacement cycles as well.

72. A gravity displacement cycle is most appropriate for liquids; however, it is rare that liquids must be sterilized within the health care facility. Liquids that must be sterile are generally supplied sterile from the manufacturer. Some medical devices, because of their design, may require a gravity displacement cycle. The device manufacturer's instructions should be consulted before selecting the cycle type, time, and temperature.

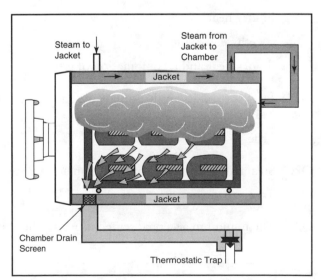

FIGURE 3-3 Steam Sterilizer—Steam Entry and Air Removal.
Source: Photo courtesy of AMSCO International, Inc.

• •

SECTION QUESTIONS

Q16. List five factors that should be considered when selecting a sterilization method. (Ref. 36)

_____

_____

Q17. Hydrogen peroxide gas plasma is used to sterilize items that can tolerate the combination of high heat and moisture. (Ref. 37)

True   False

Q18. Sterilization technologies commonly employed in the health care facility setting include (Ref. 37):

   a. steam

   b. dry heat

   c. ionizing radiation

   d. ethylene oxide

   e. ozone

   f. liquid peracetic acid

   g. hydrogen peroxide gas plasma

Q19. Items that can tolerate moisture and high temperatures are sterilized using (Ref. 37):

_____

Q20. Powders and oils may be sterilized using (Ref. 40):

   a. steam sterilization

   b. dry heat

   c. ethylene oxide

   d. dry heat and a combination of ethylene oxide

Q21. Ethylene oxide sterilization is the most common sterilization technology used for sterilization within health care facilities. (Ref. 42)

True   False

Q22. Steam at atmospheric pressure can achieve sterilization if exposure time is greatly increased. (Ref. 46)

True   False

Q23. The minimum accepted temperature at which steam sterilization may be accomplished is (Ref. 48):

   _____ °F   (_____ °C)

Q24. Steam sterilization is a function of both time and temperature. (Ref. 49)

True   False

Q25. List four advantages of steam sterilization. (Ref. 50)

_____

_____

Q26. Explain why improper preparation of items or placement within the autoclave can prevent sterilization. (Ref. 51)

_____

_____

Q27. Actual sterilization in an autoclave begins as soon as the door is closed and the button to begin the cycle is pressed. (Ref. 55)

True   False

Q28. Packages removed from the autoclave following sterilization should (Ref. 60):

   a. be immediately placed on a cool surface to reduce the temperature of the items within the package

   b. be allowed to cool for a minimum of 20 minutes

   c. not be touched during the initial cool-down period

   d. never be allowed to cool within the autoclave

Q29. All steam sterilizers can be operated with either a gravity or a prevacuum cycle. (Ref. 63)

True   False

Q30. Sterilization in a gravity displacement autoclave may be accomplished at a temperature of 250°F (121°C) or 270°F (134°C). (Ref. 67)

True   False

Q31. In a gravity displacement sterilizer, the exposure time for powered equipment may be as long as 30 minutes. (Ref. 67)

True   False

● ●

Prevacuum Sterilizer (Dynamic Air Removal)

73. The prevacuum autoclave is equipped with a vacuum pump that evacuates almost all air from the chamber prior to the injection of steam. The evacuation process takes approximately 5 minutes but may be longer, and essentially creates a vacuum within the chamber. When the steam enters the chamber, the force of the vacuum causes instant steam contact with all surfaces of the contents. Steam will penetrate almost instantly to every surface without regard to the size of the package or load.

74. Following the prevacuum phase, an exposure time of 3 to 4 minutes at 270°F to 275°F (132°C to 135°C) is the usual recommended time and temperature for accomplishing sterilization (AAMI, 2002, p. 36).

75. It is imperative that the device manufacturer's instructions be consulted before selecting cycle time and temperature. Although a 4-minute exposure time is common, required exposure times of 5, 8, and 15 minutes are not uncommon. Temperature requirements also vary from 270°F to 275°F (132°C to 135°C). In

other words, one cycle does not fit all devices. Manufacturer's instructions for sterilization should always be consulted. It should not be assumed that a 4-minute exposure at 270°F (132°C) is always adequate.

76. The advantages of a prevacuum sterilization cycle are:

   • Incorrect placement of objects within the chamber will have less impact upon air removal than in a gravity displacement cycle.

   • The entire load will heat rapidly and more uniformly than with a gravity displacement autoclave; therefore, the exposure time is shorter.

   • The autoclave may be used to a maximum capacity, allowing more supplies to be sterilized within a given time.

77. The disadvantage of a prevacuum sterilizer is that in the event of a leak, such as in the door seal, an air pocket can form and inhibit sterilization.

BOWIE-DICK TEST

78. To test whether air is effectively being eliminated from the chamber, prevacuum autoclaves are tested daily with a Bowie-Dick test. A Bowie-Dick test verifies that air removal is sufficient to achieve steam penetration of a standard load. The Association for the Advancement of Medical Instrumentation recommends this test be performed daily before the first processed load (AAMI, 2002, p. 51).

79. A commercially prepared sheet of paper with various patterns of heat-sensitive ink is used to perform a Bowie-Dick test. The sheet is placed in a specially constructed pack of towels and subjected to sterilization in an otherwise empty autoclave. A uniform color change indicates successful creation of a vacuum. (Figure 3-4)

80. A Daily Air Removal test is another commercially prepared test that may be used to test for air removal.

Steam-Flush-Pressure-Pulse Sterilizer

81. Instead of a vacuum to remove air from the chamber, a repeated sequence of steam-flush and pressure-pulses above atmospheric pressure are utilized. Because a vacuum is not drawn, a Bowie-Dick test or Daily Air Removal test is not required.

82. A variety of cycle times can be selected, based on the nature of the items to be sterilized.

83. The advantage to a steam-flush-pressure-pulse sterilizer is that sterilization is not affected in the event of an air leak into the sterilization chamber.

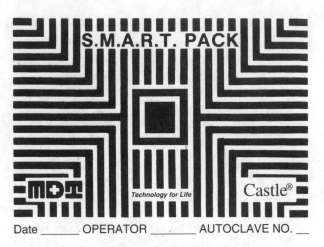

SATISFACTORY TEST

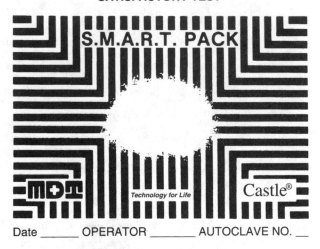

TYPICAL TEST FAILURE

FIGURE 3-4 Air Removal Test.
Source: Courtesy of MDT Biologic Company, Rochester, New York.

FLASH STERILIZATION

Overview

84. Flash sterilization is a process appropriate for steam sterilization of patient care items that are needed immediately and for which there are no replacements immediately available. Items that are flash sterilized are unwrapped. Flash sterilization is used when there is insufficient time to process in the packaged method. Flash sterilization should be reserved for instances when an item is needed immediately and a sterile replacement is not available, for example, when an item is dropped during surgery and that item is necessary to complete the surgery. Flash sterilization should not be used for routine sterilization of instruments. It

should be used only in carefully selected clinical situations and should *not* be used to sterilize implants (AORN, 2003, p. 358). Flash sterilization is discouraged by a number of standard-setting organizations (Gruendemann & Mangum, 2001, p. 199).

85. The cycle for flash sterilization is preset by the sterilizer manufacturer according to the type of sterilizer and the load contents. Flash sterilization may be performed in a gravity displacement, prevacuum, or steam-flush-pressure-pulse sterilizer.

86. Items that are flash sterilized are usually unwrapped, although a single wrapper may be used if sterilizer instructions for use indicate this is appropriate. In addition, there are some rigid containers that have been validated for flash sterilization. Drying is not a part of the flash sterilization cycle; therefore, instruments are wet at the end of the cycle.

87. Because of immediate need, items prepared for flash sterilization are often cleaned and prepared under less-than-ideal conditions. Regardless of where instruments are cleaned, the process should be consistent and in compliance with accepted standards. Often, however, the same processes and resources that are available in the sterile processing department to clean instruments may not be available in the operating room. In addition, a separate decontamination area for cleaning instruments may not exist in the operating room. A scrub sink is not appropriate for cleaning instruments.

88. Cleaning is absolutely critical to proper instrument processing. Inadequate cleaning will compromise the sterilization process.

89. A disadvantage of flash sterilization is that following sterilization, transfer of the item from the autoclave to the sterile field may be difficult because of the lack of protective packaging and because the sterilizer is located outside the actual operating room. Special containers designed for use with a flash cycle reduce the risk of recontamination during transfer from the autoclave to the sterile field. Ideally, a sterilizer used for flash sterilization opens into the actual operating room. This configuration facilitates transport without contamination.

90. Exposure times can vary by more than 30 minutes and are determined by factors such as the nature and configuration of the item, the type of sterilizer, and whether a flash container was utilized. For example, at 270°F (134°C) a 3-minute exposure is appropriate in both a gravity displacement and a prevacuum sterilizer for most metal or nonporous or nonlumened items only. However, for metal items with a lumen, a 10-minute cycle in a gravity displacement sterilizer is required. In a prevacuum sterilizer, metal items with a lumen might require only 4 minutes (AORN, 2003, p. 359). For this reason it is critical that sterilizer, container, and device manufacturer guidelines be followed.

91. Some device manufacturers do not provide instructions for flash sterilization. In this event the item should not be flash sterilized. Perioperative nurses should always refer to manufacturer's guidelines when selecting the cycle type, time, and temperature. If instructions are not available within the operating room, the perioperative nurse should consult with personnel from the sterile processing department, and in the absence of instructions the device should not be sterilized.

- -

SECTION QUESTIONS

Q32. Explain how the addition of a prevacuum or air removal period prior to sterilization shortens the sterilization cycle. (Ref. 73, 76)

_____

_____

Q33. Explain the purpose of a Bowie-Dick test. (Ref. 78)

_____

_____

Q34. The disadvantage to a steam-flush-pressure-pulse sterilizer is that in the event of an air leak into the sterilization chamber, sterilization will be adversely affected. (Ref. 83)

True   False

Q35. Describe the most appropriate use of flash sterilization. (Ref. 84)

_____

Q36. Describe two disadvantages of flash sterilization that could contribute to an item being improperly prepared for sterilization or that could contribute to the risk of contamination. (Ref. 87, 89)

_____

_____

Q37. Exposure times in all steam sterilizers should be (Ref. 90):

a. identical for all sterilizers

b. identical for all items

c. determined by the type of sterilizer

d. determined by the item being sterilized

e. determined according to manufacturer guidelines

f. determined by the skill of the sterilizer operator

• •

CHEMICAL STERILIZATION—ETHYLENE OXIDE GAS (EO)

Description

92. Ethylene oxide is a toxic gas used to sterilize items that cannot tolerate the temperature and moisture of steam sterilization. Ethylene oxide achieves sterilization by interfering with protein metabolism and reproduction of the cell.

93. A wide variety of surgical items that cannot withstand moist heat without incurring damage may be sterilized with ethylene oxide gas. Commonly gas-sterilized items are flexible and rigid endoscopes, plastic goods, instruments with electrical components, and delicate instruments with sharp edges that will dull after repeated steam sterilization.

94. The essential parameters of gas sterilization are gas concentration, temperature, humidity, and exposure time.

95. Gas concentration varies with the size of the chamber, the temperature and humidity within the chamber, and the type of gas sterilizer used.

Gas sterilizers operate at temperatures between 85°F (29°C) and 145°F (63°C). Optimum humidity levels are between 30% and 60%. Exposure times generally range from 3 to 7 hours. The sterilizer manufacturer and the device manufacturer recommendations must be followed carefully to determine exposure time.

96. Ethylene oxide supplied in a 100% concentration is packaged in small unit-dose cartridges. Because ethylene oxide is flammable and explosive when supplied in large tanks, it is mixed with inert gases such as hydrochlorofluorocarbons (HCFCs) or carbon dioxide. The selection of 100% EO or a mixture is determined by the sterilizer design.

97. In the EO sterilization cycle, the air is evacuated from the chamber and its contents, the load is preheated, and humidity is introduced. This phase is termed the *preconditioning phase*. EO is then released into the chamber, where it permeates and penetrates the load. EO sterilization operates under negative pressure. The advantage to this is that if a leak occurs, the EO will be drawn into the chamber rather than to the outside work environment.

Advantages

98. Advantages of EO sterilization are as follows:

   - EO is effective against all types of microorganisms.
   - EO does not require high heat.
   - EO is noncorrosive.
   - EO effectively penetrates large bundles and permeates all porous items.

Disadvantages

99. Ethylene oxide is a toxic gas, and the sterilization process can be complex and potentially hazardous. Because of the toxic and hazardous nature of ethylene oxide sterilization, items that can tolerate steam sterilization should not be gas sterilized.

100. Other disadvantages are as follows:

   - The sterilization cycle time is lengthy.
   - EO is highly flammable, and EO cylinders and cartridges must be carefully handled and stored.
   - The diluent HCFCs used in EO sterilization are subject to strict local, state, and federal regulations and are being phased out because they deplete the ozone layer in the atmosphere.
   - EO sterilization is more expensive than steam sterilization.
   - Toxic byproducts can form under certain conditions. For example, ethylene oxide combined with water yields the toxic byproduct ethylene glycol.
   - Because a variety of materials can absorb EO during the sterilization process, residual EO must be removed from the load contents through an aeration or detoxification process following sterilization. Aeration times in a mechanical aerator may be as short as 8 hours or longer than 24 hours. Length of aeration time is dependent upon the item, packaging, density of the load, type of sterilization and aeration system, and temperature in the aeration chamber. Items made from materials such as polyvinylchloride require the most lengthy period of aeration. Sterilizer and device manufacturer guidelines for exposure and aeration must be followed. Items should never be removed from the aerator until the aeration cycle is complete.
   - EO is regarded as a human carcinogen by the Occupational Safety and Health Administra-

   tion (OSHA). It is also recognized as having the potential to cause adverse reproductive effects in humans. In areas where EO is utilized, a sign must be posted that reads, *"Danger: ethylene oxide, cancer hazard and reproductive hazard. Authorized personnel only. Respirators and protective clothing may be required to be worn in this area"* (US Department of Labor, Occupational Safety and Health Administration, 2002, 1910. 1047 [j][1][i].

   - Exposure to EO can cause eye irritation, nausea, dizziness, vomiting, nasal and throat irritation, shortness of breath, tissue burns, and hemolysis. Insufficiently aerated items may cause patient or personnel injury.
   - Personnel working with EO must be provided personal protective equipment and instruction in the hazards associated with EO.
   - Concentrations of EO must be identified in the areas where EO sterilization occurs. Monitoring devices that produce an alarm in the event of EO exposure must be in place.
   - The OSHA standard for exposure to EO limits personnel to one part EO per million parts of air averaged over an 8-hour period. OSHA requires a monitoring program to ensure compliance with this standard. Employees that work with EO must periodically wear monitors that detect the amount of EO in the work area.
   - EO gas must be vented to the outside to avoid personnel exposure. In addition, some states have abatement requirements that add to the cost of EO processing. Abators convert waste ethylene oxide into nontoxic gases that are then vented to the outside.

101. Because of safety issues and because prolonged aeration time means instruments may be unavailable when needed, many health care facilities have significantly reduced or eliminated the use of EO by switching to newer low-temperature sterilization methods that do not have the same safety issues, lengthy process, and aeration time as EO.

LOW TEMPERATURE HYDROGEN PEROXIDE GAS PLASMA STERILIZATION

Description

102. Plasma is a state of matter that is produced through the action of a strong electric or

magnetic field. In low-temperature hydrogen peroxide plasma sterilization, a plasma state is created by the action of radio-frequency or electrical energy upon hydrogen peroxide vapor within a vacuum. (Figure 3-5)

103. Items to be sterilized are placed in a sterilizing chamber, a vacuum is established, and liquid hydrogen peroxide is injected into a cap and enters the chamber in a vaporized or gas form. Hydrogen peroxide vapor is effective in killing microorganisms. The hydrogen peroxide gas is charged with radio-frequency energy that that creates a plasma. The levels of residual hydrogen peroxide are removed, and at the end of the cycle the reactive species recombine to form oxygen and water vapor. The water vapor is in the form of humidity and cannot be felt. Packages are dry at the end of the cycle and may be used immediately or stored for future use.

Advantages

104. Advantages of low-temperature hydrogen peroxide gas plasma sterilization are as follows:

- Gas plasma offers a safe alternative to EO sterilization; no toxic chemicals are used and no aeration is required. Because there are no toxic byproducts, personal protective equip-

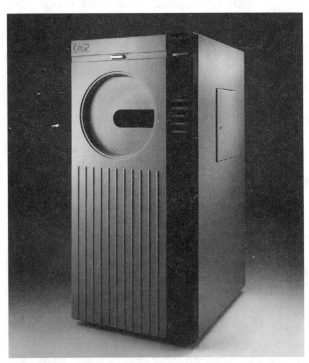

FIGURE 3-5   STERRAD® Hydrogen Peroxide Gas Plasma Sterilizer.
Source: Courtesy of Advanced Sterilization Products, Irvine, California.

ment or monitoring of the environment is not required.

- The sterilization cycle is short (about 30 minutes to over an hour depending upon the sterilizer model).
- The sterilant is compatible with most metals and plastics.
- The sterilizer is simple to operate. Cycle times are set and temperature does not require adjustment.
- There are no plumbing or other fixed requirements. Because the sterilizer connects to an electrical outlet, it can easily be relocated if the need arises.

Disadvantages

105. Disadvantages of low-temperature hydrogen peroxide gas plasma are as follows:

- Hydrogen peroxide gas plasma is not compatible with powders, liquids, textiles, and other cellulose-containing items like linen and paper.
- Packaging materials are limited to nonwoven polypropylene wraps, Tyvek® and mylar pouches, or specific container systems.
- In some hydrogen peroxide gas plasma sterilizer models, lumen restrictions prevent long-lumened devices, such as choledocoscopes, from being processed by this method.

CHEMICAL STERILIZATION—LIQUID PERACETIC ACID

Description

106. Peracetic acid solution contains acetic acid and hydrogen peroxide. Peracetic acid is acetic acid plus an extra oxygen atom. Peracetic acid disrupts protein bonds and cell systems. The extra oxygen inactivates cell systems and causes immediate cell death.

107. Liquid peracetic acid is a low-temperature, nonterminal sterilization modality that can be used for immersible items. It is used primarily for rigid and flexible endoscopes and their accessories.

108. Liquid peracetic acid sterilizers are tabletop units. The items to be sterilized are placed within a dedicated sterilizer tray and are placed into the sterilizer. The sterilant circulates through the tray, contacting all surfaces of the

items. Items with internal lumens are connected to irrigator adapters to ensure sterilant contact within the lumens.

109. For sterilization to occur, contact time is standardized at 12 minutes at a temperature of 50°C to 55°C (122°F to 131°F). A rinse period follows the contact period. Rinse time depends upon the water temperature and fill time. An entire cycle takes less than 30 minutes.

110. Following sterilization, the circulating nurse opens the sterilizer tray, retrieves the tray, transports it to the operating room, and opens it. The sterile scrub person removes the items, which are wet, from the tray and places them on the sterile field. Items that are not delivered to the sterile field are hand dried and stored for later use. Stored items are not considered sterile. (Figure 3-6)

Advantages

111. Advantages of liquid peracetic acid are:

- The sterilization cycle is less than 30 minutes and offers quick turnaround time.
- Peracetic acid is combined with anticorrosive and buffering agents that prevent corrosion of instruments and render the sterilant nontoxic to personnel and the environment.
- Peracetic acid sterilization is compatible with many materials that cannot withstand steam sterilization.

Disadvantages

112. Disadvantages of liquid peracetic acid sterilization are:

- The size of the sterilization container does not permit large loads to be sterilized. Only one flexible scope can be processed at a time.
- Only immersible items that fit within the dedicated tray may be processed.
- Items are wet at the end of the cycle.
- Sterilized items must be used immediately. The nature of the process permits point-of-use sterilization, but not sterile storage.

OTHER EMERGING STERILIZATION TECHNOLOGIES

113. Vapor phase hydrogen peroxide and ozone technology are two emerging low-temperature technologies. Vapor phase hydrogen peroxide is not yet available. Ozone has only recently been introduced to the market and is not widely used.

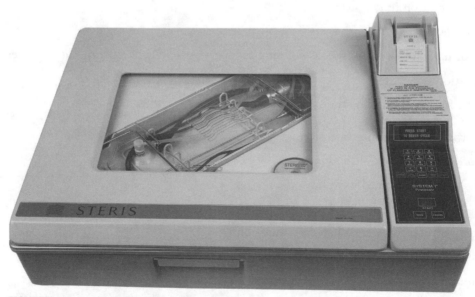

FIGURE 3-6 Steris Sterilization System. Liquid peracetic acid sterilization.
Source: Courtesy of STERIS Company, Mentor, Ohio.

. . . .

SECTION QUESTIONS

Q38. Explain when ethylene oxide sterilization is appropriate. (Ref. 92)

_____

Q39. Ethylene oxide may be supplied (Ref. 96):

    a. in a 100% concentration

    b. mixed with hydrochlorofluorocarbons

    c. mixed with sulphuric acid

Q40. List three advantages of ethylene oxide. (Ref. 98)

_____

Q41. Ethylene oxide is a known carcinogen. List six other disadvantages of ethylene oxide. (Ref. 99, 100)

_____   _____

_____   _____

_____   _____

Q42. Hydrogen peroxide gas plasma is capable of achieving sterilization. (Ref. 102, 103)

    True   False

Q43. Advantages to hydrogen peroxide gas plasma include (Ref. 104):

    a. minimal aeration time

    b. short cycle time

    c. monitoring employee exposure is not required for personnel who operate the sterilizer

    d. no aeration is required

    e. suitable for heat- and moisture-sensitive items

Q44. Liquid peracetic acid sterilization (Ref. 107, 111, 112):

    a. is appropriate for flexible endoscopes

    b. results in an unwrapped wet item

    c. results in a wrapped dry item

    d. can only be used for items that are immersible

    e. takes approximately 1½ hours

    f. permits sterile storage of processed items

. . . .

STERILIZATION—QUALITY CONTROL

Overview

114. Before an article can be considered as having been sterilized, certain parameters of time, humidity, pressure, and temperature must have been met. Chemical and mechanical process indicators and biological testing are used to monitor these parameters. Indicators provide an opportunity for a variety of personnel to check the process. The person removing the item from the sterilizer, the circulating nurse, and the scrub person all share responsibility for checking these monitors.

Mechanical Process Indicators

115. Mechanical indicators are graphs, thermometers, printouts, and gauges that record activities within the chamber during the sterilization cycle.

116. A temperature graph indicates the temperature achieved within the chamber and the length of time that temperature was sustained. A temperature graph also provides information about the time of day that the autoclave was used and the number of cycles run during a 24-hour period. Modern sterilizers employ a printout rather than a temperature graph. (Figure 3-7)

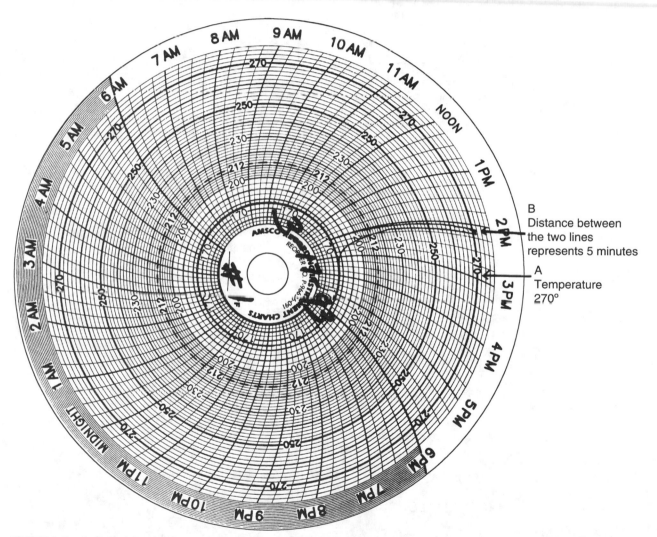

FIGURE 3-7 Autoclave Graph. The graph is affixed to a 24-hour clock device on the autoclave. The clock device and graph make one complete circle turn in 24 hours. Whenever the sterilization cycle is initiated a marking pen records the temperature achieved (A). The amount of time the temperature remained elevated is calculated by how far the graph turns before the temperature drops during the exhaust phase (B). On the above graph the sterilization cycle was initiated one time at 2:00 PM. The temperature reached slightly above 270°F and the exposure time was 5 minutes long. Note that the date and a number indicating to which autoclave the graph is attached have been written on the graph.
Source: Courtesy of AMSCO International, Inc. Markings made by author.

117. A printout record correlates the exact times, temperatures, and pressures achieved during the conditioning, exposure, and exhaust phases of the sterilization cycle. There are spaces on the printout for documentation of information such as the items in the load and identity of the operator. (Figure 3-8)

118. Gauges on the autoclave may register pressure and temperature within the jacket and the chamber. Gauges on the EO sterilizer may register temperature, gas concentration, and humidity.

119. With liquid peracetic acid, a diagnostic cycle in which electricity supply, filters, temperature, pressure, and system integrity is checked is run

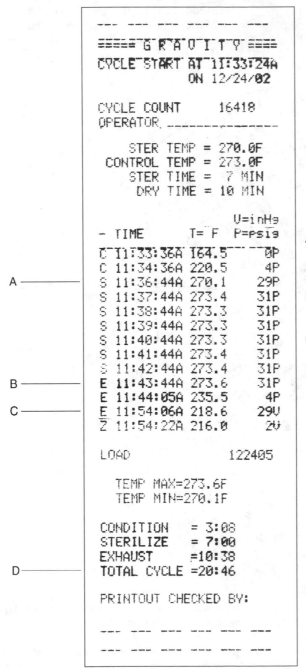

A. At 11:36 AM pressure reached 29 pounds per square inch (PSI) and temperature reached 270°, Sterilization began

B. At 11:43 AM sterilization time completed, exhaust began

C. Cycle completed at 11:54 AM

D. Total Cycle Time = 20:46

FIGURE 3-8 Printout from Gravity Displacement Cycle.
Source: Courtesy of STERIS Corporation.

at the beginning of each day, and a printout of the results is provided.

Chemical Indicators

120. Chemical indicators are impregnated with a dye or chemical that develops a visual or physical change when certain conditions have been achieved. Indicators are manufactured as tapes, strips, or labels.

121. Chemical indicators referred to as *integrators* provide results that are based on the integration of some or all of the parameters that need to be met.

122. Chemical indicators should be placed inside and outside of all packages. The chemical indicator on the outside of the package is inspected before the product is opened, and the one inside is inspected after opening. It is possible for an outside indicator to indicate the proper conditions have been achieved and an inside indicator in the same product to fail. Improper packaging is one reason an inside indicator may fail while the outside one does not. Typically the circulating nurse, or whoever obtains the instruments for a procedure, will be the person in a position to inspect the outside indicator, and the scrub person will inspect the inside indicator.

123. Five classes of indicators are as follows:

- Class 1—(process indicator): Chemical indicator intended to demonstrate that the item has been exposed to the sterilization process. Typically consists of a tape or a paper strip that changes color and distinguishes between processed and unprocessed. May be internal or external. (Figure 3-9)

- Class 2—Bowie-Dick test indicator

- Class 3—(single parameter indicator): Chemical indicator designed to react to one of the critical parameters of sterilization to indicate exposure to a sterilization cycle at a stated value of the chosen parameter.

- Class 4—(multi-parameter indicator): Chemical indicator designed to react to two or more of the critical parameters of a sterilization cycle at stated values of the chosen parameters.

- Class 5—(integrating indicator): Chemical indicator designed to react to all critical parameters over a specified range of sterilization cycles and whose performance has been correlated to the performance of the stated test organism under the labeled conditions of use (AAMI, 2002, p. 2). (Figure 3-10)

Another type of indicator that is available for steam sterilizers is an enzyme-only indicator composed of multiple interactive enzymes. A color change indicates the parameters necessary to achieve sterility have been met within the sterilizer.

124. Integrating and enzyme-based indicators provide a higher level of assurance than other

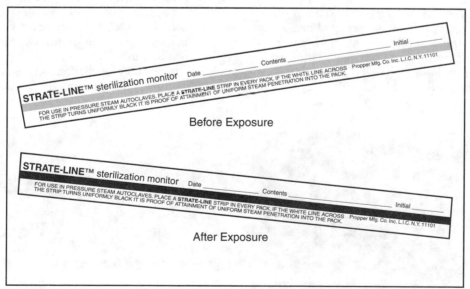

FIGURE 3-9 Chemical Indicator for Steam Sterilizers. Line turns black upon exposure to steam at 250°F.
Source: Courtesy of Propper Manufacturing Co., Long Island City, New York.

indicators. Chemical indicators, however, do not establish sterility. They are tools to determine whether conditions of sterilization have been met.

Biological Monitors

125. Biological monitoring is a process used to determine the efficacy of a sterilizer. It is the most accurate method of ensuring that the conditions necessary for sterilization have been achieved. (Figure 3-11 A & B)

126. Biological indicators (BI) are strips, ampoules, and capsules that contain a known, living, and highly resistant spore population.

127. *Geobacillus stearothermophilus* spores are used to test steam autoclaves and hydrogen peroxide gas plasma and liquid peracetic acid sterilizers. Ethylene oxide sterilizers are tested with *Bacillus atrophaeus* (formerly *Bacillus subtilis*) spores. Both are highly resistant non-pathogenic microorganisms.

128. To routinely test the ability of the sterilizer to operate effectively, one or two strips, ampoules, or capsules containing the spores are placed at a specific location within the chamber, and the sterilizer is activated.

129. Incubation of the spores follows completion of the sterilization cycle. Length of incubation varies according to the manufacturer's instructions. Growth is almost always visible within 24 hours, although the time specified for reading the results may be longer.

130. A positive (for growth) reading indicates that sterilizing conditions have not been met and requires that the sterilizer be taken out of service until the problem is corrected and a negative reading is obtained. Any items processed in the load containing a positive BI must be recalled, as well as any items processed between that load and the last load with a negative BI.

In addition, a positive BI should be reported immediately to the appropriate supervisor and the sterilizer taken out of service until the cause is determined, corrective action has been taken, and subsequent BI testing is negative.

131. A positive reading can indicate incorrect packaging, items incompatible with the process, incorrect placement within the sterilizer, or that the autoclave is malfunctioning.

132. Steam autoclaves should be tested at least weekly and preferably daily, and with every load of implantables. Liquid peracetic acid sterilizers should be tested at least weekly and preferably daily. Hydrogen peroxide gas plasma sterilizers should be tested daily. EO sterilizers should be tested with every load (AORN, 2003, p. 363).

133. Implants should not be implanted until results of biological monitoring are known and are negative for growth.

Rapid Readout Biological Monitors

134. A rapid readout enzyme-based biological indicator is another type of monitor available for testing steam and ethylene oxide sterilizers.

135. Rapid readout biological monitors for steam contain a standardized population of *Geobacillus stearothermophilus* spores. Ethylene oxide rapid readout biological monitors contain a standardized population of *Bacillus atrophaeus* spores. Fluorescence that occurs when an enzyme present within the *Geobacillus stearothermophilus* spores or *Bacillus atrophaeus* spores breaks down is noted by a color change that indicates that the conditions for sterilization have been achieved. The enzyme activity correlates to inactivation of the spores. Depending upon the product used, a result is available within 1 to 3 hours after incubating. Because these monitors contain spores, it is possible, if desired, to incu-

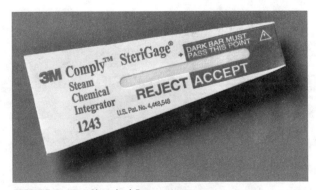

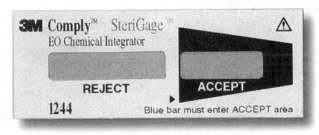

FIGURE 3-10 Chemical Integrators.
Source: Courtesy of 3M Health Care, Inc.

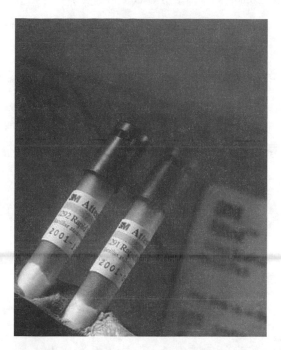
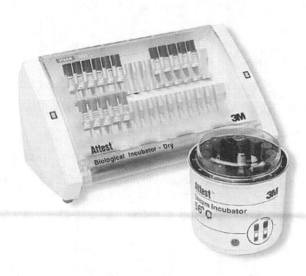

FIGURE 3-11 Biological Monitor-Capsule Containing a Known Population of Spores.
Source: Courtesy of 3M Health Care, St. Paul, Minnesota.

bate for a longer time to obtain spore testing results.

136. The benefit of a rapid readout biological indicator is that monitoring results are available soon after testing.

137. Biological monitors are not interchangeable and must be selected according to the sterilizer type and the cycle being tested.

RECORD KEEPING

138. The following records should be filed and kept as a permanent record:

- results of Bowie-Dick/air evacuation test
- sterilizer graphs and printouts, which should be initialed by the operator for verification of cycle parameters
- results of chemical and biological monitoring
- records indicating load contents and load control numbers used to designate which sterilizer was used for which items
- implantable biologic test results
- sterilizer failure results
- flash sterilization records should be traceable to the patient, procedure, and device.

SECTION QUESTIONS

Q45. A sterilizer printout is an example of a mechanical process indicator. (Ref. 115)

True   False

Q46. Select the correct answer(s). (Ref. 117, 122, 124)

a. Chemical indicators should be placed on the outside of every package to be sterilized.

b. Indicator tapes that change color when steam causes a chemical reaction to occur are a guarantee of sterility.

c. A printout record of the sterilization process displays the exact times and temperatures achieved during conditioning, exposure and exhaust phases of the cycle.

Q47. Unlike Class 1 indicators, Class 5 integrating indicators are used to guarantee sterility. (Ref. 124)

True   False

Q48. Biological monitoring of steam sterilizers (Ref. 125, 126, 130, 132):

a. ensures that the autoclave is achieving conditions necessary for sterilization

b. is accomplished with a known population of spores

c. should be conducted at least weekly

d. should be conducted after major repairs to the sterilizer

e. should be conducted with every load of implantables

Q49. What is *Bacillus atrophaeus* and what is it used for? (Ref. 127)

_____

_____

Q50. Biological monitoring of hydrogen peroxide gas plasma sterilization is accomplished with the spore *Geobacillus stearothermophilus*. (Ref. 127)

True   False

Q51. When a biological monitor that has been subject to the sterilization process results in a positive for growth result, this should be reported to the immediate supervisor. All items in that load should be re-called, as well as all items that were processed for the last week. (Ref. 130)

True   False

Q52. Hydrogen peroxide gas plasma sterilizers should be monitored with a biological indicator (Ref. 132):

a. with every load

b. daily

c. weekly

Q53. The benefit of a rapid readout monitor is that spores will grow out more quickly than with a conventional biological monitor. (Ref. 136)

True   False

• •

DISINFECTION

Overview

139. Disinfection is a process that destroys pathogenic microorganisms through the use of a liquid chemical germicide. A disinfectant is an agent that destroys vegetative forms of harmful microorganisms. Some disinfectants kill some spores; however, disinfectants do not kill high numbers of spores.

140. Chemicals used to destroy microorganisms on inanimate objects are identified as disinfectants. Chemicals used to destroy microorganisms on body surfaces are identified as antiseptics.

Levels of Disinfectants—Application

141. Disinfection is used to destroy pathogens on inanimate objects such as walls, tables, small equipment, and surgical instruments. Liquid

chemicals are used for disinfection. Disinfectants must be selected according to their intended use. Disinfectants suitable for housekeeping purposes, such as for walls and tables, are not suitable for disinfection of surgical instruments. Likewise, the most appropriate disinfecting agent for surgical instruments is not the most suitable for housekeeping.

142. Examples of disinfectants include alcohol, chlorine and chlorine compounds, formaldehyde, glutaraldehyde, hydrogen peroxide, iodophors, *ortho*-phthalaldehyde, phenolics, and quaternary ammonium compounds. Disinfectants vary in their ability to destroy microorganisms, and they are not interchangeable. Disinfectants are categorized as high-level, intermediate-level, and low-level.

143. Factors that influence the efficacy of a disinfectant include the type of chemical, concentration and temperature of the chemical, amount and type of microorganisms present, configuration of the item to be disinfected, adequacy of prior cleaning, and exposure time.

144. High-level disinfectants kill all microorganisms including vegetative bacteria forms, the tubercle bacilli, viruses, and fungi. They do not kill high numbers of spores, although some high-level disinfectants can achieve sterilization after prolonged exposure of generally 8 hours or more. Because this is impractical and provides a product that is intended for immediate use, high-level disinfectants are vary rarely used for this purpose. High-level disinfectants are only used for disinfecting instruments and medical devices; they are not used on environmental surfaces.

145. Intermediate-level disinfectants inactivate most vegetative bacteria, the tubercle bacillus, fungi, and viruses, but not necessarily bacterial spores. Low-level disinfectants kill most vegetative bacteria, some fungi, and some viruses. They do not kill the tubercle bacillus. Intermediate and low-level disinfectants are formulated to be used on environmental surfaces and are never to be used on instruments and medical devices.

146. For instrument disinfection, the most frequently used high-level disinfectants are solutions of 2% to 3.2% alkaline glutaraldehyde or 55% *ortho*-phthalaldehyde.

Glutaraldehyde

147. Glutaraldehyde is a high-level disinfectant that is also capable of sterilization. Because of the lengthy immersion period required for sterilization, glutaraldehyde is rarely used as a sterilizing agent. A 2% solution of glutaraldehyde requires an immersion period of 10 hours for sterilization to be achieved. High-level disinfection is achieved in minutes. The exact number of minutes varies with the concentration and temperature of the solution. Manufacturer's instructions and institutional policy should be consulted for exact required immersion time.

148. Items disinfected in glutaraldehyde must be thoroughly washed, rinsed, and dried prior to immersion in the disinfectant and rinsed after removal from the disinfectant.

149. Glutaraldehyde is irritating to mucous membranes and can irritate skin, eyes, throat, and nasal passages. It should be mixed in a well-ventilated room with a minimum of 10 air exchanges an hour. Local exhaust ventilation located at the level of the point of discharge is the preferred method of preventing vapor from escaping. Self-contained work stations with a fume hood should be installed where glutaraldehyde is used. Glutaraldehyde should always be stored in a closed container. Protective eyewear, nitrile gloves or a double set of latex gloves, a mask, and a repellent gown should be worn during use. Exposure varies with the activity. Mixing and discarding the solution and immersing and retrieving items from the solution are activities that pose the greatest risk of exposure.

150. The current OSHA limits for exposure are 0.2 parts of glutaraldehyde to 1 million parts of air during any part of the work day. Monitoring of the work area and employee exposure is not required by OSHA; however, monitoring should be employed when high levels of exposure are suspected.

151. Glutaraldehyde that is heated will achieve microbial kill faster than glutaraldehyde at room temperature. Some automated systems are programmed to heat glutaraldehyde. However, when glutaraldehyde is heated, the vapor pressure is raised, which in turn increases the vapors that are released into the air.

152. As with all disinfectants, glutaraldehyde must be mixed and used strictly according to manufacturer guidelines and standards of practice. Information regarding mixing instructions, use, immersion time, toxicity, and length of effectiveness can be found on the label.

Ortho-phthalaldehyde

153. *Ortho*-phthalaldehyde is a nonglutaraldehyde disinfectant widely used in operating rooms and endoscopy suites. Because it achieves disinfection faster than glutaraldehyde and because there are

no irritating odors, *ortho*-phthalaldehyde has re-placed glutaraldehyde in many facilities.

154. *Ortho*-phthalaldehyde has a very low vapor pressure, and as a result is rarely irritating to staff. There are no OSHA requirements and no monitoring requirements.

155. *Ortho*-phthalaldehyde will stain protein and items that are not thoroughly cleaned and rinsed prior to immersion. *Ortho*-phthalaldehyde will stain gray in spots where there are protein residuals.

DISINFECTION—QUALITY CONTROL

156. To avoid dilution of the disinfectant and compromise of the disinfection process, all items to be disinfected should be thoroughly cleaned, rinsed, and dried prior to immersion.

157. Date of mixing and expiration date (length of anticipated effectiveness as indicated on the label) should be indicated on the container in which the disinfectant is stored. However, one should never rely entirely on the label for expiration of the solution. A disinfectant can lose its minimum effective concentration before the expiration date. The number of times the solution is used, the amount of debris introduced into the solution, and any dilution that occurs when items are washed, rinsed, and not dried before immersion can all impact the minimum concentration and cause a solution to fail.

158. The minimum effective concentration (MEC) of disinfectant solutions should be monitored before use with indicators designed for this purpose. These indicators are usually supplied in the form of paper or plastic strips that are dipped into the solution and then observed for appropriate color change as indicated on the label. Indicators are not interchangeable, and only those supplied with a particular product should be used to test that product.

159. Chemical properties and appropriate hazard warnings should be posted.

DOCUMENTATION

160. When liquid chemical germicides are used for high-level disinfection, the following should be documented:

- results of quality control testing—performed according to manufacturer's instructions
- results of testing for minimum effective concentration
- date solution mixed/activated/opened/prepared
- expiration date—should be visible on container
- person responsible for mixing
- item disinfected
- patient on whom disinfected item is used

SECTION QUESTIONS

Q54. Antiseptics are used on (Ref. 140):

a. inanimate surfaces

b. body surfaces

Q55. All disinfectants can be used for sterilization purposes, provided immersion time is sufficient. (Ref. 144)

True   False

Q56. The high-level disinfectant glutaraldehyde is appropriate for use on (Ref. 146):

a. tabletops

b. surgical instruments

c. floors

Q57. The current OSHA limit for exposure to *ortho*-phthalaldehyde is 0.2 ppm. (Ref. 150)

    True   False

Q58. Items placed in a disinfectant should have been thoroughly cleaned and dried before immersion. (Ref. 156)

    True   False

● ●

● ● ● References

Association for the Advancement of Medical Instrumentation (AAMI). (2002). *Steam sterilization and sterility assurance in health care facilities* (ANSI/AAMI ST46: 2002). Arlington, VA: Author.

Association of periOperative Registered Nurses (AORN). (2003). Recommended practices for sterilization in perioperative practice settings. In *Standards, recommended practices, and guidelines* (pp. 351–367). Denver, CO: Author.

Favero, M., & Bond W. (2001). Chemical disinfection of medical and surgical materials. In S. S. Block, *Disinfection, sterilization, and preservation* (5th ed., pp. 881–915). Philadelphia: Lippincott Williams & Wilkins.

Gruendemann, B., & Mangum, S. (2001). *Infection prevention in surgical settings.* Philadelphia: W. B. Saunders.

Perkins, J. J. (1969). *Principles and methods of sterilization.* Springfield, IL: Charles C. Thomas.

U.S. Department of Health and Human Services, Centers for Disease Control. (1999). Bronchoscopy-related infections and pseudoinfections—New York, 1996, and 1998. *Morbidity and Mortality Weekly Report (MMWR), 18* (26), 557–560.

U.S. Department of Labor, Occupational Safety and Health Administration. (2002). Toxic and Hazardous Substances. Regulations and Standards 29R. 1910.1047.

● ● ● Suggested Reading

Gruendemann, B., & Mangum, S. (2001). Sterilization. In *Infection prevention in surgical settings* (pp. 181–205). Philadelphia: W. B. Saunders.

Phillips, N. (2003). Sterilization and disinfection. In *Operating Room Technique* (10th ed., pp. 281–323). St. Louis, MO: Mosby.

Barrett, T. (2000). Flash sterilization: What are the risks? In W. Rutala (Ed.), *Disinfection, Sterilization and Antisepsis* (pp. 70–77). Washington, DC: Association for Professionals in Infection Control.

Appendix 3-A

• •

Chapter 3 Post Test

Instructions: Fill in the blank(s), mark the correct answer(s), or answer the question as appropriate.

1. *Disinfection* means (Ref. 7, 141):

   a. the destruction of all gram-negative bacteria

   b. the destruction of all pathogenic microorganisms except spores

   c. the process used to make skin as free from bacteria as possible

2. Low-level disinfectants are capable of destroying the tubercle bacillus. (Ref. 7, 145)

   True   False

3. Sterilizers are monitored by their ability to kill a known population of spores. (Ref. 9)

   True   False

4. *Sterile* means (Ref. 10, 12):

   a. free of all living microorganisms

   b. free of all bacteria and viruses

   c. free of all viable microorganisms, including spores

5. What is the desired outcome for the patient scheduled for an invasive procedure with a nursing diagnosis of *high risk for infection?* (Ref. 13)

   _____

6. Medical devices contaminated with pathogenic microorganisms have caused patient infections. (Ref. 17)

   True   False

7. Semicritical items do not require sterilization. They do require high-level disinfection. Define a semicritical item. (Ref. 26, 27)

   _____

8. A sterility assurance level of 10^{-3} is the standard for sterilization of medical devices used in surgery. (Ref. 31)

   True   False

9. There are four sterilization technologies commonly employed in health care facilities. List three of them. (Ref. 36, 37)

   _____

10. Dry heat sterilization is appropriate for sterilizing (Ref. 40):

    a. linen

    b. powder

    c. rubber items

    d. oils

11. Select the correct answer(s). (Ref. 43, 46, 48)

    a. Steam must be subjected to pressure for it to reach a temperature high enough to accomplish sterilization.

    b. For an item to be rendered sterile, steam must contact every surface of that item.

    c. Steam at a temperature of 212°F (100°C) is sufficient to achieve sterilization.

12. One of the advantages of steam sterilization is that one cycle time is appropriate for all items. (Ref. 51, 64)

    True   False

13. If items are improperly prepared or improperly placed within the autoclave, air may become trapped and sterilization may fail to occur. Why? (Ref. 56)

    _____

14. Explain why it is inappropriate to place a warm sterilized package on a solid cold surface. (Ref. 60)

    _____

15. Explain the difference between a gravity displacement autoclave and a prevacuum autoclave. (Ref. 66, 73)

    _____

16. A prevacuum sterilization cycle provides a greater margin of safety than a gravity displacement cycle with regard to air removal. (Ref. 76)

    True   False

17. A Bowie-Dick test is a method to biologically monitor prevacuum autoclaves. (Ref. 4, 78)

    True   False

18. Sterilization will be achieved in a steam-flush-pressure-pulse sterilizer even if there is an air leak into the chamber during the cycle. (Ref. 83)

    True   False

19. When a 270°F 3-minute exposure is used on an unwrapped item, it is referred to as a _____ cycle. (Ref. 91)

20. Ethylene oxide is toxic and exposure can cause vomiting, headache, and irritation of the eyes and respiratory passages. Therefore, all porous items sterilized in ethylene oxide must go through a final aeration process. When a mechanical aerator is used this process requires a minimum of (Ref. 100):

    a. 15 minutes

    b. 1 hour

    c. 8 hours

21. The OSHA standard for exposure to ethylene oxide limits personnel to one part of ethylene oxide to _____ parts of air averaged over an 8-hour time period. (Ref. 100)

22. Hydrogen peroxide gas plasma sterilization (Ref. 104 , 105, 127):

    a. leaves no toxic residue and requires no aeration

    b. offers an alternative to ethylene oxide for sterilization of heat- and moisture-sensitive items

    c. is appropriate for linen and paper goods

    d. requires a lengthy cycle time

    e. is biologically monitored with *Bacillus atrophaeus*

23. Hydrogen peroxide gas plasma sterilization may not be used for metal instruments. (Ref. 104)

    True   False

24. Liquid peracetic acid sterilization is most appropriate for (Ref. 107):

    a. items that can tolerate immersion

    b. stainless steel surgical instruments

    c. flexible endoscopes

25. The benefit of liquid peracetic acid sterilization is that items that are not used right after sterilization can be stored in a sterile state for later use. (Ref. 112)

    True   False

26. What information can be obtained from reading an autoclave printout? (Ref. 116, 117)

    _____

27. Chemical process indicators (Ref. 121, 122, 124):

    a. are not a guarantee of sterility

    b. are used to show that parameters of sterilization have been met

    c. should be visible on the outside of every package

    d. include *Bacillus atrophaeus* and *Geobacillus stearothermophilus*

28. An integrating indicator is usually a tape that changes color to indicate exposure to one of the parameters of sterilization, and is used to distinguish between processed and unprocessed items. (Ref. 120, 123)

    True   False

29. Rapid readout biological indicators change color to indicate conditions of sterilization have been achieved. (Ref. 135)

    True   False

30. Match the technology with the biological monitor. (Ref. 127)

    _____ hydrogen peroxide gas plasma   a. *Bacillus atrophaeus*

    _____ ethylene oxide   b. *Geobacillus stearothermophilus*

    _____ steam

    _____ liquid peracetic acid

31. Steam sterilizer monitoring should be conducted (Ref. 132):

    a. at least weekly

    b. daily

    c. with every load

    d. with every implantable

    e. after major repair

32. Rapid readout biological monitors (Ref. 135):

    a. contain *Bacillus atrophaeus* or *Geobacillus stearothermopholis*

    b. cannot be incubated

    c. provide results after 1 to 3 hours of incubation that correlate to deactivation of spores

33. Results of biological monitoring, sterilizer failure records, and records indicating load contents and load control numbers that designate which sterilizer was used for which item should be kept as a permanent record. (Ref. 138)

    True   False

34. Glutaraldehyde is a high-level disinfectant that (Ref. 147, 149):

    a. is suitable for disinfection of cystoscopes

    b. can achieve sterilization in 45 minutes immersion time

    c. is irritating to mucous membranes

    d. requires the user to don protective eyewear, mask, repellent gown, and double latex or nitrile gloves during use

35. Although OSHA does not require monitoring of worker exposure to glutaraldehyde, the OSHA exposure limits are _____ parts of glutaraldehyde to 1 million parts of air during any part of the work day, and glutaraldehyde should be used in an environment where there are at least _____ air exchanges an hour. (Ref. 149, 150)

36. Items disinfected in glutaraldehyde must be (Ref. 147, 148):

    a. cleaned and rinsed before immersion

    b. dried before immersion

    c. immersed for 1 hour for disinfection to occur

    d. rinsed prior to use

37. *Ortho*-phthalaldehyde (Ref. 153, 154):

    a. disinfects in less time than glutaraldehyde

    b. has an irritating odor

    c. has a low vapor pressure resulting in no irritating odors

Appendix 3-B

• •

Competency Checklist: Sterilization and Disinfection

Under "Observer's Initials," enter initials upon successful achievement of competency.
Enter N/A if competency is not appropriate for institution.

NAME _____

	OBSERVER'S INITIALS	DATE

1. Identifies appropriate method of sterilization for item to be sterilized.   _____ _____

2. Steam sterilization

    a. sets appropriate cycle   _____ _____

    b. sets appropriate time   _____ _____

    c. sets appropriate temperature   _____ _____

    d. includes chemical process indicator or integrator in package/ visible on outside   _____ _____

    e. selects tray compatible with sterilization method   _____ _____

    f. packages correctly   _____ _____

    g. moistens lumens   _____ _____

    h. loads correctly—sterilant can exit and enter packages   _____ _____

    i. documents required information   _____ _____

    j. operates according to manufacturer's instructions   _____ _____

    k. observes graph/printout/indicator for parameters   _____ _____

    l. (flash) transports without contamination following sterilization   _____ _____

    m. (wrapped) allows package to cool before removing from autoclave   _____ _____

3. Biological monitor—steam

    a. selects appropriate monitor   _____ _____

    b. documents date, autoclave, and operator   _____ _____

    c. places biological indicator correctly within chamber (follows manufacturer's instructions for placement)   _____ _____

    d. sets appropriate cycle, time, and temperature   _____ _____

    e. incubates processed biological monitor and control according to manufacturer's instructions   _____ _____

4. Hydrogen peroxide gas plasma sterilization

    a. includes chemical process indicator   _____ _____

    b. selects tray or container appropriate for sterilization process   _____ _____

  c. packages correctly

  d. loads correctly

  e. operates sterilizer according to manufacturer's instructions

  f. documents required information

5. Biological monitor—hydrogen peroxide gas plasma

  a. selects appropriate monitor

  b. documents date, sterilizer, and operator

  c. places within chamber correctly (follows manufacturer's instructions for placement)

  d. incubates processed biological monitor and control according to manufacturer's instructions

6. Liquid peracetic acid sterilization

  a. runs diagnostic cycle

  b. loads properly—connections as appropriate

  c. documents required information

  e. operates in accordance with manufacturer's instructions

  f. transports without contamination

  g. performs biological monitor according to manufacturer's instructions

7. Disinfection

  a. identifies items appropriate for high-level disinfection

  b. prepares disinfectant according to manufacturer's instructions

  c. wears appropriate personal protective equipment during preparation of disinfectant and use

  d. performs the MEC test and documents results

  e. documents required information

8. Items are:

  a. appropriately washed and dried before disinfected

  b. rinsed after disinfected and before use

  c. handled so as to prevent contamination

OBSERVER'S SIGNATURE   INITIALS   DATE

_____

ORIENTEE'S SIGNATURE

_____

Chapter 3—Section Question Answers

Q1. False
Q2. False
Q3. False
Q4. Increased pain and suffering, delayed recovery, even death
Q5. Provides a portal of entry
Q6. Pathogenic microorganisms can cause disease. Pathogenic microorganisms can gain entry when skin integrity is interrupted.
Q7. a, b
Q8. Sterilization, disinfection
Q9. a
Q10. d
Q11. False
Q12. True
Q13. False
Q14. a
Q15. Disinfection
Q16. Compatability of the sterilization modality with the item, packaging, length of time for the process, safety, cost, availability, required equipment; configuration of the item
Q17. False
Q18. a, d, f, g
Q19. Steam
Q20. b
Q21. False
Q22. False
Q23. 250°F (121°C)
Q24. True
Q25. Readily available, economical, compatible with most devices, nontoxic
Q26. Trapped air can prevent steam contact with all surfaces
Q27. False
Q28. c
Q29. False
Q30. True
Q31. True
Q32. When air enters the chamber, the vacuum present causes instant contact with the devices
Q33. Verifies air removal—necessary to achieve steam penetration throughout the load
Q34. False
Q35. For items needed immediately for which there are no sterile replacements available
Q36. Possible inadequate cleaning of the item in the operating room, possible recontamination during transport
Q37. c, d, e
Q38. For items that cannot tolerate moisture or the high temperature of steam
Q39. a, b

Chapter 3—Section Question Answers *(continued)*

Q40. Low temperature, effective against all microorganisms, noncorrosive, good penetrator

Q41. Long cycle, diluents subject to government regulations, more expensive than steam, combined with water makes ethylene glycol, long aeration, can cause eye irritation, known carcinogen, requires personal protective equipment, environmental monitoring required, must be vented to the outside

Q42. True

Q43. b, c, d, e

Q44. a, b, d

Q45. True

Q46. a, c

Q47. False

Q48. a, b, c, d, e

Q49. A spore used to test ethylene oxide sterilizers

Q50. True

Q51. False

Q52. b

Q53. False

Q54. b

Q55. False

Q56. b

Q57. False

Q58. True

Chapter 3—Post Test Answers

1. b
2. False
3. True
4. c
5. Freedom from infection
6. True
7. An item that contacts an intact mucous membrane, does not penetrate it
8. False
9. Ethylene oxide, stream, hydrogen peroxide gas plasma, liquid peracetic acid
10. b, d
11. a, b
12. False
13. Trapped air can prevent steam contact
14. Can cause condensation, package will become damp, microorganisms can penetrate moist packages
15. Gravity—air displaced by gravity; prevacuum—air removed with pump
16. True
17. False
18. True
19. Flash
20. c
21. 1,000,000
22. a, b
23. False
24. a, c
25. False
26. Time, temperature, pressure during all phases of the sterilization cycle
27. a, c
28. False
29. True
30. b, a, b , b
31. a, d, e
32. a, c
33. True
34. a, c, d
35. 0.2, 10
36. a, b, d
37. a, c

4

Prevention of Infection—Preparation of Instruments and Items Used in Surgery: Cleaning, Packaging, and Storage

LEARNER OBJECTIVES

After reading and completing "Prevention of Infection—Preparation of Instruments and Items Used in Surgery: Cleaning, Packaging, and Storage," the learner will:

- discuss the relationship of cleaning, packaging, and storage of sterile supplies to patient outcomes of freedom from infection and freedom from injury
- describe the responsibilities of the registered nurse in relation to cleaning, packaging, and storage of sterile supplies
- discuss the decontamination process for surgical instruments, including instruments exposed to prions
- explain the role of ultrasonic cleaning in instrument decontamination
- list six criteria for packaging materials
- describe four principles of packaging
- describe three packaging materials, their use, and advantages and disadvantages of each
- define and discuss shelf life
- discuss reuse of single-use devices

• • • • • • • • • • • •
Lesson Outline

I.   DEFINITIONS
II. NURSING DIAGNOSIS—DESIRED PATIENT OUTCOMES
III. NURSING RESPONSIBILITIES
IV. PREPARATION OF ITEMS AND INSTRUMENTS FOR STERILIZATION
     A. Cleaning
         1. Intraoperative Cleaning
         2. Postoperative Cleaning
         3. Manual Cleaning
         4. Mechanical Cleaning
         5. Special Protocols for Instruments Exposed to Prions
         6. Ultrasonic Cleaning
     B. Lubrication
     C. Inspection
V.   PACKAGING MATERIALS—BARRIERS
     A. Selection Criteria
     B. Types of Packaging
         1. Overview
         2. Woven Fabric
         3. Nonwoven Materials
         4. Plastic/Paper, Plastic/Tyvek®—Pouches
         5. Rigid Containers
VI. PRINCIPLES OF PACKAGING—STEAM
     A. Instruments
     B. Other Items
         1. Basins, Bowls, Cups
         2. Rubber Goods, Tubing, Items with a Lumen, Wood Items
         3. Reusable Textiles—Linen Packs
VII. PACKAGING FOR ALTERNATE METHODS OF STERILIZATION
VIII. PACKAGE INFORMATION AND IDENTIFICATION
     A. Chemical Indicators
     B. Sealing
     C. Labels
IX. SHELF LIFE
     A. Storage Considerations
     B. Determining Factors
X.   REUSE OF SINGLE-USE DEVICES

DEFINITIONS
• •

1. **Biofilm:** A biofilm is a collection of microscopic organisms that exist in a polysaccharide matrix that adheres to a surface and prevents antimicrobial agents such as sterilants, disinfectants, and antibiotics from reaching the cells.

2. **Contaiminated:** In the operating room environment, the term *contaminated* refers to items that are not sterile. Items soiled or potentially soiled with microorganisms are considered to be contaminated. Items that were opened for surgery, whether or not they were actually used during surgery and whether or not they are known to contain microorganisms, are also considered to be contaminated. This differs slightly from the regulatory arena, in which *contaminated* refers to an item that has been in contact with an infectious agent.

3. **Decontamination:** Decontamination is the process that renders a contaminated item safe for handling.

4. **Washer-disinfector, Washer-decontaminator:** Automated processing units used to decon-

taminate instruments. Cycles within these machines vary but do include washing and rinsing and may include ultrasonic cleaning. A chemical or thermal phase within the cycle destroys specific microorganisms.

5. **Washer-sterilizer:** An automated processing unit used to decontaminate instruments. The cycle includes washing, rinsing, and sterilization. Although there is a sterilization phase at the end of the wash and rinse phase, instruments decontaminated in this manner are not ready for patient use and must be inspected and packaged in preparation for a final sterilization process.

NURSING DIAGNOSIS—DESIRED PATIENT OUTCOMES

6. The nursing diagnosis high risk for infection is appropriate for patients undergoing invasive procedures. Infection may result from contact with contaminated instruments, and injury can result when instrumentation fails to function properly. Perioperative nursing activities are directed toward the prevention of infection and injury with the goal that the patient will be free from infection and free from injury following the operation. Many perioperative nursing activities contribute to the achievement of these outcomes. Among these are cleaning, inspection, packaging, and storage of sterile supplies (surgical instruments, diagnostic devices, and other reusable patient-care items.)

NURSING RESPONSIBILITIES

7. The perioperative nurse assumes varying levels of responsibility for cleaning, packaging, and storage of sterile supplies. There is no single cleaning or packaging process that is appropriate for all supplies. The processes involved require judgment based on a solid knowledge of principles of cleaning, inspection, packaging, and storage of sterile supplies.

8. Most instrument preparation and processing is accomplished in a separate sterile processing department. Although the perioperative nurse may not provide a hands-on contribution to these processes, the nurse must be a resource for those who do. More importantly, the perioperative nurse must be able to identify that specified requirements of cleaning, inspection, packaging, and storage of supplies or instru-

ments have occurred. The perioperative nurse makes the final decision as to whether an item is fit to be entered into the sterile field for use on a patient.

9. In the event that flash sterilization or high-level disinfection is required, the perioperative nurse may assume total responsibility for cleaning, inspection, and packaging, as well as for the sterilization or disinfection process.

10. As an advocate for the patient, with the goals of freedom from infection and/or injury, the perioperative nurse must be able to ensure that all supplies, primarily instruments, used in surgery have been appropriately prepared and processed and are in working order. Desired patient outcomes may not be achieved when improperly prepared or processed supplies harbor microorganisms that can cause infection and when instruments fail to function as intended.

PREPARATION OF ITEMS AND INSTRUMENTS FOR STERILIZATION

Cleaning

11. The first and most important step in instrument decontamination is cleaning.

12. All instruments and devices intended to penetrate a mucous membrane must be subject to a sterilization process. All instruments and devices intended to contact but not penetrate an intact mucous membranes must be at least high-level disinfected.

13. Effective sterilization and disinfection are dependent on proper decontamination.

Intraoperative Cleaning

14. Contaminated instruments, including all instruments opened and/or used for a surgical procedure, should be washed as soon as possible after use to prevent blood and other debris from drying in crevices or on instrument surfaces. Dried-on debris can interfere with the sterilization or disinfection processes by preventing the sterilizing or disinfecting agent from contacting every surface of every item.

15. During the surgical procedure, instruments should be periodically wiped and/or rinsed with a wet lap sponge or immersed in sterile water to remove large particles and to prevent debris from lodging in serrations and other crevices. Instrument lumens should be kept free of debris by immersing the device to fill the lumen with sterile water or irrigating the

channels using a syringe filled with sterile water. Irrigation should take place below the surface of the water to prevent aerosolization of particles. Sterile water, not saline, should be used for cleaning items during surgery.

Postoperative Cleaning

16. Following surgery, instruments should be contained and transported to a dedicated decontamination area. The purpose of containment is to prevent personnel from contacting contaminated items during transfer. The container should be labeled to indicate that the contents are contaminated. To prevent debris from drying on instruments, a damp towel may be used to cover them during transport. An enzymatic soak solution, spray, or gel may also be applied before transport. These activities help prevent corrosion, rusting, and pitting that can occur when blood and debris are allowed to dry on instruments.

17. Instruments should not remain in water for lengthy periods of time as biofilms may form, particularly within lumens. Once formed, a biofilm can only be removed by mechanical means. Sterilization and disinfection processes are compromised in the presence of biofilms.

18. Before instruments are cleaned, the following steps should be taken:

- Box locks and other joints should be opened.
- Heavy instruments should be placed in the bottom of the tray, with lighter ones either in a separate tray or on top.
- Devices with multiple components should be disassembled.

Manual Cleaning

19. In the absence of an automated washer, instruments may be manually cleaned. Additionally, some powered surgical instruments, heat-sensitive, delicate or specialty items that cannot tolerate immersion or mechanical washing should be cleaned separately according to the device manufacturer's written guidelines.

20. Before washing with a detergent, instruments should be rinsed in cold water to remove gross debris. The detergent should be specific for instrument cleaning and should be used strictly according to the manufacturer's instructions. For example, mixing detergents to a higher concentration because of heavy debris in not appropriate and may in fact impede rinsing and interfere with the sterilization or disinfection process.

21. During manual cleaning, personnel should wear personal protective equipment, i.e., a moisture-proof gown, long cuffed utility gloves, a mask and goggles or full-face shield (AAMI, 2002, p. 20). Cleaning of immersible items should be performed below the surface of the water to prevent aerosolization of debris. Lumens and cannulated parts should be flushed while submerged. Items that cannot be immersed should be cleaned in a manner that prevents aerosolization of debris. Soft-bristled brushes or pipe cleaners may be used to remove soil from hard-to-reach places like hinges and serrations. Abrasive cleaners, scouring pads, or steel wool should not be used on surgical instruments.

Mechanical Cleaning

22. Instruments cleaned in an automated system are placed in trays with a wire open-mesh bottom. Trays are then placed in a washer-sterilizer or washer-disinfector/decontaminator where mechanical cleaning occurs.

23. Washer-sterilizers and disinfectors/decontaminators employ water and detergent to clean instruments. In a washer-sterilizer, cold water enters the chamber and mixes with detergent. Steam and air are automatically injected into the chamber to generate turbulence and agitation. The water heats and, as the chamber fills, blood and debris are loosened and lifted from the instruments. The water is flushed out through a bottom drain. Steam under pressure then enters the chamber, and the items are subjected to a sterilization cycle. Washer-sterilizers have a tendency to bake organic debris onto instruments that may not have been adequately cleaned; for this reason, decontamination is usually accomplished in a washer-disinfector/decontaminator that does not have a sterilization phase. Many facilities have replaced washer-sterilizers with washer-disinfectors/decontaminators.

24. A variety of cycles may be provided by a washer-disinfector/decontaminator. Phases in the cycle may include: cool water rinse, enzymatic soak, detergent wash, ultrasonic cleaning, hot water rinse (180°F to 195°F [70°C to 76°C]), germicide rinse, and drying.

25. Instruments that have been processed through a washer-sterilizer or washer-disinfector/decontaminator or are hand washed are considered safe to handle but are *not* ready for immediate patient use and are not considered sterile.

Special Protocols for Instruments Exposed to Prions

26. Instruments that have or are suspected to have come in contact with prions should be

cleaned and sterilized according to special protocols. A prion is an infectious protein particle. Prions are responsible for transmissible spongiform encephalopathies such as Creutzfeld-Jakob disease (CJD), a rare and fatal disease of the central nervous system. Unlike bacteria, viruses, or fungi, prions are resistant to routine sterilization and disinfection procedures.

27. Information and protocols regarding prions is evolving. The Centers for Disease Control and Prevention and the World Health Organization are two agencies that should be consulted when determining protocols for instruments exposed to prions.

28. Brain, spinal cord, and eye tissue are considered high-risk tissue for transmission of prion disease. Instruments exposed to these tissues in patients known or suspected to be infected with a prion disease require special consideration with regard to decontamination. As a guideline, the following steps should be taken for decontaminating instruments exposed, or suspected to have been exposed, to prions:

- Keep instruments moist until cleaned or decontaminated.
- Clean as soon as possible to minimize drying of tissue, blood, and body fluids on the instruments.
- Avoid mixing instruments exposed to high-risk tissue (brain, dura mater, spinal cord, eye) with instruments used on other tissue.
- Instruments exposed to high-risk tissue must be decontaminated using the following protocols:
  - For instruments that are easily cleaned:
    - After thorough cleaning, steam autoclave at 272°F (134°C) for 18 minutes in a prevacuum sterilizer or at 250°F (121°C) for 60 minutes in a gravity displacement autoclave
  - For instruments that are difficult to clean (e.g., have small lumens):
    - Discard or
    - Immerse in container filled with liquid (e.g., saline, water or phenoloic solution) to retard adherence of material to the device; drain liquid; then initially decontaminate by steam sterilization at 272°F (134°C) for 18 minutes in a prevacuum sterilization cycle or at 250°F (121°C) for one hour in a gravity cycle or,

- Soak for 60 minutes in 1 Normal sodium hydroxide (1N NaOH);
- Follow (either of these two steps) with conventional cleaning, wrapping, and sterilizing (Rutala & Weber, 2001, p. 1354)

Ultrasonic Cleaning

29. The purpose of ultrasonic cleaning is to remove and dislodge tenacious debris. High-intensity sound waves generate tiny bubbles that expand until they collapse or implode. Implosion creates a negative pressure on the surfaces of the instruments that dislodges soil that may have remained in hard-to-reach crevices. Ultrasonic cleaning is especially beneficial for items with box locks, serrations, and interstices.

30. Instrument manufacturer guidelines should be followed to determine whether ultrasonic cleaning is compatible with the instrument. If instruments of dissimilar metal are combined in the ultrasonic cleaner, etching and pitting may occur when ion transfer is caused by the cleaning process.

31. When a detergent is added to the water in the ultrasonic cleaner, it is important that both the detergent and the ultrasonic manufacturer guidelines are followed. The solution should be changed whenever the detergent solution is visibly soiled, at least daily, or more frequently if manufacturer's guidelines so indicate.

32. The lid on the ultrasonic cleaner should be closed during use to prevent aerosolization of contaminants.

33. Ultrasonic cleaning is not microbiocidal and is not a substitute for sterilization or disinfection.

34. The issue of when to use an ultrasonic cleaner is controversial. Most facilities use it prior to mechanical cleaning, while others use it after. Some facilities use it for most instruments, others only for specialty or difficult-to-clean instruments.

35. Instruments should be rinsed free of gross soil before being placed in an ultrasonic cleaner.

36. If an automated rinse phase is not included in the ultrasonic cycle, instruments should be manually rinsed with deionized water.

Lubrication

37. Instruments with movable parts should be lubricated with an antimicrobial, water-soluble lubricant that protects against rusting and staining. The lubricant must be water soluble to allow penetration of the sterilizing agent. Oils must not be used because they prevent penetration of the sterilant.

Inspection

38. Instruments are inspected for cleanliness, integrity, alignment, sharpness of edges, and function. (See Chapter 9, "Prevention of Injury—Use and Care of Basic Surgical Instrumentation.") Semicritical instruments and items intended for disinfection immediately prior to use are dried and stored in a clean, dry area. Items that do not function as intended are removed. This is a critical requirement. The opportunity to check an instrument for function immediately prior to an emergency surgery situation is limited. It is imperative that careful inspection and checking for function occur prior to packaging. The difference between whether an instrument functioned properly or failed in surgery can be the determining factor regarding patient injury.

• •

SECTION QUESTIONS

Q1. A biofilm is a collection of microscopic organisms that adhere to a surface and can only be removed by rinsing. (Ref. 1, 17)

   True   False

Q2. The difference between a washer-disinfector and a washer-sterilizer is that at the end of a washer-sterilizer cycle, instruments are patient ready. (Ref. 4, 5)

   True   False

Q3. The perioperative nurse must have a solid knowledge of principles of preparation, packaging, and storage of sterile supplies because (Ref. 7–10):

   a. the perioperative nurse must be able to identify whether items may be permitted to be placed within the sterile field

   b. the perioperative nurse is usually responsible for wrapping of supplies in preparation for sterilization

   c. infection control measures are dependent upon proper preparation and packaging of supplies

Q4. Sterile items that were opened during a surgical procedure but were not used or handled are considered contaminated. (Ref. 2, 14)

   True   False

Q5. The decontamination process (Ref. 3, 19):

   a. sterilizes instruments in preparation for surgery

   b. renders items safe for handling

   c. may be accomplished manually or by machine

Q6. The instrument cleaning process may begin during surgery when instruments that are used are rinsed and/or wiped. (Ref. 15)

   True   False

Q7. Not all instruments can be put through a mechanical cleaner such as a washer-decontaminator or washer-sterilizer. Some must be washed by hand. Give an example of a type of instrument that must be washed by hand. (Ref. 19)

Q8. List four items of protective attire that should be worn by personnel who are responsible for the decontamination of instruments. (Ref. 21)

_____

_____

_____

_____

Q9. Select the correct statement(s) regarding decontamination of instruments exposed to prions. (Ref. 28)

a. All instruments exposed to prions should be decontaminated according to routine protocols.

b. Instruments that are difficult to clean and that are suspected to have been exposed to prions should be soaked for 30 minutes in 1 Normal sodium hydroxide before sterilization.

c. Instruments that are difficult to clean and that are suspected to have been exposed to high-risk tissue in patients suspected or known to have CJD should be soaked in water to prevent debris from adhering to the devices and then initially decontaminated by sterilizing for 18 minutes at 134°C in a prevacuum sterilizer.

d. Instruments used on a patient known to have a prion disease, regardless of the tissue on which they were used, should be decontaminated by sterilizing in a gravity displacement steam sterilizer at 121°C for one hour.

Q10. An ultrasonic cleaner (Ref. 29, 31, 33, 34):

a. cleans by destroying microorganisms

b. must be used on all general surgery instruments

c. removes microorganisms by implosion

d. may be used with a detergent

e. is a substitute for sterilization

Q11. Instruments with movable parts should be lubricated with oil prior to sterilization. (Ref. 37)

True   False

• •

PACKAGING MATERIALS—BARRIERS

Selection Criteria

39. Packaging materials and systems are intended to maintain sterility of items up until their intended use.

40. Packaging material must be selected that is compatible with the sterilization process and the device manufacturer's recommendations. Certain materials are not compatible with every process; however, all materials must meet certain standard criteria as follows. Packaging must:

- permit penetration and exit of the sterilant
- allow for adequate air removal
- permit identification of the contents
- permit complete and secure enclosure of the contents
- be fluid resistant
- be intact
- resist tears and punctures
- be free of toxic ingredients
- provide a barrier to particulate matter and fluids

- provide an adequate and tamper-proof seal
- allow for aseptic delivery of contents to the sterile field
- permit labeling to identify contents
- maintain sterility of items until package is opened (AORN, 2004b, pp. 329–331; AAMI, 2002, p. 24)

Types of Packaging

Overview

41. Packaging systems include:

- woven fabrics and nonwoven materials
- paper
- plastic and paper pouches
- plastic and Tyvek pouches
- container systems

Woven Fabric

42. Muslin was the standard woven reusable wrapping material for many years. It is a reusable cotton suitable for steam and EO sterilization. To prevent the penetration of dust and airborne microorganisms, muslin wrappers with a minimum of 140 threads per square inch and consisting of two double layers (four thicknesses) was used. Although muslin permits entry and exit of the sterilant, it does not provide a tortuous path for microorganisms and does not provide a protective barrier against moisture. For these reasons, muslin has been replaced by cotton and polyester-blend fabrics that have been treated to be water repellent.

43. Packages are traditionally wrapped in two layers. In one technique, the two wrappers are folded sequentially to create a package within a package. The purpose of this technique is to provide a tortuous path to prevent microorganisms from migrating through and penetrating the material. Newer woven fabrics have been developed that provide a sufficient tortuous path and barrier without double sequential wrapping, and packages may be wrapped using a simultaneous double wrapping technique. The policy for wrapping must be driven by the ability of the wrap to maintain items in a sterile state. Institutional policy may or not require double sequential wrapping.

44. Packages are secured with pressure-sensitive tape that also serves as a chemical indicator. Chemical indicator tape must be selected that is specific to the intended sterilization method.

45. Woven wrappers do not exhibit "memory," a characteristic that causes a material to return to the state in which was originally folded or placed.

46. Woven fabrics should be laundered between use to prevent superheating and deterioration of the fabric. They should be maintained at room temperature (i.e., 68°F to 73°F [20°C to 23°C]) and at a relative humidity of 30% to 60% (AAMI, 2002, p. 25). They must be inspected between uses for pinholes and tears that must be repaired with heat-sealed patches. Woven fabrics may produce lint. They lose their water repellency over time and must be retreated or discarded. A method should be in place to determine and monitor useful life.

47. Woven wrappers are compatible with steam and EO sterilization but may not be used with hydrogen peroxide gas plasma.

Nonwoven Materials

48. Nonwoven wrappers are made of a combination of cellulose and/or other synthetic materials. Nonwoven wrappers are single use; disposable; almost entirely lint free; resist tearing; and provide an excellent barrier against dust, airborne microorganisms, and moisture.

49. Items wrapped in nonwoven material are wrapped according to manufacturer recommendations. Some nonwoven wraps require two layers and sequential wrap. Others require a single wrap only that is equivalent to a sequential double wrap. The deciding factor in whether one or two layers or sequential wrapping is required is the degree of barrier provided by the wrapper.

50. Nonwoven wrappers eliminate the need for washing, inspecting, and patching. Quality is consistent because wrappers are used only once and then discarded.

51. Nonwoven cellulose-based wrappers are not compatible with hydrogen peroxide gas plasma sterilization. Polypropylene wrappers must be used for hydrogen peroxide gas plasma.

52. Nonwoven wrappers may display undesirable memory, as wrapper edges try to return to their original fold when packages are opened. This creates the potential for contamination of package contents when a wrapper edge that has been handled folds back into the package and contacts the sterile contents.

53. Some nonwoven packaging materials may require a longer sterilization time than woven packaging materials. This information must be supplied by the manufacturer.

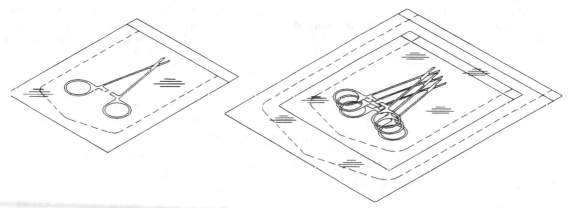

FIGURE 4-1 Examples of single- and double-packaging with paper/plastic pouches.

54. Nonwoven wrappers are compatible with steam and EO. Nonwoven, noncellulose-based wrappers are compatible with hydrogen peroxide gas plasma sterilization.

Plastic/Paper, Plastic/Tyvek®—Pouches

55. Combination plastic and paper and combination plastic and Tyvek® (material made from high-density polyethylene fibers) pouches or peel packs may be used to wrap items in preparation for sterilization. The plastic/paper combination is appropriate for steam or EO sterilization. Tyvek plastic combinations are used with EO and hydrogen peroxide gas plasma sterilization. With both types of pouches, the plastic film is fused to the paper or Tyvek so that one side is clear and the other opaque.

56. Advantages of combination plastic and paper or Tyvek wrappers are that they are inexpensive, permit visualization of the contents, are lint free, provide an effective barrier against airborne microorganisms, and are suitable for packaging a limited number of small items.

57. Disadvantages are a tendency to display memory, and the paper and plastic combination provides little resistance to punctures.

58. Items packaged in pouches are single- or double-pouched depending on manufacturer guidelines and individual institutional policies. Where double pouching is used, the inner pouch should fit into the outer pouch without being folded (AAMI, 2002, p. 31). (Figure 4-1)

59. Where double pouching is used, they should be positioned so that plastic faces plastic and paper faces paper (AAMI, 2002, p. 31). The sterilant penetrates the paper or Tyvek portion of the pouch, while the plastic portion allows the item to be viewed.

60. Pouch packages should be processed in a vertical position.

Rigid Containers

61. Rigid containers are rectangular receptacles made from aluminum, stainless steel, heat-resistant plastics, or a combination. The lid and bottom contain perforations that are sealed with a bacterial filter or a valve system that allows entry and exit of the sterilant. The lid and base are held together by a latch or a lock and key. (Figure 4-2)

62. Advantages of rigid containers are that they are durable and protect instruments from damage. They are more resistant than other packaging materials to contamination during storage. Containers eliminate the necessity for a wrapper.

63. Disadvantages include weight and potential for residual condensation. Containers can weigh up to 10 pounds. Condensation on the inner or outer surfaces following steam sterilization is sometimes a problem.

64. Containers must be washed prior to filling. The gaskets, valves, and filters should be checked and changed according to the manufacturer's recommendation. The filters and valves must be inspected for integrity before and after sterilization.

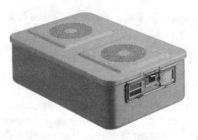

FIGURE 4-2 Instrument Container
Source: © Courtesy of Aesculap, Inc. Used with permission.

65. Information on compatibility with sterilization technologies and cycles, arrangement of instruments within containers, sealing, labeling, exposure times, and cleaning instructions must be obtained from the manufacturer. In addition, the manufacturer should be requested to supply data that support shelf-life claims.

• •

SECTION QUESTIONS

Q12. Packaging materials must (Ref. 40):

    a. be compatible with the sterilization process

    b. resist tears and punctures

    c. be impervious to penetration of microorganisms

    d. be made of muslin

    e. maintain sterility of items for six months

Q13. Select the correct statement(s). (Ref. 42, 45, 46, 48, 50, 52)

    a. Muslin wrap is rarely used today.

    b. Wrappers may be either single or double, provided they provide a barrier to the passage of microorganisms.

    c. Woven wrappers exhibit memory.

    d. Woven wrappers must be laundered between use.

    e. Nonwoven polypropylene wrappers are single-use items.

Q14. List three advantages of paper and plastic or Tyvek and plastic wrappers. (Ref. 56)

_____

Q15. Containers (Ref. 61–64):

    a. must be wrapped in polypropylene

    b. are more resistant to contamination than other packaging materials

    c. can permit condensation on their inner surface following steam sterilization

    d. must be washed between use

• •

PRINCIPLES OF PACKAGING—STEAM

Instruments

66. Instruments and other items are arranged in sets and are placed in a tray with a perforated or mesh bottom or other specially designed container that permits steam to penetrate and also prevents air from being trapped. A non-linting absorbent towel may be placed in the bottom of the tray to help absorb condensate that is formed during sterilization and to help speed the drying process.

67. A critical factor in arranging instruments and other items is to place them so that all surfaces of each item will be exposed to the sterilant.

68. Joints and hinges of instruments must be opened and detachable parts disassembled (AORN, 2004a, p. 312). Racks, pins, or stringers may be used to assist in arranging instruments and to secure them in an open position.

69. To prevent damage, heavy instruments are placed on the bottom of the tray, and delicate instruments are placed on top.

70. There is no standard weight limit for instrument sets. The weight should be based on the design and density of individual instruments, distribution of the metal mass, the ability to achieve dry sets at the end of the sterilization process, and consideration for personnel who must lift the set. To facilitate achievement of necessary temperature and adequate drying, the weight of the instrument set should be determined by the container and the manufacturer's instructions. Instrument sets that are too heavy may concentrate too much metal mass and prevent the achievement of sufficient temperature during steam sterilization processes for sterilization to occur.

71. Paper/plastic pouches should not be used within wrapped sets or containers because pouches cannot be positioned to ensure adequate air removal, steam contact, and drying (AAMI, 2002, p. 31).

Other Items

Basins, Bowls, Cups

72. Basins, bowls, and cups can be nested one inside the other if they are separated by a porous material such as gauze or an absorbent towel. The porous material permits sterilant entry, contact of the sterilant with all surfaces, and exit of the sterilant.

73. Nested items should be placed facing in the same direction to prevent air pockets, allow circulation of the steam, and permit condensate to drain out.

Rubber Goods, Tubing, Items with a Lumen, Wood Items

74. Rubber sheeting or other impervious material is not folded on itself. In preparation for steam sterilization, it is covered with a porous material, such as gauze, of the same size, loosely rolled, and then wrapped. This allows steam contact with the entire surface of the rubber or other impervious material.

75. Items with a lumen, such as ventricular and irrigation needles, must be cleaned and the lumen rinsed with distilled water. During steam sterilization, the moisture in the lumen will become steam as the temperature rises, and it will displace the air in the lumen. Sterilization of the lumen can then be achieved.

76. Rarely are items made of wood used in surgery today; however, they deserve special mention as resin can be forced out of wood during steam sterilization, condense onto other items, and cause a tissue reaction when contacted by a mucous membrane. Therefore, wood items should be individually wrapped and not included in sets with other instruments.

Reusable Textiles—Linen Packs

77. Textile packs should be composed of materials that permit air removal, steam penetration, and drying. Size and density of textile packs should be determined in consultation with the textile manufacturer. There are many materials used in the manufacture of textiles, and no one guideline is appropriate for all. Prior to sterilization, linen must be hydrated by laundering and must be stored at a humidity level of 30% to 60% and room temperature of 68°F to 73°F (20°C to 23°C). Linen that is not laundered or stored under these conditions may be dehydrated and subject to superheating during the steam-sterilization process. Superheating occurs when the temperature of the fabric exceeds the temperature of the surrounding steam. Superheating destroys cloth fibers and causes linen to deteriorate.

78. Reusable textiles have a limited life and after repeated use will lose their barrier qualities. For this reason, a wrapper should not be utilized beyond its intended life. A tracking or marking system to indicate the number of uses should be in place where reusable textiles are utilized.

PACKAGING FOR ALTERNATE METHODS OF STERILIZATION

79. Cleaning and packaging for ethylene oxide (EO) sterilization is the same as for steam sterilization, with some exceptions.

80. Items prepared for gas sterilization **must** be dry. Ethylene oxide in contact with water forms ethylene glycol. This is a toxic acid residue that can be avoided if items are dry before EO sterilization. To ensure drying, items with a lumen should be blown dry.

81. Oil-based lubricants must be removed. Ethylene oxide cannot penetrate the film left by these lubricants.

82. For hydrogen peroxide gas plasma, all items must be thoroughly dry. Cellulose-based material, such as gauze, linen, or towels, absorb hydrogen peroxide and could adversely affect the sterilization process. They should not be included within the load. Polypropylene wrap must be used to wrap sets. Paper and cloth may not be used. Trays and containers compatible with this technology may be used. Manufacturer's guidelines must be followed when selecting trays and containers.

PACKAGE INFORMATION AND IDENTIFICATION

Chemical Indicators

83. Chemical indicators vary in their ability to detect sterilizing conditions. Class 1 indicators, usually a heat-sensitive tape, label, or strip, are used on the outside of a package. Class 1 indicators demonstrate that the package was exposed to a sterilization process and serve to distinguish processed from unprocessed devices. A chemical indicator should be visible on the outside of all packages. Pouch packaging often includes an external indicator as part of the pouch.

84. Chemical indicators should also be placed in all packages, either in the center or in the area most difficult to sterilize. The Association of Perioperative Registered Nurses and the Association for the Advancement of Medical Instrumentation recommend that a monitoring device be included in each package to be sterilized and that when the indicator is not visible from the outside of the package, a separate process indicator be used on the outside of the package (AORN, 2004c, p. 379; AAMI, 2002, p. 43.)

85. Although Class 1 indicators may be used internally, Class 3, 4, or 5 indicators are more appropriate because they measure one or more of the sterilization parameters that must be achieved for sterilization to occur. (See Chapter 3 for a discussion of chemical indicators.) For steam sterilization, these include time, temperature, and moisture. For EO sterilization, these include time, temperature, gas concentration, and relative humidity. The parameters for hydrogen peroxide gas plasma are hydrogen peroxide concentration, pressure, time, and temperature. All indicators do not measure all parameters. Internal indicators should be placed in an area within the package that is the least accessible to the sterilant.

86. Chemical indicators do not guarantee sterility. They demonstrate only that the items have been exposed to the physical conditions within the chamber that are monitored by the indicator.

87. The perioperative nurse must understand the nature of the indicator used and be able to immediately interpret the reading to determine whether or not an item has been subjected to the requirements for sterilization.

88. Where there is no visible indicator, the package must be considered contaminated.

Sealing

89. All items intended for sterilization must be securely sealed.

90. Pressure-sensitive tape is used for woven and nonwoven wrappers. Plastic and paper and plastic and Tyvek pouches may be either heat sealed or sealed with pressure-sensitive tape. Most pouches are available with a self-seal feature. Self-seal often provides the most secure seal. When heat sealers are used, it is important that the temperature be appropriate to the type of pouch being sealed. Incorrect temperature may result in a weak or incomplete seal.

91. To prevent damage or loss of package integrity, heat seals must not permit resealing once opened.

Labels

92. Items packaged for sterilization should be clearly labeled with the contents, initials of the package assembler, and lot control number. The lot control number indicates the sterilization date, sterilizer used, and the cycle or load number. Lot control numbers, in conjunction with computerized instrument tracking systems, facilitate inventory control, stock rotation, and sterilization failure or sterilizer failure.

93. Indelible, nonbleeding, nontoxic labels, felt-tip ink pens, or very soft lead pencils may be used to mark packages (AORN, 2004b, p. 332).

SHELF LIFE

Storage Considerations

94. Sterilized items should be stored in a well-ventilated, limited-access area with controlled temperature and humidity.

95. Sterile items should be stored in an area separate from clean items. They should not be stored under or next to sinks or other areas where they might become wet. The area should be clean and dust free.

96. Packages should not be bent or crushed or crammed together.

97. To reduce dust accumulation, wire mesh shelving may be preferable to closed shelving.

98. Closed cabinets are best for items that are used infrequently. Cabinets and shelves should permit adequate cleaning and air circulation. Storage cabinets and shelves should be far enough away from floors, ceiling fixtures, vents, sprinklers, and lights to prevent con-

tamination. Shelves should be at least 18 inches below the ceiling, 2 inches from outside walls, and 8 to 10 inches above the floor (AAMI, 2002, p. 37).

Determining Factors

99. *Shelf life* is the amount of time an item may be considered sterile. Theoretically, if an item is not contaminated during storage, it will remain sterile indefinitely. Shelf life is related to the events that can occur that will cause an item to become contaminated. A small percentage of institutions have policies that require that an expiration date be placed on stored items, after which time the item is no longer considered sterile and must be reprocessed. The expiration date is only a guideline to indicate how long the package has been on the shelf. Contamination may occur long before the expiration date. For example, a package sterilized on June 26, 2003 with an expiration date of December 26, 2003 may become contaminated because of improper storage conditions at any time between June and December, in which case the expiration date has no meaning. Actual shelf life is event related, not time related. Events are what determine shelf life. A package is sterile until an event happens to render that package unsterile. Only proper packaging, handling, and storage can prevent contamination. The poorer the quality of the wrapper, the poorer the storage conditions, the more a package is handled, and the longer it is stored, the greater the possibility is for an event to occur that will cause contamination.

100. Most institutions have eliminated the use of expiration dates and have identified the parameters that must be achieved to consider a package sterile. Before any package is opened for surgery, it must be visually inspected to determine whether sterility appears to have been maintained. A stain, a pinhole, or a tear are several obvious examples of contamination and would preclude using the item in surgery.

101. Shelf life is determined by many factors. These include the following:

    - type and configuration of packaging material—items packaged in rigid containers may have a longer shelf life than items packaged with woven and nonwoven materials
    - use of dust covers—dust covers can extend shelf life
    - conditions of storage—dust, temperature, humidity, and traffic can affect shelf life
    - number of times a package is handled before use—the more handling, the greater the risk of contamination
    - whether stored on open or closed shelves—closed cabinets reduce risk of contamination

102. Commercially prepared items usually do not indicate an expiration date and are considered sterile provided the package is intact. Expiration dates on commercially prepared items may indicate that the integrity of the device or material will be compromised after the indicated date, and the item should not be used once this date has been reached.

REUSE OF SINGLE USE DEVICES

103. Commercially prepared items labeled as single-use are sometimes opened for a surgical procedure and not used. In the past some facilities chose to repackage and sterilize these items to be used again. In addition to reprocessing single-use devices that have been opened but not used, many facilities reprocessed devices that were opened and used because it "appeared" that the device could be reused without a problem occurring. This was seen as a method to reduce the expenditures for surgical supplies. Until 2000, when the Food and Drug Administration (FDA) published "Enforcement Priorities for Single-Use Devices Reprocessed by Third Parties and Hospitals," there were no regulations associated with reprocessing of single use devices (U.S. Food and Drug Administration, 2000).

104. Under current FDA regulations, any hospital that chooses to reprocess single-use class III devices (devices that carry a significant risk in the event of failure) that have been opened and used will be held to the same standard as the original manufacturer of that item. The requirements for the original manufacturer are extremely stringent and virtually impossible for a hospital to achieve. Regulations regarding opened and unused devices and devices other than class III are evolving and will probably further restrict reprocessing of single-use devices. The perioperative nurse in the operating room should never attempt to reprocess a single-use item. When there is a question regarding the appropriateness of reprocessing a single-use device, the item should be sent to the sterile processing department for a decision as to whether or not to reprocess.

• •

SECTION QUESTIONS

Q16. It is important for instruments to be in a closed position during sterilization. (Ref. 68)

True   False

Q17. Select the correct statements. (Ref. 66, 68, 70, 71)

a. Instruments should be assembled prior to sterilization.

b. The weight of instrument sets should not exceed 17 pounds.

c. Paper and plastic pouches should not be packaged within instrument sets.

d. A towel must be placed in the bottom of instrument sets.

Q18. Explain why it is necessary to separate nested items with a porous material in preparation for steam sterilization. (Ref. 72)

_____

_____

Q19. Prior to steam sterilization, items with a lumen must have the lumen (Ref. 75):

a. flushed with tap water

b. flushed with distilled water

c. blown dry

Q20. Why must linen be laundered prior to sterilization? (Ref. 77)

_____

Q21. Water in combination with ethylene oxide forms _____, which is toxic. Therefore, items to be sterilized in ethylene oxide must be dried. (Ref. 80)

Q22. Packaging for hydrogen peroxide gas plasma sterilization may be (Ref. 82):

a. cloth

b. paper

c. polypropylene

Q23. Chemical indicators placed in the center of packages determine whether sterilization has occurred. (Ref. 86)

True   False

Q24. All chemical indicators measure all sterilization parameters. (Ref. 85)

True   False

Q25. List three pieces of information that should be indicated on packages prepared for sterilization. (Ref. 92)

_____

Q26. Shelf life is determined by factors such as (Ref. 101):

    a. the method of sterilization used

    b. the packaging material used

    c. conditions of storage

    d. number of times a package is handled

• •

• • • References

Association for the Advancement of Medical Instrumentation (AAMI). (2002). *Steam sterilization and sterility assurance in health care facilities* (ANSI/AAMI ST 46). Arlington, VA: Author.

Association of Perioperative Registered Nurses (AORN). (2004a). Recommended practices for cleaning and caring for surgical instruments and powered equipment. In *Standards, recommended practices and guidelines* (pp. 309–317). Denver, CO: Author.

AORN. (2004b). Recommended practices for selection and use of packaging systems. In *Standards, recommended practices and guidelines* (pp. 329–334). Denver, CO: Author.

AORN. (2004c). Recommended practices for sterilization in perioperative practice settings. In *Standards, recommended practices and guidelines* (pp. 373–381). Denver, CO: Author.

Rutala, W. A., & Weber, D. J. (2001). Creutzfeldt-Jakob disease: Recommendations for disinfection and sterilization. *Clinical Infectious Diseases, 32,* pp. 1348–1356.

U.S. Food and Drug Administration. (2000). *Enforcement priorities for single use devices processed by third parties and hospitals.* Retrieved February 24, 2004, from www.fda.gov/cdrh/Reuse/reuse-documents html

• • • Suggested Reading

Truscott, W. (2003). Sterile packaging and storage. In J. Ninemeier (Ed.), *Central service technician manual* (6th ed., pp. 195–231). Chicago: International Association of Healthcare Central Service Material Management.

Appendix 4-A

• •

Chapter 4 Post Test

Instructions: Fill in the blank(s), mark the correct answer(s), or answer the question as appropriate.

1. Sterilization is the most important step in instrument decontamination. (Ref. 11)

   True   False

2. Contaminated instruments and items include (Ref. 14):

   a. items opened and used during surgery

   b. visibly soiled items

   c. items opened for surgery, not used, and no visible debris

3. An enzymatic spray can be used on contaminated instruments to prevent adherence of debris. (Ref. 16)

   True   False

4. Instruments that are heavily soiled may need to be manually washed or brushed. Washing and brushing should be done beneath the surface of the water to prevent (Ref. 21):

   _____

5. The temperature of a hot water rinse in an automated washer-disinfector is usually in the range of 180°F to 195°F (70°C to 76°C). (Ref. 24)

   True   False

6. After decontamination, instruments are considered safe for patient use. (Ref. 25)

   True   False

7. Protocols for difficult-to-clean instruments used in the brain of a patient known or suspected to have Creutzfeld-Jakob disease include but are not limited to the following (Ref. 28):

   a. discard instrument(s)

   b. soak for 1 hour in 1N NaOH, follow with conventional cleaning, wrapping and sterilizing

   c. sterilize for 18 minutes in a gravity displacement sterilizer

   d. soak for 1 hour in 1N NaOH and then sterilize for 1 hour in a prevacuum sterilizer

8. Ultrasonic cleaning (Ref. 29, 30, 33):

   a. kills microorganisms

   b. may be used in place of disinfection

   c. removes debris from instruments

   d. may be used for all instruments

9. Instrument lubrication must be water soluble. (Ref. 37)

   True   False

10. Packaging materials should be compatible with the sterilization process. List six additional considerations when selecting packaging materials. (Ref. 40)

_____

_____

11. Packages may be single- or double-wrapped, depending upon the barrier qualities of the wrapper. (Ref. 43)

    True   False

12. Combination Tyvek and plastic are appropriate for both hydrogen peroxide gas plasma sterilization and for steam sterilization. (Ref. 55)

    True   False

13. When items are double-pouched, the inner pouch should (Ref. 58, 59):

    a. not be folded

    b. be folded to fit inside the outer pouch

    c. be positioned so that the plastic side of the pouch is in contact with the paper or Tyvek® side of the pouch

    d. be positioned so that the plastic side of the pouch is in contract with the plastic side of the outer pouch

14. Pouches should be processed in a vertical position. (Ref. 60)

    True   False

15. Explain why rubber sheeting or other impervious material is covered with a porous material and loosely rolled in preparation for steam sterilization. (Ref. 74)

_____

16. Items sterilized with hydrogen peroxide gas plasma can be wrapped in polypropylene wrap. (Ref. 82)

    True   False

17. A chemical indicator should be visible on the outside of all packages. (Ref. 83)

    True   False

18. Shelf life is a guarantee that items will remain sterile until the expiration date. (Ref. 99)

    True   False

19. A hospital that reprocesses class III single-use items that were opened and used in surgery will probably be in violation of FDA regulations. (Ref. 104)

    True   False

Appendix 4-B

• •

Competency Checklist: Cleaning, Packaging, and Storage

Under "Observer's Initials," enter initials upon successful achievement of competency.
Enter N/A if competency is not appropriate for institution.

NAME _____

	OBSERVER'S INITIALS	DATE
1. Items are rinsed/wiped/irrigated during procedure.	_____	_____
2. Contaminated instruments are contained during transportation to decontamination area.	_____	_____
3. Enzymatic soak solution, spray, or gel is applied before transport to the decontamination area.	_____	_____
4. Personal protective equipment is worn during washing procedures.	_____	_____
5. Manual washing is accomplished below the surface of the water.	_____	_____
6. Decontamination equipment is operated according to manufacturer's instructions.	_____	_____
7. Ultrasonic cleaner is operated according to manufacturer's instructions.	_____	_____
8. Instruments are lubricated with water-soluble lubricant.	_____	_____
9. Instruments are inspected for:		
a. cleanliness	_____	_____
b. function	_____	_____
10. Instruments are packaged appropriately:		
a. appropriate tray/container	_____	_____
b. disassembled	_____	_____
c. opened	_____	_____
d. delicate on top of heavy	_____	_____
e. nested items separated with porous material and placed facing same direction	_____	_____
f. instruments dried	_____	_____
g. lumens rinsed for steam	_____	_____
h. lumens dried for ethylene oxide and hydrogen peroxide gas plasma	_____	_____
i. chemical process indicator/integrator placed within package	_____	_____
j. appropriate wrapping material selected	_____	_____
k. no pouches within tray/container	_____	_____

l.   process indicator visible on outside of package   _____   _____

m. seal is secure   _____   _____

n.   labeled with contents, lot number, initials   _____   _____

11. Rigid containers are used appropriately:

a.   container washed between uses   _____   _____

b.   gaskets, valves, filters checked prior to placement of instruments or sterilization   _____   _____

c.   items packaged in container system according to manufacturer's guidelines   _____   _____

OBSERVER'S SIGNATURE   INITIALS   DATE

_____

ORIENTEE'S SIGNATURE

_____

Chapter 4—Section Question Answers

Q1. False
Q2. False
Q3. a, c
Q4. True
Q5. b, c
Q6. True
Q7. Powered surgical instruments, delicate instruments, heat-sensitive instruments, instruments that cannot tolerate immersion
Q8. Long cuffed utility gloves, moisture-proof gown, mask, goggles (or full-face shield)
Q9. c
Q10. c, d
Q11. False
Q12. a, b, c
Q13. a, b, d, e
Q14. Permit visualization of the item, inexpensive, lint free, effective barrier, suitable for small items
Q15. b, c, d
Q16. False
Q17. c
Q18. Permits entry and exit of the sterilant and contact of the sterilant with all surfaces
Q19. b

(continues)

Chapter 4—Section Question Answers *(continued)*

Q20. Must be hydrated to prevent superheating
Q21. Ethylene glycol
Q22. c
Q23. False
Q24. False
Q25. Contents, lot control number, initials of person who packaged items
Q26. b, c, d

Chapter 4—Post Test Answers

1. False
2. a, b, c
3. True
4. Aerosolization of debris
5. True
6. False
7. a, b
8. c
9. True
10. Permit penetration and exit of the sterilant, allow for adequate air removal, permit identification of the contents, be fluid resistant, be intact, resist tears and punctures, be free of toxic ingredients, provide a barrier, allow for aseptic delivery to the sterile field, permit labeling, maintain sterility, permit secure and complete enclosure, provide adequate seal
11. True
12. False
13. a, d
14. True
15. Allow steam contact
16. True
17. True
18. False
19. True

5

Prevention of Infection—Aseptic Practices: Attire, Scrubbing, Gowning, Gloving, Draping, Prepping, Creating and Maintaining a Sterile Field, and Sanitation

---

LEARNER OBJECTIVES

After reading and completing "Prevention of Infection—Aseptic Practices: Attire, Scrubbing, Gowning, Gloving, Draping, Prepping, Creating and Maintaining a Sterile Field, and Sanitation," the learner will:

- describe the impact of a surgical site infection
- discuss the relationship of aseptic practice to the prevention of infection
- identify the perioperative nurse's responsibility with regard to aseptic practice
- identify four sources of infection
- list the precautions for contact-, airborne-, and droplet-transmitted infections
- describe the purpose and technique of a surgical prep
- list the desired characteristics of topical antimicrobial agents
- describe two processes for surgical hand antisepsis
- describe open and closed gloving technique
- identify restricted, semirestricted, and unrestricted areas of the operating room
- describe appropriate attire within restricted, semirestricted, and unrestricted areas
- define and discuss the term *surgical conscience*

- discuss six guidelines for draping
- list the desired characteristics of surgical gowns and drapes
- discuss four techniques to help maintain a sterile field
- list recommended air exchanges per hour, temperature, and humidity in the operating room
- describe the process for cleanup of small and large spills
- identify items that should be cleaned between cases, at the end of the day, and periodically
- describe appropriate traffic patterns relative to movement around a sterile field
- state one nursing diagnosis related to a surgical incision

• • • • • • • • • • • • •

Lesson Outline

I.   NURSING DIAGNOSIS—DESIRED PATIENT OUTCOMES
   A.   Overview
II. NURSING RESPONSIBILITIES
III. PATHOGENIC MICROORGANISMS
IV. SOURCES OF INFECTION (ENDOGENOUS)
   A.   Patients
V.   SOURCES OF INFECTION (EXOGENOUS)
   A.   Personnel
   B.   Environment
   C.   Equipment
VI. STANDARD AND TRANSMISSION-BASED PRECAUTIONS
VII. CONTROL OF SOURCES OF INFECTION
   A.   Control of Patient Sources of Infection—Skin Prep
   B.   Control of Personnel Sources of Infection
      1. Attire
      2. Scrubbing, Gowning, and Gloving
         a. Definitions
         b. Traditional Surgical Hand Antisepsis (Traditional Scrub Procedure)
         c. Use of Alcohol-Based Hand Rubs
         d. Gowning and Gloving Procedure
         e. Assisting Others to Gown and Glove
   C.   Creating a Sterile Field
      1. Draping
      2. Draping Guidelines
      3. Standard Drapes
   D.   Maintaining a Sterile Field
   E.   Control of Environmental Sources of Infection
      1. Traffic Patterns
      2. Operating Room Environment
      3. Operating Room Sanitation
      4. Additional Considerations—Cleaning and Scheduling

NURSING DIAGNOSIS—DESIRED PATIENT OUTCOMES

Overview

1. A surgical incision creates an opportunity for microorganisms to enter the body and for infection to result. As a result, a common nursing diagnosis for the patient undergoing surgical intervention is high risk for surgical site infection.

2. Infection may be evidenced by fever, erythema, tenderness, induration, cellulitis, purulent drainage, abscess, or dehiscence. The desired patient outcome is for the patient to exhibit none of the signs or symptoms of infection.

3. Surgical site infection (SSI) is the third most frequently reported nosocomial infection and accounts for 14% to 16% of all nosocomial infections among hospitalized patients (Mangram, Horan, Pearson, Silver, & Jarvis, 1999, p. 251).

4. Surgical site infections are defined as superficial incisional, deep incisional, or organ/space. Superficial incisional infection involves only the skin or subcutaneous tissue. It is the most common surgical site infection and is usually diagnosed after patient discharge. Removal of sutures or staples and/or drainage of the area is the usual treatment. Deep incisional infection involves deep soft tissue, e.g., fascia and/or muscle. Deep incisional SSIs occur less frequently than superficial incisional SSIs, usually follow more extensive surgeries, and are usually diagnosed prior to discharge. Prolonged hospitalization or rehospitalization for management of surgical site complications is common for deep incisional infections. Organ/space infection involves the visceral cavity or anatomic structures not opened during the procedure. These infections are most severe and require prolonged hospitalization, often with multiple reoperations. Organ/space SSI infection is associated with long-term morbidity and death.

5. In addition to delayed wound healing, the patient with an SSI will experience discomfort or pain and a possible loss of earning capacity. The economic impact of an SSI is also significant in terms of healthcare costs. Studies estimate the increased cost for care of the patient with an SSI range from $2,714 to $30,000 for an infected joint and an increased hospital stay from 4 to 14 days (Fry, 2002, p. S41).

6. The National Nosocomial Infections Surveillance report for 1986–1996 described an SSI rate of 2.6% for over 500,000 operations at reporting hospitals (Fry, 2002, p. S39). The actual rate may be significantly higher, however, because more than 70% of all surgery is ambulatory; infection is often not noted until after the patient has left the healthcare facility; and the infection may not be reported.

7. The number of variables that can influence the SSI rate is significant and beyond the scope of this chapter. Prevention of SSI in the OR involves multiple interventions but focuses primarily on adherence to aseptic practices related to attire, scrubbing, gowning, gloving, prepping, draping, maintaining a sterile field, and sanitation of the suite. If these are not performed in accordance with accepted principles, the patient's risk of developing an SSI may increase.

NURSING RESPONSIBILITIES

8. *Asepsis* refers to the absence of pathogenic organisms. Asepsis in the operating room, also referred to as *aseptic technique*, refers to the practices by which contamination with microorganisms is prevented. Although it is impossible to eliminate all microorganisms in the surgical environment, strict adherence to aseptic technique is a most important measure in preventing the patient and staff from acquiring an infection.

9. The perioperative nurse is responsible for creating and maintaining a sterile field and for monitoring aseptic practice of all members of the surgical team. Appropriate implementation of this responsibility requires an understanding of infection sources, transmission modes, and the methods of reducing or eliminating microorganisms in the surgical setting. The perioperative nurse must have in-depth knowledge of principles and practices associated with attire, scrubbing, gowning, gloving, prepping, draping, maintaining a sterile field, and operating room sanitation.

10. The responsibility for reducing the number of microorganisms in the operating room to the lowest level possible is shared by all members of the surgical team and personnel employed in the department. However, the perioperative nurse assumes major responsibility for ensuring that each patient is provided with as aseptic an environment as possible and that risk for SSI is reduced to its lowest potential. The perioperative nurse continuously monitors all aspects of the environment in the operating room to ensure adherence to aseptic principles and compliance with aseptic practice.

PATHOGENIC MICROORGANISMS

11. *Pathogenic microorganisms* are microorganisms that cause disease. The pathogens most commonly associated with SSI are *Staphylococcus aureus, Staphlyococcus epidermidis,* coagulase-negative staphylococci, and *Enterococcus* spp. An increasing proportion of SSIs are caused by microorganisms resistant to antibiotics. A common example is methicillin-resistant *S. aureus* (MRSA). SSIs caused by microorganisms resistant to antibiotics are particularly problematic, as they are difficult and sometimes impossible to resolve.

12. The more virulent the microorganism, the greater the potential for infection. More virulent strains of bacteria or bacteria with an endotoxin in the outer cell membrane require a smaller inoculum to cause an infection than less virulent strains.

SOURCES OF INFECTION (ENDOGENOUS)

Patients

13. Endogenous sources of infection arise from within the body. The patient is a source of endogenous infection because of the large number of microorganisms normally found on the patient's skin, mucous membranes, and hollow viscera. In fact, the majority of SSIs are caused by the patient's own flora. However, if these microorganisms remain in their normal environment and if their numbers are not altered by external factors, they will not cause infection.

14. The skin is the first line of defense against the entry of microorganisms into the body. By incising the skin, a portal of entry for pathogenic microorganisms is created, and the patient is immediately exposed to the risk of infection. In addition, certain factors or conditions, if present, may significantly impact a patient's risk for developing an SSI. These may include, but are not limited to, extremes of age; poor nutritional status; obesity; a compromised immune system; preexisting disease, especially diabetes; presence of preexisting infection; burns; and use of nicotine.

15. Length of surgery, type of procedure, surgical technique, and an extended preoperative hospital stay can also increase risk of SSI. Colonization of the patient with hospital-associated microbes is likely when the patient has extensive preoperative hospitalization.

16. Geriatric and neonate patients have an increased risk of postoperative surgical site infection. Impaired healing in the aged is often related to inadequate circulation due to atherosclerosis or the presence of coexisting disease. Delayed healing increases the opportunity for surgical site infection. The premature infant has increased susceptibility to infection due to immature globulin synthesis, antibody formation, and cellular defense. The smaller the neonate, the less resistance there is to infection. Invasive procedures increase the risk of infection.

17. Poor nutritional status, such as frequently accompanies drug or alcohol addiction, can delay wound healing and increase risk for infection. Obesity is a risk factor because less blood is supplied to fatty tissue and avascular tissue is susceptible to infection.

18. Defense mechanisms are impaired in the immunocompromised patient. Patients receiving radiation therapy, chemotherapy, corticosteroids, or who have AIDS are immunocompromised. Additional stress is placed on the immune system of patients with chronic conditions such as diabetes, cancer, and cardiac and respiratory diseases.

19. The presence of infection anywhere in the body significantly increases the risk of an SSI and is always a contraindication for elective surgery. Whenever possible, surgery should be postponed until a preexisting infection is resolved.

20. The first line of defense is the patient's skin. When it is destroyed, such as with a burn, the patient is susceptible to infection.

21. Smoking decreases the delivery of oxygen to the tissues. This delays wound healing, which may result in an SSI.

22. The risk of infection increases with the length of exposure of internal tissues to the environment, the presence of implants, and the amount of ischemic tissue present. Although necessary, catheters and drains can increase the risk of infection because they provide a pathway for pathogenic microorganism migration. The longer these are left in place, the greater is the risk for infection.

23. There are multiple sources for infection; however, for an infection to occur, the following must be present:

- pathogens of sufficient virulence
- a sufficient quantity of pathogens
- a susceptible host
- a portal of entry
- a mode of transmission

SOURCES OF INFECTION (EXOGENOUS)

Personnel

24. Exogenous sources of infection are from outside the body and include the environment and personnel.

25. Personnel are a major source of microorganisms in the operating room. The greater the number of personnel in the operating room, the greater the number of microorganisms.

26. The skin of all persons in the area is a potential source of infection. Cells and surface organisms are constantly being shed from skin surfaces. Certain body areas such as the head, neck, axilla, hands, groin, legs, and feet harbor an especially large number of microorganisms. Hair is a major source of *Staphylococcus*. The number of microorganisms present in hair is related to its length and cleanliness.

27. Talking, coughing, and breathing release numerous organisms into the environment.

28. Jewelry, artificial nails, cracks in nail polish, and cosmetic detritus may harbor millions of microorganisms. Artificial nails may increase bacterial and fungal colonization of the hands even after a surgical scrub. Higher numbers of gram-negative microorganisms have been cultured from the fingertips of personnel wearing artificial nails than from personnel with natural nails, both before and after hand washing (Pottinger, Burns, & Manske, 1989, p. 340). Healthcare workers who wear artificial nails are more likely to harbor pathogens, especially gram-negative bacilli and yeasts, than are those with natural nails (Mycek, 2004, p. 34). The effect of nail polish on the number of microorganisms found on the fingernails of personnel after a surgical hand scrub has been questioned, and one study found no significant difference between polished, unpolished, damaged, or undamaged nails in the number of microorganisms found on fingernails (Baumgardner, Maragos, Walz, & Larson, 1993, p. 87).

Environment

29. The operating room is not sterile. Organisms are present in the air, on dust particles, and on dirt in the environment.

30. The walls, floors, overhead lights, light tracks, cabinets, door handles, and other stationary fixtures in the operating room may harbor microorganisms and are therefore potential sources of infection.

Equipment

31. All instruments, supplies, and equipment that come in contact with air and personnel become potential sources for infection because personnel transfer organisms to whatever instruments, supplies, or equipment they touch.

32. Whenever dust particles in the air settle on instruments or supplies, the organisms on those dust particles are also deposited on those items.

STANDARD AND TRANSMISSION-BASED PRECAUTIONS

33. Standard and Transmission-Based Precautions are methods of infection control that can be used to prevent the transmission of pathogens and protect the patient and the healthcare worker from exposure to pathogenic microorganisms found in blood and body fluids and on non-intact skin and mucous membranes. Standard Precautions should be used in the care of all patients.

34. Standard Precautions include the use of personal protective equipment (PPE) and prompt and frequent hand washing. PPE includes use of gloves when touching blood, body fluids, secretions, excretions, and contaminated items, and use of masks, eye protection, and gowns during procedures with the potential to generate splashes of blood, body fluids, secretions, and excretions. Shoe and leg covering may also be used as needed. Hand washing should be done after touching blood, body fluids, secretions, excretions, and contaminated items whether or not gloves are worn.

35. Transmission-Based Precautions are used in addition to Standard Precautions for patients who are known or suspected to be infected with epidemiologically important and highly transmissible pathogens (AORN, 2004d, p. 363).

36. There are three types of Transmission-Based Precautions: Airborne, Droplet, and Contact Precautions. Airborne Precautions are appropriate against pathogens, such as rubeola, TB, or varicella, that are transmitted by the airborne route. Airborne Precautions include use of respiratory protection and special air handling and ventilation. Persons susceptible to airborne pathogens should wear respiratory protection, and infected patients should wear a mask during transport. Droplet Precautions are appropriate for protection against pathogens, such as influenza and mumps, that are transmitted through droplets. Droplet Precautions include wearing a mask within 3 feet of an infected patient and positioning other patients at least 3 feet from infected patients.

Infected patients should wear a mask during transport. Contact Precautions are appropriate for protection against pathogens that are transmitted by direct or indirect contact. Contact Precautions include the use of gloves and gowns and cleaning and disinfecting patient equipment.

37. *Universal Precautions* was defined by the Centers for Disease Control in 1987. It is a set of precautions designed to prevent transmission of human immunodeficiency (HIV), hepatitis B (HBV), and other bloodborne pathogens. Blood and certain body fluids of all patients are considered potentially infectious for bloodborne pathogens. Universal precautions have been incorporated into Standard and Transmission-Based Precautions. Because operating-room personnel are often exposed to large amounts of blood, they tend to be more familiar with the term "universal precautions." Universal precautions apply to blood and other body fluids containing visible blood, semen, and vaginal secretions. Universal precautions requires that blood and body fluids of all humans (patients and personnel) be considered infectious and that the same safety precautions be taken whether or not the patient is known to have a bloodborne infectious disease. The practice of universal precautions is a method of infection control that protects both the patient and operating-room personnel. Standard Precautions apply to blood, all body fluids, secretions, and excretions except sweat, regardless of whether or not they contain visible blood, nonintact skin, and mucous membranes (CDC, 1997). Standard Precautions is more comprehensive and should be adhered to by all personnel providing healthcare.

38. In 1992, the Occupational Safety and Health Administration established mandatory universal precautions practice standards. The three critical components of universal precaution standards are (1) use of personal protective barriers, (2) proper hand washing, and (3) precautions in handling sharps.

39. The standards include but are not limited to the following (Johnson & Johnson, 1992, pp. 4-10):

- Employers must list job classifications, tasks, and procedures in which employees have occupational exposure to blood or other potentially infectious body fluids.

- Gloves must be worn when direct contact with blood or other potentially infectious body fluids is expected to occur.

- Masks with face shields or protective eyewear with side shields must be worn when splashes, splattering, or aerosolation of blood and body fluids is anticipated.

- Gowns, appropriate to the procedure being performed, must be worn when aerosolation or splattering of blood or other body fluids is anticipated. Gowns must not permit passage of blood or body fluids.

- Personal protective equipment (gloves, masks, face shields, gowns, and so forth) is provided by the employer at no cost to the employee.

- Hands and other skin surfaces must be washed as soon as feasible if contaminated with blood or body fluids.

- Contaminated needles are not recapped or removed unless required by a specific procedure. If recapping or removal is required, it must be accomplished with a mechanical device.

- Sharps are deposited in rigid, leak-proof, puncture-resistant containers that must be readily accessible.

- A written schedule of cleaning and appropriate disinfection of equipment and the environment must be implemented and maintained.

- Contaminated laundry is placed in labeled or color-coded laundry bags that prevent leakage.

- Infectious waste containers must be closable, prevent leakage, and be labeled or color coded as potentially infectious.

- The employer must provide a hepatitis B vaccination and a postexposure follow-up program. A preexposure vaccine must be offered free of charge.

- Training and education programs must be made available to all employees who may be exposed to blood or other body fluids that are potentially contaminated with hepatitis B virus (HBV) or HIV.

In addition, OSHA revised the Bloodborne Pathogens Standard (29 CFR 1910.1030) in 2003 to include the requirement that employers identify, evaluate and implement safer medical devices. The revision also requires that nonmanagerial healthcare workers must be involved in evaluating and choosing safer needle devices. A sharps injury log must be maintained as well.

SECTION QUESTIONS

Q1. Surgical site infections are the most frequently reported nosocomial infection. (Ref. 3)

True   False

Q2. There are three categories of surgical site infection. They are (Ref. 4):

_____

Q3. Postoperative surgical site infection (Ref. 2, 4, 5, 6, 7):

    a. is related to implementation of proper aseptic technique

    b. is a major cause of extended hospital stay

    c. is usually evident prior to discharge

    d. that results in an organ/space SSI is associated with long term morbidity and death

    e. may be evidenced by dehiscence

Q4. The perioperative nurse assumes major responsibility for monitoring the aseptic practice of all team members. (Ref. 10)

True   False

Q5. A compromised immune system can influence the risk of postoperative surgical site infection. List six additional endogenous factors that can influence and increase the risk of postoperative surgical site infection. (Ref. 14, 15, 16, 17, 18, 19)

_____

_____

_____

_____

Q6. Operating room personnel represent an exogenous source of infection. (Ref. 24, 25)

True   False

Q7. Hair is a potential source of infection and is a major source of _Streptococcus_. (Ref. 26)

True   False

Q8. Talking is a source of contamination. (Ref. 27)

True   False

Q9. Personnel who wear nail polish will have more microorganisms on the tips of their fingers after scrubbing than personnel who do not wear nail polish. (Ref. 28)

True   False

Q10. A patient infected with a pathogen transmitted through droplets should wear a mask during transport to the operating room; however, personnel caring for the patient are only required to wear a mask if within _____ feet of the patient. (Ref. 36)

Q11. Standard Precautions (Ref. 37, 38):

a. protects patients

b. protects personnel

c. should be practiced for all patients

d. includes hand washing

e. includes precautions in handling sharps

f. is mandated by OSHA

● ●

CONTROL OF SOURCES OF INFECTION

40. Infection prevention in the operating room includes adherence to aseptic practices in relation to surgical attire, sterilization of instruments and equipment, staff and patient skin preparation, creation and maintenance of a sterile field, and control of the environment. A major responsibility of the perioperative nurse is to implement and ensure practices that are designed to prevent infection.

41. Some aseptic practices are mandated by regulatory bodies such as the Occupational Safety and Health Administration (OSHA). Others are derived from standard-setting bodies such as the Association of Registered periOperative Nurses (AORN) and the Association for Advancement of Medical Instrumentation (AAMI).

42. Regardless of the source of the aseptic practices, they are only as good as the surgical conscience of the individual practitioner. A *surgical conscience* is an inner commitment to adhere strictly to aseptic practice, to report any break in aseptic practice, and to correct any violation, whether or not anyone else is present or observes the violation. A surgical conscience mandates a commitment to aseptic practice *at all times*.

43. Aseptic practice is the method used to prevent contamination from microorganisms. The Association of Operating Room Nurses has identified recommended practices to prevent contamination from microorganisms. The purpose of these practices is to prevent contamination of the open wound and to create and

maintain a sterile field that is isolated from the surrounding unsterile area. Adherence to these practices contributes to providing a safe environment for the patient that minimizes potential for surgical site infection. The AORN recommended practices are critical components of infection control and are addressed throughout this chapter.

Control of Patient Sources of Infection—Skin Prep

44. Efforts to reduce patient sources of infection are aimed at lowering the number of bacteria on the skin prior to surgery and reducing potential bacterial contamination from within the patient during surgery. Although the skin cannot be sterilized, the incision site and the area immediately surrounding it should be as free of microorganisms as possible prior to surgery.

45. Hair at the incision site should be removed only when its presence interferes with the intended procedure (Mangram et al., 1999, p. 266). Preoperative hair removal has been associated with increased risk of surgical site infection (Cruise and Foord, 1980, pp. 27–40; Winston, 1992, p. 320). If hair must be removed, it should be done immediately prior to the operation (Mangram et al., 1999, p. 266).

46. Before hair is removed from the surgical site, the patient's skin should be assessed for the presence of rashes, moles, warts, or other conditions. Trauma to these can provide an opportunity for the colonization of pathogenic microorganisms.

47. The preferred method of hair removal is with electric clippers. Clippers decrease the poten-

tial for nicks in the skin that can provide a portal of entry for microorganisms. Hair removal is also accomplished with a depilatory cream or with a razor.

48. Depilatory creams are infrequently used because of potential irritation to the skin and because they tend to be messy.

49. When shaving is the method used to remove hair, it should be performed wet and as close as possible to the time of surgery to prevent microorganism growth in nicks and scratches that may be left by the razor. The incidence of postoperative surgical site infection increases in relation to the length of time before surgery that the shave is performed (Olsen, MacCallum, & McQuarrie, 1986, p. 182). A wet shave also helps to control potential dispersal of the shaved hair.

50. To prevent airborne dispersal of hair and possible contamination of the sterile field, hair removal should be performed outside the room where surgery will be performed.

51. The operative site and the immediate surrounding area is cleaned and an antiseptic applied prior to surgery. The objective of skin cleansing is to remove dirt and skin oils, to reduce the number of microorganisms on the skin to a minimum, and to prevent further microbial growth throughout the procedure.

52. The patient may be instructed to shower or bathe with an antimicrobial soap the night before surgery and/or just prior to surgery. Whether or not this is done, the patient's skin will be cleaned again with an antiseptic agent just prior to surgery.

53. The choice of antiseptic agent depends on the condition of the patient's skin, patient allergies, the intended incision site, and surgeon and hospital preference.

54. Acceptable antiseptic products should have the following properties:

- cleans effectively
- reduces microbial count rapidly
- has a broad spectrum of activity
- is easy to apply
- is nonirritating and nontoxic
- provides residual protection

55. The most common antimicrobial agents include iodophors, chlorhexidine gluconate, and alcohol preparations in concentrations of 60%–90%.

56. The duration of the prep should be based on the manufacturer's recommendation and studies on the effectiveness of the antimicrobial agents.

57. Prior to the skin prep, the patient should be assessed for allergies or sensitivities to prep solutions. An alternate antimicrobial solution should be chosen if allergies or sensitivities are noted.

58. The area prepped should include the incision site and a substantial area surrounding it. Anticipated additional incision sites and potential drain sites must also be prepped. (Figures 5-1, 5-2, 5-3, 5-4, 5-5, 5-6, 5-7)

59. The following guidelines should be adhered to when performing the skin prep:

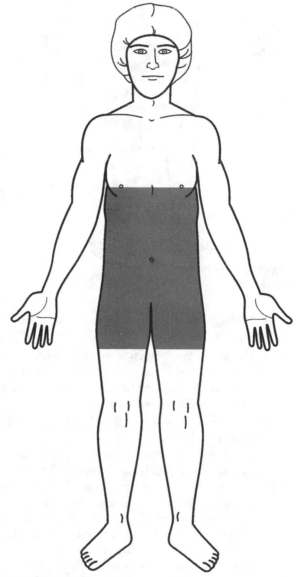

FIGURE 5-1 Abdomen Prep.
Source: Courtesy of Gina Beckman.

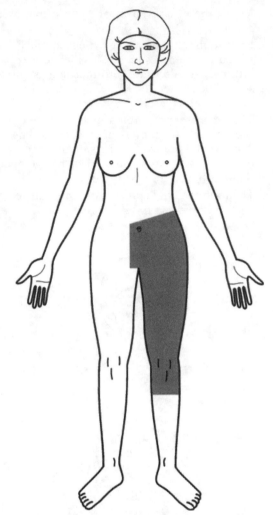

FIGURE 5-2   Hip Prep.
Source: Courtesy of Gina Beckman.

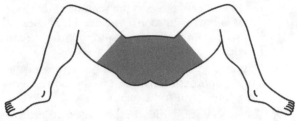

FIGURE 5-3   Perineum Prep.
Source: Courtesy of Gina Beckman.

scrub with an iodophor soap and depends upon manufacturer's instructions. The area is blotted with a sterile towel, and an antiseptic paint solution applied. Some commercially prepared prep sets include both a soap preparation for cleansing the area and an antiseptic solution to be applied after cleaning. Controversy exists over whether sterile gloves and a sterile prep kit are more effective than clean gloves or a clean prep

- If the patient is awake, an explanation is given regarding the prep.
- Unnecessary exposure of the patient is avoided. To retain patient dignity and to prevent unnecessary heat loss, only the area to be prepped is exposed.
- The prep is performed using mechanical friction. The prep begins at the incision site and progresses outwardly to the periphery. A widening circular motion is preferable to a back-and-forth motion. A back-and-forth motion can cause bacteria to be dragged from the unprepped areas back to the clean center portion of the prepped area. The process is repeated several times. The length of the skin scrub may vary from 1 minute for an alcohol wipe to a 5-minute or longer

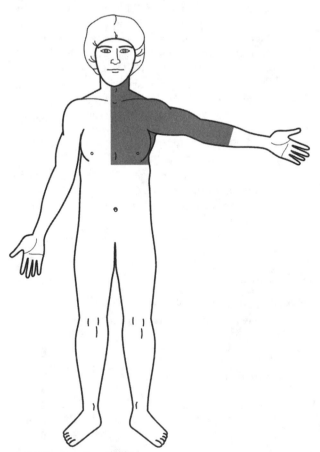

FIGURE 5-4   Shoulder Prep.
Source: Courtesy of Gina Beckman.

to absorb excess fluid, to prevent saturation of drapes or linens, and to prevent pooling.

- The dirtiest areas are prepped last. Movement in all areas is from clean to dirty. In cases where skin is intact and open wounds and body orifices are not part of the area to be prepped, the prep begins at the proposed line of incision. In cases where potentially contaminated areas are included in the prep area, the prep begins at the surrounding skin area. The umbilicus is cleaned separately with cotton-tip applicators. A colostomy or stoma is covered until the surrounding area is prepped and then prepped with a separate sponge. In a perineal prep, the vagina and/or

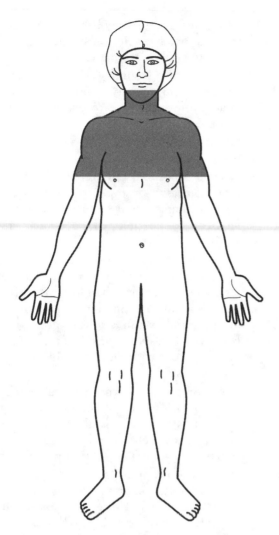

FIGURE 5-5 Head and Neck Prep.
Source: Courtesy of Gina Beckman.

kit. Insufficient research data exists to determine effect on patient outcomes.

- A sponge or applicator used to prep an area is never reapplied to an area previously prepped. The sponge or applicator should be discarded once the periphery is reached so that bacteria from adjacent non-prepped areas are not inadvertently transferred to the prepped area.
- Prep solutions are not allowed to pool under the patient or flow under a tourniquet cuff or electrocautery dispersive electrode. Prep solutions that are allowed to pool have the potential to cause chemical burn. Folded towels should be placed at the periphery area

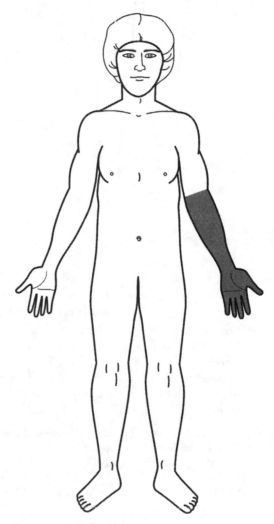

FIGURE 5-6 Hand Prep.
Source: Courtesy of Gina Beckman.

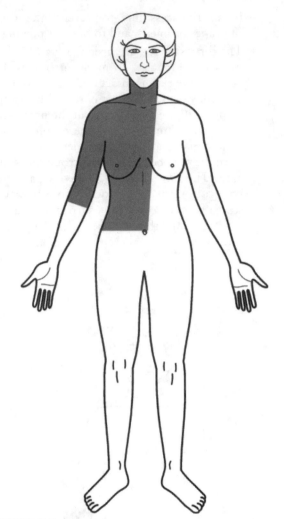

FIGURE 5-7   Breast Prep.
Source: Courtesy of Gina Beckman.

anus is prepped last with a separate sponge. In a shoulder prep, the axilla is prepped last.

- For unusual wounds or incision sites when it may be difficult to know where to begin, nursing judgment must be used to decide upon the prep process that will result in reducing the number of microorganisms at the incision site to the lowest level possible.

60. In addition to the previous guidelines, the following considerations should be noted:

- Eyes are washed with cotton balls with a nonirritating solution. The prep is begun at the nose and continues toward the cheeks.

Warm sterile water may be used to rinse off the solution. The solution should not be allowed to pool on the patient's eyes.

- For traumatic wounds, large amounts of irrigating solution may be used prior to and in addition to the prep to remove dirt and debris.
- Normal saline should be used to prep burned or denuded skin.
- When it is necessary to prep a limb, an additional person or apparatus is needed to hold the limb securely so the entire circumference can be prepped adequately and safely.
- The brush part of the sponge/brush may be useful for areas such as hands and feet. Care must be taken when using the brush part to avoid irritating tender skin or creating scratches and a portal of entry for bacteria. Care should also be taken to prevent aerosolization of prep solutions and skin debris.
- Warm prep solutions are preferable. They may help maintain body temperature and are more pleasing to the awake patient. Care must be taken not to overheat and possibly compromise the efficacy of the prep solution.
- During certain preps, such as for a malignant breast tumor, prepping must be gentle to prevent potential spread of cancer cells. A gentle technique should also be used when prepping fragile skin sites.
- If alcohol or alcohol-based prepping agents are used, the surgery should not begin until the solution on the patient has dried. Equipment used in surgery may produce a spark with the potential to ignite volatile prep solutions.

61. Documentation of the skin prep should include the following:

- assessment of the skin at the operative site
- hair removal, if performed, including site, method, time, and person who removed hair
- patient skin allergies or sensitivities
- prep agents or solution
- name of person performing the prep
- patient response to prep, i.e., allergic reaction

• •

SECTION QUESTIONS

Q12. Define what is meant by *surgical conscience*. (Ref. 42)

_____

_____

Q13. The goal of the patient skin prep is to (Ref. 44):

  a. sterilize the skin

  b. lower the number of bacteria on the patient's skin

  c. reduce the potential for bacterial contamination from the patient

Q14. Regarding hair at the incision site (Ref. 45–50):

  a. Hair at the incision site should always be removed.

  b. When hair is removed, a shave with a razor is the preferred method.

  c. When hair is removed, it should be removed at least 12 hours prior to surgery.

  d. A depilatory is not appropriate for hair removal.

  e. Hair removal should not be done in the actual operating room.

Q15. List four desirable properties of a skin prep product. (Ref. 54)

  _____   _____

  _____   _____

Q16. The area prepped should include the incision site and no more than 2 inches around it. (Ref. 58)

  True   False

Q17. The skin prep (Ref. 59):

  a. begins at the dirtiest area and progresses toward the incision

  b. begins at the incision site and progresses to toward the periphery

  c. must last at least 6 minutes

  d. should always be performed vigorously

Q18. Documentation of the skin prep should include (Ref. 61):

  a. the agent used

  b. method of hair removal

  c. time the prep was performed

  d. length of time for the prep

• •

Control of Personnel Sources of Infection

Attire

62. Personnel who work in the surgical suite are required to change into special operating room or surgical attire designed to interfere with the passage of microorganisms from personnel to the patient and the environment and from patient to personnel.

63. Appropriate surgical attire in the operating room suite includes hats or hoods, scrub outfits (commonly referred to as "scrubs"), and shoe covers (optional).

64. Hats or hoods are worn so that head and facial hair is completely covered. Hair is a gross contaminant and major source of bacteria. It attracts and sheds bacteria in proportion to its length, oiliness, and curliness. To prevent contamination of scrubs from hair or dandruff, a hat or hood should be the first item of apparel donned. Hair should not be combed once scrubs are donned. A hat or hood should be worn in areas where supplies are processed and stored. Hats are usually disposable (single use). Reusable hats should be laundered when soiled and between each wearing. Hats should be removed and deposited in a designated receptacle before leaving the operating room suite.

65. Scrubs are either a one-piece cover-up, such as a dress, or a two-piece shirt and pants set. Pants may be designed with stockinette cuffs to prevent shedding. To prevent shedding, the shirt must fit close to the body or be tucked into the pants. Scrubs may be made of a tightly woven reusable fabric that minimizes shedding, or they may be disposable. Reusable scrubs should be freshly laundered. Controversy exists over whether home laundering rather than hospital laundering is acceptable. Proponents of healthcare facility laundering cite controlled load mix, detergent, cycle time, and water temperature as reasons to mandate laundering in the healthcare facility. However, there are no well-controlled studies that have evaluated scrub suit laundering as a risk for a surgical site infection and no data to support improved patient outcomes as a result of mandatory healthcare facility laundering. Many healthcare facilities do permit home laundering of scrubs with the exception of grossly contaminated scrubs. The occupational Safety and Health Administration mandates that garments penetrated by blood or other potentially infectious materials be removed immediately or as soon as feasible (OSHA 1910.1030 [d][3][vi]). In this event, the facility must supply a fresh scrub suit.

66. In addition to scrubs, unscrubbed or nonsterile team members should wear a warm-up jacket with long sleeves to prevent shedding from bare arms. Operating rooms are cool, and warm-up jackets also serve to keep personnel warm. Warm-up jackets should be snapped or buttoned to prevent the edges from inadvertently coming into contact with and contaminating sterile supplies. Warm-up jackets may be reusable or disposable.

67. Hospital policy dictates whether scrubs are to be removed when leaving the operating room suite and fresh ones donned upon reentry or if cover gowns or lab coats must be worn over scrubs outside the operating room. Changing of scrubs or use of cover gowns has not been shown to influence the risk of surgical site infection (Pfaff, 1993, p. 627). Surgical attire should be changed or removed when it becomes visibly soiled or wet. Fresh scrub attire should be worn each day.

68. High-filtration masks are worn in areas specifically designated according to hospital policy and should be worn in the presence of open sterile supplies (AORN, 2004e, p. 224). Masks contain droplets expelled from the mouth and nasopharynx during talking, sneezing, and coughing. Whether masks reduce risk of infection when worn by personnel who are not scrubbed and who are in forced ventilation systems is not clear and requires further research. For this reason, policies on wearing of masks may vary.

69. Masks should cover the nose and mouth completely and securely. Most masks contain a small malleable metal strip that should be pinched to conform to the nose to provide a secure, proper fit. The mask should be tied securely at the back of the head in a manner that prevents venting, which can allow unfiltered exhaled air to escape from the sides.

70. Masks with face shields or splash guards, or masks worn with protective eyewear, such as goggles or glasses with side shields, are worn whenever splashes, sprays, or aerosols of potentially infectious agents, such as blood, are anticipated.

71. Masks are either on or off and should not be left to dangle from the neck or be folded and placed in a pocket for future use. Masks should be removed and discarded after use and when they become wet. Masks should be removed and discarded by handling only the ties. Masks that have been worn are contaminated with droplet nuclei. Handling of the face portion of the mask after use can transfer microorganisms from the mask to the hands;

therefore, only the ties should be handled. Masks should be disposed of in a designated receptacle. Hands should be washed after mask removal.

72. Shoe covers are usually optional and have not been shown to contribute to reducing surgical site infection rates. Shoe covers may be worn to protect personnel footwear from becoming soiled. Shoe covers are considered personal protective equipment and, as such, OSHA requires that they be worn in situations when gross contamination can be anticipated (OSHA 1910.1030 [d][3][xi]). Various length high-top shoe covers that cover the shoe and lower leg are appropriate when contact with copious or potentially infectious fluids is anticipated to occur on the legs and shoes of personnel.

73. Shoe covers should be removed and deposited in a designated receptacle before leaving the operating room suite. Removal of shoe covers can permit transfer of microorganisms from the shoe covers to the hands. Hands should be washed after shoe cover removal.

74. Although wearing of jewelry has not been shown to impact on surgical site infection rates, jewelry easily harbors bacteria and therefore should be confined or removed. Confinement of jewelry also reduces the potential for it to fall onto the sterile field.

75. Nails should be short and clean. Artificial nails should not be worn. Long nails may puncture protective gloves or scratch a patient during transfer. Although the impact of artificial nails on surgical site infection rates is unknown, healthcare workers who wear artificial nails are more likely to harbor gram-negative pathogens on their fingertips than those who have natural nails. In addition, artificial nails have been implicated in several infection outbreaks outside of the operating room (CDC, 2002, p. 31). Available data suggest that chipped nail polish or polish worn more than 4 days harbors greater numbers of bacteria than natural nails or freshly polished nails (Pottinger, Burns, & Manske, 1989, p. 340).

76. Other attire worn to protect personnel from infectious agents includes gloves, liquid-resistant aprons, and gowns.

77. Personnel who scrub for surgery are referred to as "members of the sterile team" or "scrubbed persons." In addition to wearing appropriate operating-room attire, scrubbed persons must wash their hands and forearms by performing surgical hand antisepsis, commonly referred to as scrubbing, prior to donning a sterile gown and sterile gloves.

Scrubbing, Gowning, and Gloving

DEFINITIONS

78. **Alcohol-based hand rub**—A product containing alcohol intended for application to the hands for the purpose of reducing the number of microorganisms on the hands. Alcohol-based hand rub products are available as rinses, gels, and foams and are usually formulated to contain 60% to 95% alcohol. Alcohol-based hand rubs do not require the use of a scrub sponge/brush or sponge. Some, but not all, alcohol-based hand rubs have been cleared by the FDA as surgical hand antiseptics and may be used for cleaning hands in preparation for gowning and gloving for surgery.

Anatomical timed scrub—A scrub procedure using a sponge/brush and an antimicrobial surgical scrub agent, whereby a specified amount of time is allocated for scrubbing each surface of the fingers, hands, and portion of the arms with the antimicrobial scrub agent. Brushes are no longer recommended.

Antimicrobial soap—Soap containing an antiseptic agent

Antimicrobial surgical scrub agent—A product intended for surgical hand antisepsis.

Antiseptic agent—An antimicrobial substance applied to the skin to reduce the number of resident and transient microbial flora.

Antiseptic hand wash—A hand wash performed with a product formulated with an antiseptic agent.

Counted stroke scrub—A scrub procedure using a sponge/brush and an antimicrobial surgical scrub agent, whereby a prescribed number of strokes is specified for scrubbing each surface of the fingers, hands and arms.

Hand hygiene—Refers to hand washing, antiseptic hand wash, antiseptic hand rub, or surgical hand antisepsis

Handwashing—Washing hands with plain soap (soap without an antimicrobial) and water

Resident microorganisms—Microorganisms that are permanent residents of the skin

Surgical hand antisepsis—Antiseptic hand wash or antiseptic hand rub performed prior to surgery by surgical personnel to eliminate transient microorganisms and reduce resident hand flora. Products used for surgical hand antisepsis may be used in place of the traditional brush/sponge and antimicrobial surgical scrub agent.

Surgical hand antiseptic agent—An antimicrobial product formulated to significantly reduce the number of microorganisms on skin. Surgical hand antiseptic agents are broad spectrum and should exhibit both persistence and cumulative effect that prevents or inhibits proliferation or survival of microorganisms.

Transient microorganisms—Microorganisms found on the skin that are easily removed with a soap and water hand wash or with an antimicrobial hand rub agent

79. Hand hygiene is often considered the single most important step in prevention of infection. Operating room personnel, like all healthcare personnel, should perform hand hygiene before and after patient contact, before donning gloves, and after removing them.

80. Hand hygiene, other than in preparation for surgery, requires washing hands with either plain or antimicrobial soap and water or application of an alcohol-based skin rub. When hands are visibly soiled or contaminated with proteinaceous material, **hand washing** must precede application of an alcohol-based hand rub.

81. Hand hygiene prior to donning sterile gown and gloves in preparation for surgery is referred to as "surgical hand antisepsis." Surgical hand antisepsis, traditionally referred to as "scrubbing," has traditionally required that personnel scrub their hands and arms with a sponge/brush or sponge using an antimicrobial surgical scrub agent while adhering to either an anatomical timed scrub procedure or a counted stroke method procedure. Traditional antimicrobial scrub agents are detergent-based products containing alcohol, iodine/iodophors, chlorhexidine gluconate, triclosan, or parachlorometaxylenol. Provodine-iodine and chlorhexidine gluconate products are most common.

82. Alcohol-based products in combination with other products, i.e., chlorhexidine gluconate, that add a persistent characteristic have been shown to be rapid and effective, and as a result, many facilities have changed their policies and procedures related to surgical hand antisepsis.

83. Surgical hand antisepsis requires hand washing followed by application of an alcohol-based antiseptic hand rub cleared by the Food and Drug Administration for use as a surgical hand antiseptic agent; or handwashing followed by application of an antimicrobial scrub agent (typically applied using a sponge/brush) cleared by the Food and Drug Administration for use as a surgical hand antiseptic agent.

Regardless of whether an alcohol-based antiseptic hand rub or a sponge/brush and surgical hand antiseptic hand agent is used, the hands should first be washed. Hands should also be washed after removing gloves (AORN, 2004f, pp. 294, 296).

84. Surgical hand antisepsis is an activity performed immediately prior to gowning and gloving in preparation for surgery. The purpose of surgical hand antisepsis is to remove dirt, skin oils, and transient microorganisms; to reduce the amount of resident microorganisms on the nails, hands, and lower arms to as low a level as possible; and to prevent growth of microorganisms for as long as possible. This is accomplished through mechanical washing and chemical antisepsis.

85. Mechanical washing is the removal of dirt, oils, and microorganisms by means of friction. Antisepsis is the prevention of sepsis by the exclusion, destruction, or inhibition of growth or multiplication of microorganisms from body tissues and fluids.

86. The objective of the surgical hand antisepsis is to prevent the transfer of microorganisms from personnel to patients and from patients to personnel in the event of glove tears or gown penetration.

87. Prior to performing surgical hand antisepsis, all jewelry must be removed from hands and arms. All other jewelry must also be removed or be completely contained. Hands and arms should be examined for cuts and other lesions that could ooze serum, which is a medium for microbial growth and serves as a potential means of transmission of microorganisms into the patient. Persons with cuts and abrasions should not function in the scrub role.

88. Personnel with respiratory infections should not function in the scrub role.

89. Surgical hand antiseptic agents should meet the following criteria:

- broad spectrum of activity (effective against gram-negative and gram-positive organisms)
- rapid acting
- noniritating
- not dependent upon a cumulative effect (the first application is as effective as subsequent applications); however, should demonstrate a cumulative effect
- significantly reduces microorganisms on the skin
- persistent activity—rapid growth of microorganisms inhibited

TRADITIONAL SURGICAL HAND ANTISEPSIS
(TRADITIONAL SCRUB PROCEDURE)

90. Surgical hand antisepsis should be performed according to hospital policy, which should specify the agent and the method to be used. Manufacturer's recommendations and supporting literature regarding use of the agent should be incorporated into policy.

91. Historically, scrub policies called for an anatomical scrub or a timed scrub. In either method, the scrub should include cleaning and scrubbing of all surfaces of each nail, finger, hand, and arm to 2 inches above the elbow.

92. Anatomical scrubs may indicate the number of strokes to be applied to each area to be scrubbed. The entire surface to be scrubbed is broken into specified areas with a specified number of strokes for each area. For example, each finger has four surfaces, each of which is scrubbed a specified number of times.

93. Timed scrubs specify the length of time a scrub should last and may specify how long the scrub should last on each specified surface. The number of strokes and time may both be incorporated into a scrub policy.

94. Scrub policies have traditionally called for a 5-minute or longer scrub, although recent studies suggest that, depending upon the formulation of the surgical hand antiseptic agent, shorter times are equally effective (CDC, 2002 p. S20).

95. Basic steps in the traditional scrub procedure (scrub sponge/brush and antimicrobial surgical scrub agent) include the following:

- Individually packaged commercially prepared product intended for traditional surgical hand antisepsis is selected. Product usually contains a sponge/brush combination impregnated with antimicrobial surgical scrub agent and a nail cleaning tool.
- The faucet is turned on with water set at a comfortable temperature.
- Hands and forearms are washed with soap and running water.
- The packaged sponge/brush containing nail cleaner is opened.
- Nail cleaner and sponge/brush are removed from the package.
- The sponge/brush is held in one hand; and under running water the nail cleaner is used to clean nails and subungual spaces on the other hand.
- The process is repeated with the opposite hand.
- The nail cleaner is discarded.
- Nails and hands are rinsed.
- The sponge/brush, if it is impregnated with antimicrobial agent, is moistened. If it is not impregnated with antimicrobial surgical agent, an antimicrobial agent is added to the hands, usually from a foot-pump container.
- The arms are held in a flexed position with the fingertips pointing upward. Throughout the scrub, the hands are held up and away from the body. The elbows are flexed and the hands held higher than the elbows. Water and cleanser flow from the fingertips (the cleanest area) to the elbow and into the sink.
- Using circular motion and pressure adequate to remove microorganisms but not sufficient to abrade skin, the nails, fingers, hands, and arms are methodically scrubbed, beginning with the fingertips and continuing through the foreams. Care is taken not to splash water onto surgical attire. Wet surgical attire can cause the transfer of microorganisms from personnel to the sterile gown worn during surgery.
- The scrub sponge/brush is discarded.
- The hands and arms are rinsed. Arms are flexed with hands above elbows as the scrubbed person enters the operating room.
- Care should be taken throughout the procedure to prevent splashing of surgical attire.

USE OF ALCOHOL BASED HAND RUBS

96. Alcohol-based hand rub products have been widely used in Europe for some time and are becoming increasingly popular in the United States. They have been shown to save time and reduce costs, are more effective than products used in the traditional scrub method, and because of added emollients are gentle to the hands (CDC, 2002, pp. 13, 19, 21). Policies and procedures for using an alcohol-based hand rub vary; however, it is critical that manufacturer's instructions for use are followed. The procedure should include the following:

- Hands and forearms are washed with soap and running water.
- The nails and subungual areas of both hands are cleaned with a nail cleaner.
- Hands and forearms are rinsed and thoroughly dried with a clean towel.

- Instead of scrubbing according to the traditional scrub, an alcohol-based hand rub product cleared by the FDA for use as a surgical hand antiseptic is applied to hands and forearms.

- Amount of product applied and procedure for use must be strictly in accordance with manufacturer's instructions.

- Hands and forearms are rubbed until dry.

97. Alcohol-based hand rub products do not take the place of washing and mechanical action when hands are visibly soiled or contaminated with proteinaceous material.

98. Product selection and policies and procedures for surgical hand scrub should be determined in conjunction with the end users, operating room managers, and the healthcare facility infection control practitioner/committee.

GOWNING AND GLOVING PROCEDURE

99. A gown package containing a sterile towel and sterile gown is opened on a small table, separate from the instrument or back table, within the operating room. The gown and towel are packaged so that when it is opened the towel is on top of the gown. The gown is folded inside out and from bottom to top in such a manner that the top inside portion of the gown is directly beneath the towel. The towel and gown may be reusable or single use/disposable.

100. If the traditional scrub procedure was performed, the hands and arms must be thoroughly dried before the gown is donned. If the hands and arms are not thoroughly dried, contamination of the gown may occur by strikethrough from organisms contained in moisture on the skin.

101. The scrub person grasps the sterile towel and lifts it straight up and away from the gown without dripping water on the gown or the sterile field. The scrub person steps away from the sterile field and allows the towel to unfold without contacting the scrub attire. If the towel contacts an unsterile surface, the towel is considered contaminated and a new sterile one is used.

102. The top half of the towel is held in one hand while the opposite hand and forearm are dried. To decrease the risk of contamination, a rotating motion beginning at the hand and working toward the elbow is used for drying. When the first hand and forearm are dry, the lower half of the towel that is unused is grasped with the dry hand, and the opposite hand and forearm are then dried. Care is taken not to return to an area that is already dried.

103. Sterile gowns may be reusable or disposable. The gown should be constructed of a material that provides a barrier to prevent the passage of microorganisms from the surgical team to the patient and from the patient to the surgical team. Gown manufacturer's data should be obtained to verify that the materials used in gowns provide a protective barrier against transfer of microorganisms and fluids.

104. Gowns should be fire retardant, as lint free as possible, free from tears or holes, and fluid resistant or fluid proof. Fluid-*proof* gowns are coated or laminated with an impervious film that does not permit penetration of fluids. Fluid-*resistant* gowns provide an effective barrier and do not permit ready penetration of liquids. The barrier quality of gowns varies. For procedures where little or no exposure to blood or body fluids is anticipated, a gown with minimal barrier protection is acceptable. Fluid-resistant gowns should be worn whenever splashes or spraying of blood or other infectious fluids is anticipated. Where large amounts of fluid are anticipated, fluid-proof gowns should be worn.

105. Other desirable characteristics are as follows. Surgical gowns should:

- maintain their integrity
- be durable—resistant to tears, punctures and abrasions
- be lint free or low linting
- be appropriate to the methods of sterilization available within the healthcare facility
- have limited memory—flexible enough to conform loosely to the wearer's body
- have a favorable cost-benefit ratio (AORN, 2004c, p. 286)

106. Reusable gowns eventually lose their barrier qualities with repeated laundering. Quality monitoring should be in place to ensure that only gowns of appropriate quality are used.

107. The cuffs are stockinette and fit tight to the wrist. Gowns may or may not be wraparound style and are held closed with cotton tapes, snaps, or Velcro fasteners.

108. The scrubbed person dons the sterile gown using the following procedure:

- The sterile gown is grasped by the inside neckline and lifted away from the gown wrapper.
- Holding the gown by the neck edge, the scrub person moves away from areas of possible contamination and lets the gown unfold downward.

- The scrub person locates the armholes, and both arms are simultaneously inserted into the sleeves. If a closed-gloving technique is intended to be utilized, the arms are inserted into the gown only until the hands reach the proximal edge of the cuff. If an open-gloving technique is intended, the arms are inserted into the gown until the hands advance through the cuffs.

- The gown is fastened in the back at the neckline and the waist by a nonsterile team member.

- Gloves are donned.

- After gloving is completed, the scrubbed person extends a paper tab attached to one of the gown ties to another team member (sterile or unsterile). The scrub person then pivots away from the other team member, causing the gown to wrap around the scrub person. The scrub person then grasps the tie and pulls it, releasing it from the paper tab. The scrub person then ties the gown securely in front. If a tab is not included with the gown, the scrub person may attach a sterile instrument to the end of one tie and hand it to an unsterile team member who utilizes the instrument in the same manner as a paper tab. (Figure 5-8)

109. Sterile gloves are a barrier that is intended to prevent passage of microorganisms from the scrubbed person to the patient and from the patient to the scrubbed person.

110. Gloves should be selected according to desired strength, durability, and compatibility. Extra-strength specialty gloves are available and should be used for procedures, such as bone and joint surgeries, where there is high risk of percutaneous blood exposure.

111. Latex-free gloves must be used when personnel or the patient have latex allergies. Hypo-allergenic and powder-free gloves should be chosen for personnel sensitive to glove chemicals and powders.

112. Sterile gloves that have powders or talc on them should be wiped with sterile water or saline prior to the surgical incision. Powders and talc can incite an inflammatory response and delay healing if introduced into the wound (Ellis, 1990, p. 521).

113. Closed gloving is a method of donning sterile gloves whereby the scrubbed hands remain inside the gown sleeve until the glove cuff is secured over the gown cuff.

114. Closed gloving is begun with the hands inside the sleeves. Using the right hand that is still inside the right cuff, the scrub person grasps the left glove by the glove's everted cuff.

115. The left forearm is extended with the palm facing up and the hand still inside the sleeve. The left glove is then placed palm side down on the upturned left sleeve, palm to palm, thumb to thumb, with the fingers of the glove pointing toward the scrubbed person's body. Using the

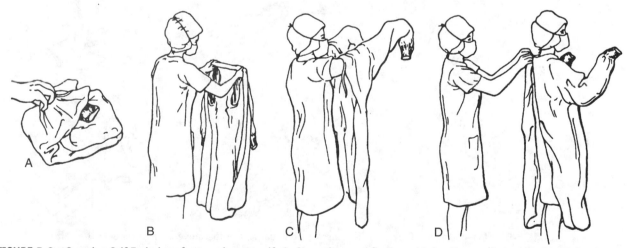

FIGURE 5-8 Gowning Self Technique for gowning oneself. **A,** Grasp the gown firmly and bring it away from the table. It has been folded so that the outside of the gown faces away. **B,** Holding the gown at the shoulders, allow it to unfold gently. Do not shake the gown. **C,** Place hands inside the armholes and guide each arm through the sleeves by raising and spreading the arms. Do not allow hands to slide outside cuff of gown. **D,** The circulator will assist by pulling the gown over the shoulders and tying it.
Source: Reprinted with permission from S.S. Fairchild, *Perioperative Nursing: Principles and Practice*, 2nd ed., p. 155, © 1993, W.B. Saunders Company. Original illustration permission—J.R. Fuller, *Surgical Technology: Principles and Practice*, 2nd ed., p. 45, © 1986, W.B. Saunders Company.

left thumb and index finger, the glove cuff is grasped through the stockinette cuff and the glove is held in place. The fingers of the left hand must not extend beyond the stockinette cuff to grasp the glove. Using the sleeve-covered right hand, the cuff of the left glove is then stretched over the open end of the left sleeve. The glove should totally encompass the stockinette portion of the sleeve. The sleeve-covered right hand is then used to exert an even pull on the left sleeve of the gown, causing the left hand to slide into the glove.

116. To glove the right hand, the right glove is grasped with the already gloved left hand and placed on the right sleeve, palm to palm, thumb to thumb, with glove fingers pointing toward the scrub person's body. With the use of the right thumb and index finger, the right glove cuff is grasped through the stockinette cuff and held in place. The fingers of the right hand must not extend beyond the stockinette cuff to hold the glove in place. Using the gloved left hand, the right glove is stretched

over the open end of the right sleeve. The left hand is then used to pull lightly and evenly on the right sleeve, causing the right hand to slide into the right glove. (Figure 5-9)

117. In the open-glove technique, the scrub person extends the hands through the stockinette cuff of the sleeves when donning the gown. During gloving, the surgically clean hand touches only the inside of the sterile glove and never contacts the exterior of the glove.

118. The glove package is opened by a nonscrubbed person on a clean, dry surface. Using the right hand, the scrub person grasps the everted cuff of the left glove and slides the fingers and thumb of the left hand into the glove, leaving the everted cuff of the glove over the hand and below the cuff of the gown sleeve. The scrub person then slips the fingers of the left gloved hand under the everted cuff of the right glove and slides the fingers and hand into the right glove. The everted glove cuff is brought up and over the cuff of the gown. Care is taken to prevent the sterile gloved hand from touching the

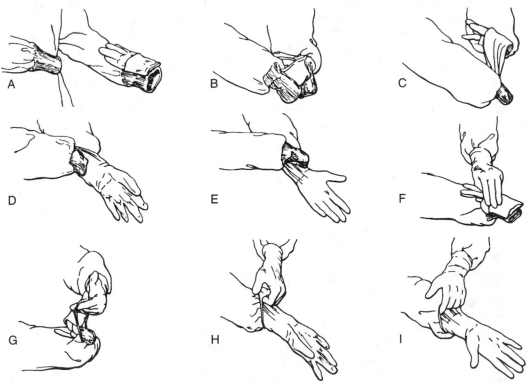

FIGURE 5-9 Closed Gloving. Gloving self—closed technique. **A,** Lay the glove palm down over the cuff of the gown. The fingers of the glove face toward you. **B and C,** Working through the gown sleeve, grasp the cuff of the glove and bring it over the open cuff of the sleeve. **D and E,** Unroll the glove cuff so that it covers the sleeve cuff. **F,G,H, and I,** Proceed with the opposite hand, using the same technique. Never allow the bare hand to contact the gown cuff edge or outside of glove.
Source: Reprinted with permission from J.R. Fuller, *Surgical Technology: Principles and Practice,* 2nd ed., p. 46, © 1986, W.B. Saunders Company.

skin of the wrist or hand. In the final step, using the gloved right hand, the everted cuff of the left glove is brought over the stockinette cuff of the left sleeve. (Figure 5-10)

119. Although both the closed- and the open-glove techniques are acceptable during initial gloving, the closed-glove technique is often preferred. In the open-glove technique there is a greater chance of the scrub person's bare hands contacting the outside of the sterile glove, thereby causing it to become contaminated.

Assisting Others to Gown and Glove

120. After the scrub person has donned a gown and gloves, he or she assists other team members to gown and glove.

121. The scrub person extends a towel to a newly scrubbed person, being careful not to touch that person's hands. The towel should be presented by placing one end over the outstretched hand of the newly scrubbed person.

This step is not necessary if an alcohol-based hand rub product was used.

122. The scrub person then grasps the folded gown at the neck edge, lifts it away from the sterile field, and allows it to unfold. Keeping the hands on the outside of the gown and using the neck and shoulder area of the gown to form a protective cuff over the gloves, the scrub person offers the inside of the gown to the newly scrubbed team member.

123. The newly scrubbed person will don the gown by inserting the arms into the sleeves and extending the hands through the stockinette cuff of the gown. A nonsterile team member will then secure the gown at the neck and waist area. (Figure 5-11)

124. The scrub person will then glove the newly scrubbed team member. The sterile glove is grasped under the everted edge and held so the thumb of the glove is in opposition to the thumb of the person being gloved. The cuff is then stretched open wide. The newly gowned person then advances a hand into the glove. The cuff of the glove must be stretched wide enough and high enough to cover the stockinette gown cuff entirely. This procedure is repeated to glove the other hand.

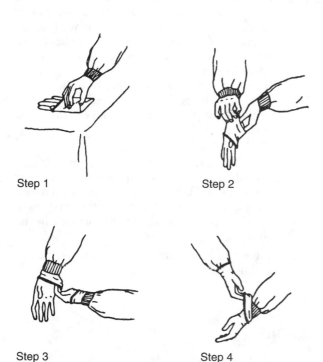

Step 1   Step 2

Step 3   Step 4

FIGURE 5-10 Open Gloving. Open-glove technique. Step 1, The glove is picked up by the top surface of the folded-down cuff. Step 2, The glove is held by the inner surface and pulled onto the left hand. Step 3, The right glove is picked up by grasping the glove under the folded-down cuff with gloved left hand. the glove is pulled onto the hand and the cuff of the glove flipped up and over the cuff of the gown. Step 4, With the gloved right hand the turned-down cuff of the left glove is flipped up and over the cuff of the gown.
Source: Operating Room Technologies for the Surgical Team, Crooks, Little, Brown. Used by permission of Lippincott Williams & Wilkins.

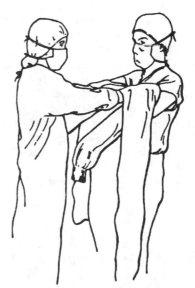

FIGURE 5-11 Gowning Others. Using the outside of the gown neck and shoulder area to form a protective cuff over her gloves the scrub person offers a gown to the newly scrubbed team member.
Source: Reprinted with permission from S.S. Fairchild, *Perioperative Nursing: Principles and Practice,* 2nd ed., p. 160, © 1993, W.B. Saunders Company. Original illustration permission—J.R. Fuller, *Surgical Technology. Principles and Practice,* 2nd ed., p. 48 © 1986, W.B. Saunders Company.

125. Wearing a second pair of gloves over the first is known as *double gloving*. Double gloving has been shown to reduce hand contact with the patient's blood and/or body fluids during surgery and is widely practiced (Mangram et al., 1999, p. 262). Double gloving is indicated for surgical procedures where risk of percutaneous exposure to bloodborne pathogens is high. Individual institutional policies, sound judgment, and knowledge of surgical procedures should influence the decision of whether or not to wear two pairs of gloves.

126. If a team member's glove becomes contaminated, that person steps back from the sterile field and extends the contaminated hand to a nonsterile team member who dons protective gloves and removes the sterile team member's contaminated glove by grasping the outside of the glove approximately 2 inches below the top of the glove and pulling the glove off inside out. Care must be taken that the gown cuff not be pulled down or slip down over the hand because the gown cuff is considered contaminated once the original gloves are donned. The scrub person may reglove the team member in the same manner as previously performed, or the open-glove technique can be used to reglove without assistance.

127. If a team member's gown becomes contaminated, a nonsterile team member dons protective gloves and unfastens the gown at the neck and waist, grasps it in front at the shoulders, and pulls it forward and off over the scrubbed person's hands, which are still gloved. The gown should come off inside out. The nonsterile team member then removes the sterile team member's gloves, and the scrub person regowns and regloves the sterile team member or the sterile team member may regown and reglove without assistance. The contaminated gown should always be removed *before* the gloves are removed. This prevents microorganisms and debris that may be found on the gown from being dragged across unprotected, ungloved hands.

128. The closed-glove technique is not acceptable for changing a contaminated glove. During initial gowning and gloving, the scrubbed, but not sterile, ungloved hand passes through the gown cuff, causing the cuff to be considered contaminated. In the closed-glove technique, the cuff contacts the sterile glove; therefore, the new sterile glove would be contaminated by the contaminated cuff.

129. At the completion of surgery, the gown and gloves are removed. The gown is removed **first**. It is grasped near the neck and sleeve and brought forward over the gloved hands, inverting the gloves as it is removed. The gown is folded so the contaminated outside surface is on the inside. It is deposited in a designated linen basket or waste receptacle.

130. Gloves are removed so that bare skin does not contact the contaminated external glove. The gloved fingers of one hand are placed under the everted glove cuff of the opposite hand and pulled off. The fold on the remaining glove is grasped with the bare fingers of the opposite hand and the glove is pulled off. This technique must be performed carefully to prevent bare skin from contacting the contaminated glove surface. Gloves are deposited in a designated waste receptacle.

131. After gloves are removed, hand hygiene is performed. If desired, an antimicrobial product may be used. Hand hygiene lessens the chance of contamination of the hands that may have occurred from an invisible hole or tear in the glove.

132. Gown and gloves are not worn outside the operating room.

• •

SECTION QUESTIONS

Q19. Warm-up jackets keep personnel warm but their main purpose is (Ref. 66):

_____

Q20. Scrub attire (Ref. 65):

a. should be changed when it becomes wet

b. should be laundered between wearings

c. may be laundered either at home or a hospital laundry

Q21. OSHA mandates the wearing of surgical masks in areas where surgical supplies are stored. (Ref. 68)

True   False

Q22. Shoe covers (Ref. 72):

a. decrease risk of infection

b. protect personnel footwear

Q23. The purpose of surgical hand antisepsis is (Ref. 84):

a. to sterilize the hands of the scrubbed person

b. to remove dirt and skin oils

c. to remove transient microorganisms

d. to reduce the number of resident microorganisms

e. to prevent growth of microorganisms for as long as possible

Q24. Surgical hand antisepsis (Ref. 77, 81, 83):

a. is performed by team members who function in the scrub role

b. must always be performed with a sponge/brush

c. may follow a timed anatomical protocol or a counted stroke protocol

d. is performed before and after donning gloves

e. should always last 6 minutes or more

Q25. Surgical hand antisepsis is performed for the purpose of removing all transient and resident micro-organisms and to prevent regrowth of microorganisms for as long as possible. (Ref. 84)

True   False

Q26. During the traditional surgical scrub, the hands are held away from the body and higher than the elbows. (Ref. 95)

True   False

Q27. Alcohol-based hand rubs (Ref. 78, 97):

a. are formulated as rinses, gels, and foams

b. eliminate the need to wash hands

Q28. Repeated laundering will cause a fluid-proof gown to lose its barrier qualities over time. (Ref. 106)

True   False

Q29. Explain when it is good practice for the scrub person to wipe his/her sterile gloves with sterile water prior to the surgical incision. (Ref. 112)

_____

_____

_____

Q30. Regarding gloving (Ref. 119, 125, 127, 128, 129):

a. During initial gloving, the open and closed-gloving techniques are both acceptable.

b. When a glove becomes contaminated and a new one is donned, the closed-glove technique is preferable.

c. Wearing two pairs of gloves is acceptable practice.

d. At the completion of surgery, the sterile team members should remove their gloves only after they remove their gowns.

Creating a Sterile Field

Draping

133. Drapes serve as a barrier to prevent the passage of microorganisms between sterile and nonsterile areas. Sterile drapes are used to create a sterile surface around the incision site that may be used for sterile supplies and equipment. This area is referred to as the *sterile field*.

134. The sterile field includes the patient, furniture, and other equipment that is covered with sterile drapes. (Figure 5-12) The sterile field is isolated from unsterile surfaces and items. Only sterile items are placed on a sterile field.

135. Sterile drapes are positioned over the patient in such a way that only a minimum area of skin around the incision site is exposed.

136. Frequently draped furniture includes instrument or "back" tables, the Mayo stands, and the ring stands. (Figure 5-13)

137. Drapes may be reusable or single use/disposable. Criteria for drapes are that they be:

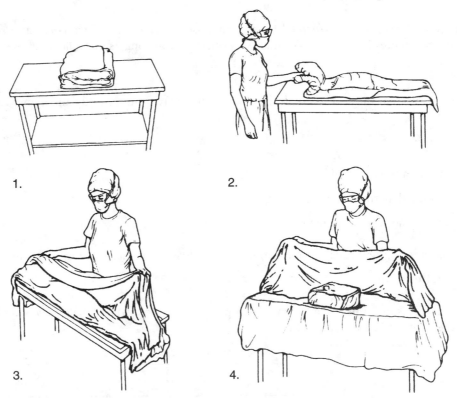

FIGURE 5-12   Draping a Table.
Source: Reprinted with permission from S.S. Fairchild, *Perioperative Nursing: Principles and Practice*, pp. 235–236, Little, Brown & Company.

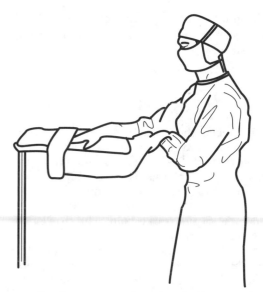

FIGURE 5-13 Draping the Mayo stand.

- resistant to blood and liquid penetration and provide an effective barrier to prevent passage of microorganisms from nonsterile to sterile areas
- durable—resistant to tears
- lint free or low linting to reduce airborne contamination or shedding into the operative site—microorganisms and dust particles may settle on airborne lint and shed into the operative site
- flame resistant
- memory free—easily conform to body and equipment contours
- comfortable

138. As with gowns, drapes may be fluid resistant or fluid proof. Materials that are liquid resistant have varying degrees of resistance.

139. Single use/disposable drapes are more common than reusable drapes; however, both are appropriate for creating a sterile field. Reusable drapes are manufactured in a variety of fabrics with varying degrees of barrier effectiveness. All reusable drapes will, over time, lose their barrier qualities with repeated laundering and sterilizations. Laundering and steam sterilization swell fibers, and drying shrinks them. This reduces the tightness of the fibers and causes ultimate loss of barrier effectiveness. A quality monitoring program should be in place to ensure drape integrity and barrier effectiveness. The program may include tracking the number of times a drape has been laundered. All reusable drapes must be routinely inspected for tears and punctures.

140. Single use/disposable drapes are composed of nonwoven natural and synthetic materials and also are manufactured with varying degrees of barrier effectiveness. These fabrics include a fluid-proof polyethylene film laminated between the fabric layers at strategic locations of the drape, usually around the drape fenestration. Nonwoven drapes are available in a variety of configurations and are commercially packaged and sterilized. They are designed for one-time use and are not resterilized.

141. Clear plastic drapes with or without adhesive backings are available in various sizes. They are available plain or impregnated with iodophor. These incise drapes are applied directly over the skin at the operative site. They may be partially applied over the drapes, in which case they assist in keeping the drapes in place without the use of towel clips. The incision is made through the plastic drape. Some plastic drapes include a fluid collection pouch to collect fluids. These may prevent the accumulation of moisture under the drapes where bacteria can proliferate and contaminate the wound.

142. Plastic drapes are useful for draping irregular body areas such as joints, eyes, and ears. Plastic drapes may be used to seal off a contaminated area such as a stoma.

143. Impervious polyvinyl drapes are available for equipment, such as portable C Arm and X-ray equipment, and for specialty needs such as to seal off the perineal area, to cover a tourniquet, or to contain body fluids and irrigation.

Draping Guidelines

144. The following guidelines should be followed during draping:

- Only sterile drapes that are intact are used for draping. All defects must have been patched with a vulcanized heat seal patch.
- Drapes should be handled as little as possible.
- Drapes are gently placed. They are not flipped or shaken. Shaking and flipping causes air currents that are a vehicle for dust, lint, and other particles.
- Drapes are carried folded to the operating table and held higher than the OR table.
- Draping is done from the operative site to the periphery.

- Once a drape is placed, it is not moved or repositioned. Drapes that are placed incorrectly are removed by an unscrubbed person.
- When draping, a cuff is formed from the drape to protect the sterile gloved hands of the person draping.
- A towel clip with points that has been positioned through a drape will have its points contaminated and must not be removed until completion of the procedure. Nonpenetrating towel clips do not interrupt the integrity of drapes and should be used when possible
- Whenever the sterility of a drape is in doubt, it is considered contaminated and is not used. (Figure 5-14)

Standard Drapes

145. The amount, type, and size of drapes that are selected for a procedure require careful planning. Selection factors will include the type of procedure to be performed, the amount of area around the incision that should be included in the sterile field, and furniture and equipment that will be draped. Cost considerations require that variety and amount of drapes be kept to a minimum.

146. Standard drapes include:

- flat sheets used to drape instrument tables and areas of the patient
- Mayo stand covers
- towels used to drape the operative site
- fenestrated drapes with openings of various sizes and configurations to drape for specific procedures or specialities (typical types include but are not limited to abdominal laparotomy, chest/breast, head and neck, total hip joint, and extremity); fenestrations are generally reinforced with an impervious barrier; the fenestrated drape is large enough to cover the entire patient and the operating table with sufficient material to extend over the foot of the table, the ether screen at the head of the table, and the arm boards
- aperture drape—a small clear fenestrated plastic drape frequently used in eye and ear procedures
- equipment drapes—clear plastic drapes that cover X-ray machines, microscopes, and other equipment
- stockinette drape used to drape feet and hands

- leggings—part of drape set intended for surgery with the patient in the lithotomy position

Maintaining a Sterile Field

147a. *Scrubbed personnel function within a sterile field* (AORN, 2004b, p. 367).

Personnel in the sterile field should wear sterile gowns and gloves. Surgical gowns and gloves establish a barrier that minimizes the passage of microorganisms between nonsterile and sterile areas. Once donned, the gown is considered sterile in front from the chest to the level of the sterile field. The sleeves are considered sterile from 2 inches above the elbow down to the top edge of the cuff. The neckline, shoulders, axilla, and cuffed portion of the sleeves may become contaminated by perspiration and therefore are not considered sterile. The back is considered nonsterile because it cannot be under constant observation by the scrubbed person. The cuffs are considered contaminated once the hands have passed through them.

b. *Sterile drapes should be used to establish a sterile field* (AORN, 2004b, p. 367).

To create a sterile field, sterile drapes are placed on the patient and on all furniture and equipment that will be part of the sterile field. Sterile drapes are a barrier to the passage of microorganisms, isolate the sterile field from the surrounding environment, and minimize passage of microorganisms between sterile and nonsterile areas.

c. *Items used within a sterile field should be sterile* (AORN, 2004b, p. 368).

Items used during surgery are wrapped and sterilized prior to surgery. On occasion, unwrapped items may be taken directly from the autoclave following sterilization and dispensed to the sterile field.

Sterility of items must be ensured by the person dispensing them to the sterile field and by the person accepting them. The circulating nurse should check the integrity of the wrapper, the expiration date (if there is one), and the color of the indicator tape. The chemical indicator or integrator inside the package is checked by the scrub person to ensure that items were exposed to the sterilant or, depending upon the type of indicator used, that parameters of sterilization were attained during the sterilization process. If an item is taken directly from the autoclave, the circulating nurse must ensure that the proper technique is used to transfer items to the sterile field.

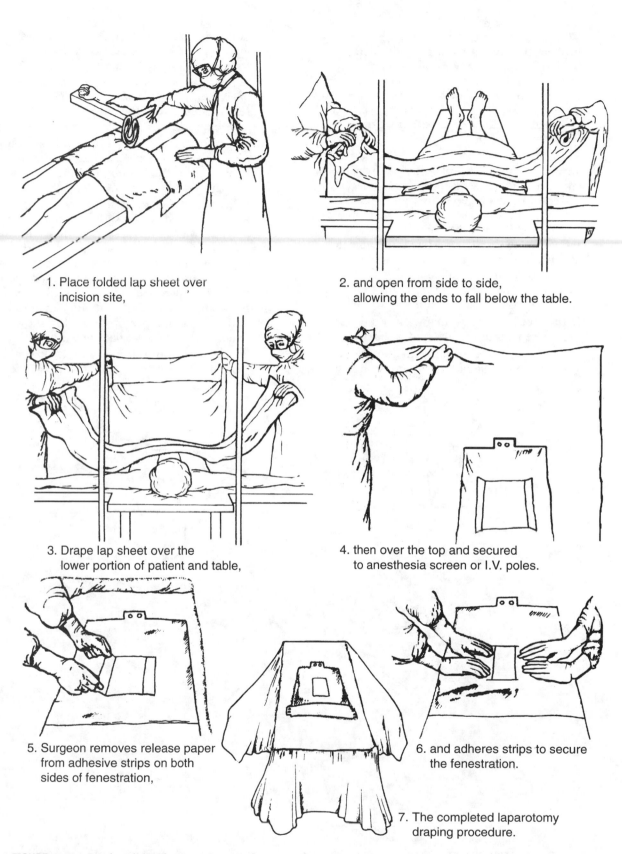

1. Place folded lap sheet over incision site,

2. and open from side to side, allowing the ends to fall below the table.

3. Drape lap sheet over the lower portion of patient and table,

4. then over the top and secured to anesthesia screen or I.V. poles.

5. Surgeon removes release paper from adhesive strips on both sides of fenestration,

6. and adheres strips to secure the fenestration.

7. The completed laparotomy draping procedure.

FIGURE 5-14 Draping the Patient.
Source: Reprinted with permission from S.S. Fairchild, *Perioperative Nursing: Principles and Practice*, p. 248, Little, Brown & Company.

Whenever the integrity of a sterile barrier is broken, the contents must be considered unsterile. Wrappers, gowns, gloves, and drapes are all examples of sterile barriers. Examples of sterile barriers that have been permeated are a tear or hole in a wrapper or glove; a wet, scorched, or stained wrapper; or a barrier that looks questionable.

The contents of wet or stained wrappers may have been subject to strike-through, which occurs when liquids soak through a barrier from a sterile to an unsterile area and vice versa. Strike-through provides for passage of microorganisms through the barrier, and therefore the contents must be considered contaminated. When strike-through occurs, it may not be noticed initially and the item may dry. Therefore, items contained in wrappers that are stained should be considered contaminated.

If the sterility of any item is in doubt, it is considered contaminated and is discarded.

Items that become contaminated must not be permitted on the sterile field. Items, such as suc-tion and cautery, that remain on the drapes during the procedure are secured to prevent them from sliding below the level of the sterile field.

d. *Items introduced to a sterile field should be opened, dispensed, and transferred by methods that maintain sterility and integrity* (AORN, 2004b, p. 368).

Several techniques may be used by unscrubbed personnel to dispense sterile items onto the sterile field while maintaining the sterility of the field.

When dispensing an item to the sterile field, the unscrubbed person should open the wrapper flap that is furthest away first and the wrapper flap that is closest last. All wrapper edges should be secured to prevent accidental contamination of the scrub person or sterile field with a wrapper edge. If an item cannot be carefully placed or easily flipped onto the field, the scrub person must lift the item straight up out of the package. (Figure 5-15) Sterile gowns and drapes and other similar items may be placed onto the sterile field;

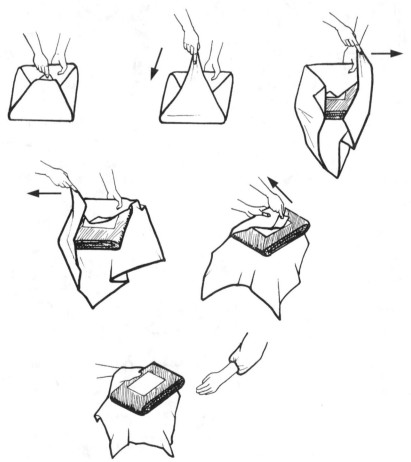

FIGURE 5-15   Opening a Package. Circulating nurse passes sterile item to scrub person by opening package and bringing wrapper back over hand to form a protective barrier.

however, the portion of the unscrubbed person's hand that may extend over the sterile field is covered by an everted portion of the sterile wrapper.

Heavy, awkward, or sharp items should not be tossed onto the sterile field because they may roll off the edge of the sterile field, displace other items from the sterile field, or penetrate the sterile barrier. These items should be opened on a separate table or stand or received directly by the scrub person. (Figure 5-16)

Sterile basins into which sterile solutions will be poured are placed at the edge of the table or are held by the scrub person. This decreases the risk of splashing the sterile field and creating the potential for strike-through. Because the edge of the bottle is considered contaminated once the cap is removed, the cap should not be replaced. Solutions remaining within a bottle or container should not be used. Drops may have contacted the unsterile outside of the bottle or container during initial pouring and could contaminate solutions if they are subsequently poured. Therefore the entire contents of the bottle should be poured into the receptacle. (Figure 5-17)

Boundaries between sterile and unsterile are not always clearly defined, and good judgment and keen observation are needed to ensure that only sterile items are introduced to the sterile field.

e. *A sterile field should be maintained and monitored continuously* (AORN, 2004b, p. 368).

A sterile field should be set up as close to the time of surgery as possible. The longer ster-

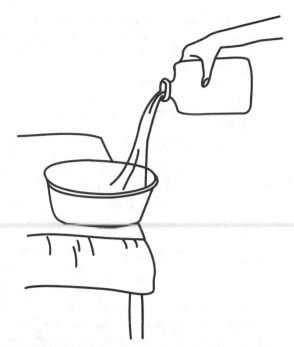

FIGURE 5-17   Pouring Liquid. Sterile basin is placed at edge of table allowing only sterile lip of bottle to extend over the edge of basin while solution is poured.

ile items are open to the environment, the greater opportunity there is for contamination to occur.

Covering a sterile field to prevent contamination is a questionable practice. It is difficult to remove a cover without causing contamination to occur. Removing a single cover requires that a portion of the cover that has been below the level of the sterile field be drawn up over the top of the sterile field. This can cause contamination. Some institutional policies may permit covering using two drapes. Each drape is positioned to cover half of the sterile field and to meet in the middle, where an everted cuff is formed from each drape. Using the cuffs, each drape is removed from the center outward rather than up and over the field. This is not an AORN recommended practice, however, and where it is practiced strict guidelines should be provided on application and technique.

Once a sterile field has been created, it should be monitored by all team members for possible contamination. For this reason the sterile field should not be left unattended.

Only sterile items should be permitted into the sterile field. Furniture and equipment such as Mayo stands, tables, and tanks that will be part of the sterile field must be covered with a sterile barrier.

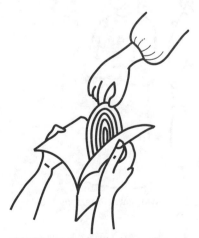

FIGURE 5-16   Retrieving an Item. Large or awkward items are presented directly to the scrub person, who is careful not to touch the wrapper.

Talking should be kept to a minimum in the presence of a sterile field. Talking can produce droplets with the potential to contaminate the sterile field.

f. *All personnel moving within or around a sterile field should do so in a manner that will maintain the sterile field* (AORN, 2004b, p. 368).

The surgical team must be aware of sterile and unsterile items within the operating room and move in a manner that does not cause sterile items or fields to become contaminated.

Scrubbed persons touch only sterile items and areas. Scrubbed persons remain as close to the sterile field as possible and do not wander about or leave the room. Scrubbed persons face the sterile field. When scrubbed persons move or change places with each other, they do so face to face or back to back and maintain a safe distance apart. (Figure 5-18)

The scrubbed person should not change levels from standing to sitting and the reverse. Changing levels can cause the lower portion of the gown, which is considered contaminated, to be drawn close to or in contact with the sterile field and increases the risk of sterile-field contamination. The only time scrubbed persons should sit is when the entire procedure is performed at this level.

The patient is the center of the sterile field. All additional sterile equipment is grouped around the patient within view of the scrub person.

Unscrubbed persons contact only unsterile items. Unscrubbed persons keep a safe distance from the sterile field to prevent accidental contamination. Determining a safe distance requires astute judgment. Unscrubbed persons who approach the sterile field do so by facing the sterile field. Unscrubbed persons do not walk between two sterile fields.

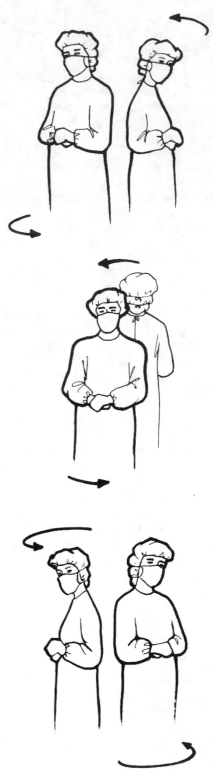

FIGURE 5-18   Back to Back. Two gowned persons shown passing each other back to back.

● ●

SECTION QUESTIONS

Q31. Explain how drapes assist in the creation of a sterile field. (Ref. 133)

_____

_____

Q32. Explain why it is important for drapes to be as lint free as possible. (Ref. 137)

_____

_____

Q33. If a drape is incorrectly placed on the patient, it must be carefully repositioned by the scrub person. (Ref. 144)

True   False

Q34. Explain why a towel clip that has been positioned through a sterile drape is not removed until after surgery. (Ref. 144)

_____

_____

Q35. Before an item is dispensed to the sterile field, the scrub person and the person dispensing the item are always responsible for checking the item to ensure that parameters of sterilization have been met. (Ref. 147c)

True   False

Q36. If the wrapper of a sterile packaged item has a stain on it (Ref. 147c):

a. and the wrapper is intact and the chemical indicator indicates it has been sterilized, the item may be dispensed to the sterile field

b. and the wrapper is dry and intact and the chemical indicator indicates it has been sterilized, the item may be dispensed to the field

c. it is considered contaminated and not dispensed to the sterile field

Q37. Define *strike-through*. (Ref. 147c)

_____

_____

Q38. Sterile setups should be (Ref. 147e):

    a. covered if surgery is delayed

    b. monitored for possible contamination

    c. prepared as close to the time of surgery as possible

    d. used within one hour of setup

Q39. It is proper aseptic technique for two scrubbed persons to pass each other back to front. (Ref. 147f)

    True   False

• •

Control of Environmental Sources of Infection

Traffic Patterns

148. To reduce potential contamination from outside sources, the operating room suite is usually located away from major traffic areas within the facility.

149. The operating room itself is divided into three areas that are defined by the activities that occur within each area. These areas are restricted, semirestricted, and unrestricted.

150. The restricted area is where surgical procedures are performed and sterile supplies are stored. This area includes the operating and procedure rooms, scrub-sink areas, substerile area where the autoclave may be located, and the clean core where sterile supplies are stored. Scrub attire and hair covering is required in the restricted area. A long-sleeved cover-up jacket that is buttoned or snapped closed is recommended as well. A mask is required in the presence of open supplies or scrubbed persons (AORN, 2004g, p. 397). The patient is not required to wear a mask except when transmission-based airborne or droplet precautions are necessary.

151. The semirestricted area includes storage for clean and sterile supplies, instrument-processing areas, and corridors leading to restricted areas. A long-sleeved cover-up jacket that is buttoned or snapped closed is recommended as well. Depending on the design of the suite, lounges may be included in the semirestricted area. Scrub attire and hair covering are required in the semirestricted area. Only authorized personnel and patients are permitted in this area.

152. The unrestricted area is where operating room personnel interface with outside departmental personnel and includes locker rooms, patient reception areas, and areas where supplies are received. Street clothes are permitted in the unrestricted area.

153. Movement from unrestricted to restricted areas should be through a transition zone such as a locker room, office, or holding area.

154. Numbers of personnel and the movement of personnel within the suite during surgery is kept to a minimum. The organisms most frequently associated with surgical site infection are *S. epidermidis* and *S. aureus*, organisms that are found on skin. The higher the number of personnel in the operating room, the higher the number of these microorganisms. It is possible for these organisms to be shed and to settle on dust particles in the air. Airborne contaminants may contribute to the risk of surgical site infection.

155. Items that are considered contaminated, soiled, or dirty should not be transported through the same corridors as clean and sterile items. The flow of supplies should be from the clean core to the operating room and from the operating room to a peripheral corridor, and not back into the clean or sterile area. For example, supplies for a procedure should be taken from the clean core into the operating room, and after the procedure all instruments and/or other contaminated items should exit the operating room into a peripheral corridor where they are transported to an area for discard or transported to a decontamination area. In healthcare facilities where design does not permit this, for example, where there is only one door into the operating room, contaminated, soiled, or dirty items should be contained/covered and transported to the decontamination area at times other than when clean or sterile items are transported through the same area.

156. Items delivered to the operating room from sources outside the healthcare facility should be removed from packing and external shipping

cartons before being permitted into the operating room. Outside shipping cartons may harbor insects and dirt collected during transport.

157. Items and supplies prepared or selected for surgical cases that are delivered to the operating room from departments within the healthcare facility should be transported in closed or covered carts to reduce the potential for contamination.

Operating Room Environment

158. The operating room is considered a clean environment. The design of the operating room, its location within the healthcare facility, limited access, traffic patterns, and policies and procedures for control and cleaning of the environment help to maintain its cleanliness.

159. The operating room has a separate ventilation and air filtration system. All air is filtered through a two-filter system. Filters are designed to remove dust and aerosol particles from the air. All flow is from ceiling to floor.

160. Air is directed into the operating room under positive pressure. The air pressure is higher in each operating room than in the hallways so that the more contaminated hallway air is not pulled into the room. (The exception to positive-pressure air flow is for rooms specifically designed for procedures that should be performed in a negative-pressure environment, such as a bronchoscopy on a patient with tuberculosis.) Because of this pressure difference, doors to each operating room must be kept closed to prevent disruption of the air flow.

161. To maintain the cleanest air possible, a majority of operating rooms adhere to the standards identified by the American Institute of Architects, which require an air flow rapid enough to change the total volume of air in each operating room a minimum of 15 times per hour with at least 3 exchanges of outside air (Mangram et al., 1999, p. 267). (This standard will be reviewed in 2005.) Many newer facilities are ventilated with 20 to 25 changes per hour. Ventilation systems must comply with local, state, and national regulations, which may vary in the requirement for the number of air exchanges per hour and the number of fresh air exchanges required.

162. Laminar air-flow systems may be found in some operating rooms. A laminar air-flow system is an unidirectional ventilation system in which filtered, bacteria-free, "ultraclean" air is circulated over the patient from a filtered outlet and returned through a receiving air inlet. Air is filtered through high efficiency particulate air (HEPA) filters that remove all particles equal to or greater than 0.3 microns with an efficiency of 99.7%. Laminar air flow systems can deliver upwards of 200 air exchanges an hour. Only sterile items are permitted within the area across which the filtered air flows. Laminar air flow systems are used most often for procedures such as total joint replacement.

163. Room temperature is maintained between 68°F and 73°F (20°C and 23°C). This is comfortable enough for the surgical team yet will inhibit bacterial growth. Relative humidity is maintained at 30% to 60%. Higher humidity can provide an opportunity for mold growth, and lower humidity can result in excessive amount of dust that can carry bacteria (American Institute of Architects, 2001).

Operating Room Sanitation

164. Operating-room sanitation practices play a significant role in creating a surgical environment for patient and personnel that is clean and contains a minimum of microorganisms. Pathogenic microorganisms can survive on many environmental surfaces, and in fact, the inanimate environment may serve as a reservoir for certain pathogens such as methicillin resistant staphylococcus aureus (MRSA) (Cozad, 2003, p. 244). Adherence to specified cleaning practices is essential to control and minimize the numbers of pathogens present in the suite.

165. Although cleaning and housekeeping protocols may vary among healthcare institutions, cleaning procedures are generally carried out prior to the beginning of the day's schedule, during the procedure, between procedures, at the end of the daily schedule, and periodically, e.g., weekly or monthly. Only products registered with the Environmental Protection Agency (EPA) as hospital-grade disinfectants should be used for cleaning inanimate surfaces in the operating room.

166. Persons responsible for cleaning and who, in the course of their work, have the potential to contact contaminated items, blood, or body fluids must practice Standard Precautions by wearing personal protective attire that is appropriate to the task to be performed. Such attire includes gloves, masks, eyewear, and gowns.

167. Prior to the first procedure of the day, furniture, equipment, and surgical lights should be damp-dusted with a lint-free cloth moistened with an EPA-registered hospital-grade disinfectant. Particular attention should be paid to horizontal surfaces because dust and lint that transport microorganisms settle on these sur-

faces. Equipment from other areas, such as X-ray machines and tourniquet devices that are necessary for the procedure, are damp-dusted before they are brought into the room.

168. If possible, patients known to have a latex allergy should be scheduled as the first case of the day. Latex products used during the day may remain cause latex particles to remain airborne for a period of time and damp-dusting may not be sufficient to remove all traces of latex protein.

169. Throughout the procedure, an effort is made to confine and contain contamination to as small an area around the patient and sterile field as possible. During the procedure, spills or splashes of blood and body fluids may occur in the immediate vicinity of the sterile field. These should be promptly cleaned and disinfected with a soft absorbent cloth and an EPA-registered germicide with a tuberculocidal claim or an EPA-registered germicide with an HIV or Hepatitis B claim. A 1:100 dilution of bleach may be used for small spills on nonporous surfaces. Spills or splatters of other organic debris, such as patient tissue, should also be promptly cleaned.

170. When a spill consists of greater than 10 ml of blood or other potentially infectious material, the spill should first be absorbed with a soft cloth and then cleaned with a germicide (AORN, 2004a, p. 274). Spill kits should be available for large spills of body fluids.

171. Persons responsible for cleanup should wear personal protective equipment, such as gown and gloves, appropriate to the activity.

172. Disposable items that become contaminated should be discarded into leak-proof and tear-resistant containers to prevent contact with the environment and with personnel who are responsible for handling operating-room waste. Sponges are deposited into a plastic-lined bucket. They are counted as soon as possible and sealed in an impervious receptacle. They are not left to hang over the sides of the bucket where they can drip onto the floor. Blood, body secretions, and other fluids from the sterile field are collected in leak-proof containers.

173. Specimens should be placed in clean leak-proof containers. Upon receipt of the specimen from the sterile field, the container is sealed and, if necessary, the container is wiped with an EPA-registered hospital-grade germicide. Care is taken to prevent contamination of supporting specimen documents and other records.

174. Contaminated reusable items that fall or are removed from the sterile field should be wiped with a germicide and placed in an impervious

container. Gloves must be worn by persons who handle contaminated items.

175. All items that come in contact with the patient or the sterile field are considered contaminated and, if single use/disposable, should be discarded according to local, state, and national waste regulations, which specify what constitutes infectious waste. Disposable items contaminated with infectious waste are deposited in leak-proof containers or bags that are color-coded, tagged, or labeled so as to be immediately recognizable as hazardous waste. Examples of such waste are gowns, gloves, sponges, and suture threads.

176. Infectious waste fluids may be poured down a drain connected to a sanitary sewer if regulations permit, or the collection container must be sealed and placed in a leak-proof container or bag that is color coded and tagged or labeled so as to be immediately recognizable as hazardous waste.

177. Disposal and treatment of infectious waste is significantly more costly than disposal and treatment of noninfectious waste. For this reason, noninfectious waste should not be placed into hazardous-waste bags/containers. This is also the reason it is important to know the definition of infectious waste in the area in which one practices, and to deposit only those items that meet the definition of *infectious* into the hazardous-waste bag or container. Not all items contaminated with blood are defined as infectious waste. Some regulations define infectious waste as items contaminated with blood or other materials that if compressed would release blood or other infectious material.

178. Noninfectious disposable items are deposited into receptacles not designated for infectious waste, are sealed, and are removed from the room.

179. Sharp items, such as needles, staples, and scalpel blades, are considered infectious waste. They are deposited in a designated leak-proof, puncture-resistant sharps container identified with a biohazard label. Sharps containers are sealed and exchanged by designated personnel when they become full.

180. Reusable linen that is identified as infectious is placed in a closeable bag that is color coded, tagged, or labeled as infectious waste. When contaminated linen is wet, it should be placed in a bag that prevents leak-through. Reusable noninfectious items are transported, cleaned, and disinfected or sterilized according to healthcare facility policy.

181. All instruments opened for a procedure, *whether or not they were actually used,* are

considered contaminated and must be appropriately cleaned and processed. They should be placed in designated closed carts and transported to instrument cleaning areas. Where designated carts are not available, the instruments should be covered and transported.

182. Furniture, including operating lights, linen hamper frames, the OR bed and mattress, suction canisters, and other equipment used during the procedure, is wiped with an EPA-registered hospital-grade germicidal agent. Kick buckets are cleaned and relined. Patient transport vehicles, including straps, railings and other attachments, are also wiped with an EPA-registered hospital-grade germicidal agent.

183. After each procedure, any equipment or furniture that is visibly soiled is cleaned with an EPA-registered hospital-grade germicide. Walls, doors, push plates, handles, cabinets, lights, and other areas that are visibly soiled are cleaned. Visible soiled areas on the floor are cleaned with an EPA-registered hospital-grade germicidal agent. If visibly soiled, a 3- to 4-foot area of the floor around the operating room table should be cleaned with an EPA-registered hospital-grade germicidal agent. A clean mop head should be used for each cleanup, and the mop should not be dipped into the solution once the mop has been used. If the used mop is not dipped into the solution, the solution may be used for subsequent cleanups, provided a clean mop head is also used. A clean mop head should be used for each room/patient procedure. Individual institutional policies for cleaning the floor may vary, and floor cleaning may not be necessary after all procedures.

184. At the conclusion of the day's schedule, operating and procedure rooms, scrub-utility areas, corridors, furnishings, and equipment should be terminally cleaned.

185. Areas that should be cleaned with an EPA-registered hospital-grade germicidal agent at the conclusion of the day include but are not limited to:

- surgical lights and tracks
- ceiling-mounted equipment
- scrub sinks
- faucet heads
- horizontal surfaces
- furniture
- drawer, door, and cabinet handles
- push plates
- vent face plates

- furniture castors and wheels
- cabinet and operating room doors
- kick buckets and other trash receptacles
- utility carts
- refillable soap dispensers
- floors in the operating room, scrub sink area, and corridor (AORN, 2004a, p. 276)

186. Reusable cleaning equipment is disassembled, cleaned, and dried prior to storage.

187. Many items and areas within the operating room are cleaned periodically. Cleaning may be weekly, monthly, or as otherwise indicated in the policies of the institution. Each facility should have written policies that address cleaning schedules, techniques, and persons responsible for the following—including but not limited to:

- lounges, locker areas, offices
- holding areas
- cabinet shelves
- walls
- ceilings
- air conditioning vents, grills, filters
- ice machines
- sterilizers
- restrooms

188. Every facility should also have a cleaning schedule for the cleaning of anesthesia equipment. The anesthesia department is generally responsible for cleaning and caring for its own equipment. The Association of periOperative Registered Nurses has written guidelines for cleaning and processing anesthesia equipment.

Additional Considerations—Cleaning and Scheduling

189. Under the concept that all recipients of healthcare, i.e., all surgical patients, are considered infectious and the potential for cross infection exists for all procedures, no special cleaning technique is required after procedures on patients known to be infected with HIV or other infectious microorganisms. Routine cleaning, however, must be adequate and thorough.

190. At one time it was believed that patients known to be infected with HIV, hepatitis, or other infectious diseases should be scheduled as the last patient of the day to prevent possible cross-contamination with other patients who would subsequently be brought into the room where surgery had been performed on the known infected patient. Because every

surgical patient is considered infectious, because standard precautions are practiced, and because cleaning practices should be consistent across patients and procedures, there is no need to schedule known infected patients as the last procedure for the day.

191. The exception to this is for patients with airborne-transmitted infectious diseases. These patients should be scheduled when personnel and patient traffic is minimal and exposure is therefore reduced. Scheduling as the last case of the day may be appropriate for these patients.

• •

SECTION QUESTIONS

Q40. Scrub attire is required in the semirestricted area of the operating room. (Ref. 151)

True   False

Q41. Explain why supplies are removed from their external shipping cartons before being permitted entry into the operating room. (Ref. 156)

_____

Q42. Air flow in the operating room (Ref. 159, 160, 161):

a. flows from ceiling to floor

b. is directed into the room under positive pressure

c. to be effective requires that operating room doors be closed

d. is filtered before it enters the room

e. must have a minimum of 10 air exchanges an hour

Q43. A patient with a latex allergy should be scheduled as the last case of the day whenever possible. (Ref. 168)

True   False

Q44. Describe the procedure for cleaning up a spill of 30 ml of blood. (Ref. 170)

_____

_____

Q45. When a specimen is received from the sterile field and placed in a specimen container, the container should be sealed and sterilized before it is transported to the laboratory. (Ref. 173)

True   False

Q46. Under no circumstances should infectious waste fluids be poured down a drain. (Ref. 176)

True   False

Q47. Infectious waste is deposited in specially marked color-coded bags. Explain why it is prudent to include only infectious waste in these bags and to exclude noninfectious waste. (Ref. 177)

_____

Q48. Instruments that were opened for a procedure but not used should be transported to the instrument cleaning area in a closed or covered cart. (Ref. 181)

True   False

Q49. Insert the correct letter(s). (Ref. 182–188)

a—between cases, b—terminal cleaning, c—periodic cleaning

_____ scrub sinks

_____ locker areas

_____ OR bed

_____ kick buckets

_____ visibly soiled area of the floor

_____ walls

_____patient transport vehicle

_____surgical lights

_____sterilizer

_____ceiling

_____floor

_____ceiling-mounted equipment

• •

• • • References

American Institute of Architects Committee on Architecture for Health (with assistance from the US Department of Health and Human Services). (2001). Guidelines for construction and equipment of hospital and medical facilities. Washington, DC: AIA Press. In: AORN. *Frequently asked questions*. Retrieved February, 2004, from www.aorn.org/Practice/faq4.htm

Association of periOperative Registered Nurses (AORN). (2004a). Recommended practices for environmental cleaning in the surgical practice setting. In *Standards, recommended practices, and guidelines* (pp. 273–280). Denver, CO: Author.

AORN. (2004b). Recommended practices for maintaining a sterile field. In *Standards, recommended practices, and guidelines* (pp. 367–372). Denver, CO: Author.

AORN. (2004c). Recommended practices for selection and use of surgical gowns and drapes. In *Standards, recommended practices, and guidelines* (pp. 285–290). Denver, CO: Author.

AORN. (2004d). Recommended practices for standard and transmission based precautions in the perioperative practice setting. In *Standards, recommended practices and guidelines* (pp. 361–365). Denver, CO: Author.

AORN. (2004e). Recommended practices for surgical attire. In *Standards, recommended practices, and guidelines* (pp. 223–227). Denver, CO: Author.

AORN. (2004f). Recommended practices for surgical hand antisepsis. In *Standards, recommended practices, and guidelines* (pp. 291–297). Denver, CO: Author.

AORN. (2004g). Recommended practices for traffic patterns in the perioperative practice setting. In *Standards, recommended practices, and guidelines* (pp. 397–399). Denver, CO: Author.

Baumgardner, C., Maragos, C., Walz, J., & Larson, E. (1993). Effects of nail polish on microbial growth of fingernails. *AORN Journal, 58*(1), 84–89.

Centers for Disease Control and Prevention (CDC). (2002). Guideline for hand hygiene in healthcare settings: Recommendations of the healthcare infection control practices advisory committee and the HICPAC/SHEA/APIC/IDSA hand hygiene task force. *MMWR Morbidity and Mortality Weekly Report, 51* (RR-16), 1–44 retrieved Oct 17, 2004 from www.cdc.gov/mmwr/preview/mmwrhtml/rr5116a1.htm

CDC Hospital Infection Control Practices Advisory Committee. (1997, February). *Evolution of isolation practices*. Retrieved July 3, 2004, from www.cdc.gov/ncidod/hip/ISOLAT/isopart1.htm

Cozad, A. (2003). Disinfection and the prevention of infectious disease. *American Journal of Infection Control, 31*(4), 243–254.

Cruise, P., & Foord, R. (1980). The epidemiology of wound infection: A 10 year prospective study of 62,939 wounds. *Surgical Clinics of North America, 60,* 27–40.

Ellis, H. (1990). The hazards of surgical glove dusting powders. *Surgery, Gynecology & Obstetrics, 171*(6), 521–527.

Fry, D. (2002). The economic costs of surgical site infections. *Surgical Infections, 3*(Supplement), 37–43.

Johnson & Johnson Medical, Inc. (1992). *Bloodborne infections: A practical guide to OSHA compliance*. Arlington, TX: Author.

Mangram, A., Horan, T., Pearson, M., Silver, L. & Jarvis, W. (1999). Guideline for prevention of surgical site infection, 1999. *Infection Control and Hospital Epidemiology, 20*(4), 247–278.

Mycek, S. (2004). Nail down infection control. *Materials Management in healthcare, 13*(3), 34.

OSHA. (1910.1030) *Bloodborne pathogen standard.* Retrieved October 16, 2004 date of document Jan. 18, 2001, from http://www.osha.gov/pls/oshaweb/owadisp.show_document?p_table=STANDARDS&p_id=10051www.OSHA.gov

Olsen, M., MacCallum, J., & McQuarrie, D. G. (1986). Preoperative hair removal with clippers does not increase infection rate in clean surgical wounds. *Surgery, Gynecology and Obstetrics, 162,* 182.

Pfaff , S. J. (1993). Infection control and prevention. In N. Burden (Ed.), *Ambulatory surgery nursing*. Philadelphia: W. B. Saunders.

Pottinger, J., Burns, S., & Manske, C. (1989). Bacterial carriage by artificial versus natural nails. *American Journal of Infection Control*, Dec. 17(6), 340–341.

Wade, J. J., & Casewell, M. W. (1991). The evaluation of residual antimicrobial activity on hands and its clinical relevance. *Journal of Hospital Infection*, June, 18 Suppl B:23-8.

Winston, K. R. (1992). Hair and neurosurgery. *Neurosurgery, 31*(2), 320–329.

Appendix 5-A

· ·

Chapter 5 Post Test

Instructions: Fill in the blank(s), mark the correct answer(s), or answer the question as appropriate.

1. Organ/space surgical site infection is associated with long-term morbidity and mortality. (Ref. 4)

   True   False

2. The overall rate of surgical site infection is just under 10%. (Ref. 6)

   True   False

3. Two pathogens most commonly associated with surgical site infection are (Ref. 11):

   _____

4. The patient who sustains a surgical site infection cannot be the source of that infection. (Ref. 13)

   True   False

5. Explain why the patient who has sustained severe burns is at increased risk of infection. (Ref. 14)

   _____

6. The premature infant is at increased risk for surgical site infection. (Ref. 16)

   True   False

7. For infection to occur, there must be pathogens of sufficient virulence present and a sufficient quanity of pathogens. List 3 other requirements for infection to occur. (Ref. 23)

   _____   _____   _____

8. Match the PPE with the type of precautions. (Ref. 34, 36, 37, 39)

   a. mask   _____ Contact Precautions

   b. gloves   _____ Airborne Precautions

   c. gown   _____ Droplet Precautions

   d. eye protection   _____ Universal Precautions

9. Standard Precautions mandates that the employer provide a hepatitis B vaccination and postexposure program for persons whose occupation poses a risk of exposure to bloodborne pathogens. (Ref. 39)

   True   False

10. With regard to infection prevention (Ref. 45, 47, 49):

    a. a dry shave of the operative site is preferable

    b. a wet shave of the operative site is preferable

    c. no shave is preferred unless hair interferes with the intended procedure

    d. if hair is removed, removal with electric clippers is preferred

11. Prep solutions should provide residual protection against growth of microorganisms. (Ref. 54)

    True   False

12. Wearing of warm-up jackets is advisable for unscrubbed personnel in restricted areas. (Ref. 66, 150)

    True   False

13. Use of cover gowns or lab coats and frequent changing of scrub attire is a practice that has been shown to reduce the rate of surgical site infection. (Ref. 67)

    True   False

14. One mask may be worn for consecutive cases provided it is not permitted to dangle from the neck between cases. (Ref. 71)

    True   False

15. Shoe covers are optional and never necessary. (Ref. 72)

    True   False

16. Choose the correct statement(s). (Ref. 80, 81, 84, 88, 89, 97)

    a. Hands should be washed prior to performing surgical hand antisepsis.

    b. Provodine-iodine and chlorhexidine gluconate are appropriate products to use for surgical hand antisepsis.

    c. Surgical hand antisepsis requires mechanical washing and chemical antisepsis.

    d. Persons with respiratory infections should double mask when scrubbing.

    e. Products used for surgical hand antisepsis should have persistent activity.

    f. Alcohol-based hand rub products take the place of hand washing unless hands are visibly dirty or contaminated with proteinaceous material.

    g. Surgical hand antiseptic products cleared by the FDA may be used instead of scrubbing with a scrub sponge/brush and an antimicrobial agent in preparation for gowning and gloving for surgery.

17. A person with a cut on the hand (Ref. 87):

    a. should not function in the scrub role

    b. may scrub if two pairs of gloves are worn

    c. may scrub if the cut is appropriately bandaged

18. A scrub that lasts less than 5 minutes cannot be effective. (Ref. 94)

    True   False

19. During the scrub, the water should (Ref. 95):

    a. run from the elbows down the arms and flow off the fingertips

    b. run from the fingertips down the arm and flow off the elbows

20. The scrub person's sterile gown should be opened on the same table as the sterile instruments. (Ref. 99)

    True   False

21. For initial gloving closed gloving by the scrub person is a preferred technique to prevent contamination; however, the open-glove technique should be used in the event that the scrub person's glove becomes contaminated and the scrub person must reglove. (Ref. 119, 128)

    True   False

22. If the surgeon's glove becomes contaminated during surgery (Ref. 126):

    a. the scrub person should remove the contaminated glove and reglove the surgeon

    b. the unscrubbed person should remove the surgeon's glove and the scrub person should reglove the surgeon, or the surgeon may use the open glove technique to reglove without assistance

23. If the gown of a sterile team member becomes contaminated and a new gown is donned (Ref. 127):

    a. the team member should first remove gloves, then gown, and then regown and reglove

    b. the team member should first remove gown, then gloves, and then regown and reglove

    c. the team member should keep gloves on, remove gown, and then regown as there is no need to change gloves since only the gown was contaminated

24. Following surgery, it is necessary to perform hand hygiene after glove removal. (Ref. 131)

    True   False

25. Reusable drapes should (Ref. 139, 144):

    a. be tracked for number of times used because laundering will reduce barrier effectiveness over time

    b. be inspected after each use

    c. have defects repaired with a vulcanized heat seal patch

26. Explain why the back of the sterile gown and the cuffed portion of the sleeve are not considered sterile once the gown is donned. (Ref. 147a)

    _____

    _____

27. Under no circumstances should an item be used in surgery if it appears that the wrapper may have been subject to strike-through. (Ref. 147c)

    True   False

28. A wrapped heavy item, such as a surgical drill, may be tossed on to the sterile field by the unscrubbed person as long as the portion of the unscrubbed person's hand that extends over the sterile field is covered by a sterile wrapper. (Ref. 147d)

    True   False

29. After pouring sterile solutions into a container on the sterile field, solution that remains in the bottle may be used at a later time provided the bottle is promptly recapped. (Ref. 147d)

    True   False

30. If a scrubbed person is asked during surgery to move to the other side of the table, the scrub person should (Ref. 147f):

    a. move to the other side while facing the sterile field

    b. pivot away from the sterile field, keep back to the sterile field, and move to the other side

    c. pass other scrubbed persons at the sterile field in a back-to-back manner

31. In restricted areas in the presence of open sterile supplies, the following attire should be worn by non-scrubbed personnel (Ref. 150):

    a. hat

    b. scrub clothes

    c. mask

    d. shoe covers

32. Explain why it is so important to limit access to the operating room and to limit the number of personnel in the operating room during surgery. (Ref. 154)

    _____

    _____

33. Temperature of the operating room should be between _____ and _____ degrees and humidity should be between _____ and _____ %. (Ref. 163)

34. Small spills of blood that occur in the vicinity of the sterile field during surgery (Ref. 169):

    a. should be left untouched until the end of surgery when the floor can be cleaned

    b. should be vigorously wiped with a detergent germicide

    c. should be promptly cleaned with an FDA-registered chemical germicide

    d. may be cleaned using a 1:1000 dilution of bleach

35. When single-use items are opened for a procedure, whether or not they are used during the procedure, they should be deposited in color-coded biohazard-waste bags designated for infectious waste. (Ref. 177)

    True   False

36. All items that were opened for a procedure, whether or not they were actually used during the procedure, are considered contaminated. (Ref. 181)

    True   False

Appendix 5-B

· ·

Competency Checklist: Asepsis

Under "Observer's Initials," enter initials upon successful achievement of competency.
Enter N/A if competency is not appropriate for institution.

NAME _____

	OBSERVER'S INITIALS	DATE

Standard and Universal Precautions

1. Blood and body fluids of all patients are considered infectious.   _____ _____

   Standard Precautions are practiced as follows:

   a. gloves worn when direct contact with blood and body fluids is expected   _____ _____
   to occur

   b. masks and protective eyewear worn when aerosolization or splattering   _____ _____
   of blood and body fluids is anticipated

   c. gowns worn that provide a barrier appropriate to the procedure   _____ _____

   d. needles not recapped   _____ _____

   e. sharps deposited in sharps containers   _____ _____

   f. infectious waste correctly identified   _____ _____

   g. infectious waste deposited in designated container   _____ _____

   h. contaminated laundry deposited in designated laundry bags   _____ _____

Skin Prep

2. Skin condition and sensitivities are assessed and assessment is documented.   _____ _____

3. Prep is implemented as follows:

   a. awake patient is informed   _____ _____

   b. unnecessary exposure is avoided   _____ _____

   c. prep begins at incision site and continues outward to periphery   _____ _____

   d. prep progresses from clean to dirty and not in reverse   _____ _____

   e. prep solutions are not permitted to pool   _____ _____

   f. dirtiest areas are prepped last   _____ _____

4. Prep is documented for:

   a. skin assessment   _____ _____

   b. solution used   _____ _____

   c. person performing prep   _____ _____

   d. if hair removed—site, method, time and person   _____ _____

e. person who performed prep   _____ _____

f. patient response to prep   _____ _____

Attire

5. Hat/hood is worn so that all head and facial hair is covered.   _____ _____

6. Surgical attire that becomes visibly soiled is removed and fresh attire donned.   _____ _____

7. Mask

a. covers nose and mouth and does not permit venting   _____ _____

b. is not left to dangle around the neck   _____ _____

c. changed between cases   _____ _____

8. Appropriate attire is worn in restricted and semirestricted areas.   _____ _____

Surgical Scrub

9. Jewelry is removed.   _____ _____

10. Scrub includes all surfaces of nails, subungual areas, hands, and arms to 2 inches above the elbow.   _____ _____

11. Timed anatomical, stroke count scrub, or alcohol rub procedure adheres to institutional policy.   _____ _____

Gowning and Gloving

12. Hands are dried without contamination of towel.   _____ _____

13. Gown is donned correctly and without contamination.   _____ _____

14. Open gloving is performed correctly and without contamination.   _____ _____

15. Closed gloving is performed correctly and without contamination.   _____ _____

16. Assistance in gowning and gloving other team members is performed without contamination.   _____ _____

17. At end of procedure, gown is removed before gloves.   _____ _____

18. Gloves are removed in manner so that bare skin does not contact contaminated glove.   _____ _____

19. Hand hygiene performed after gown and glove removal.   _____ _____

Draping

20. Equipment is draped without contamination:

a. back table   _____ _____

b. Mayo stand   _____ _____

c. ring stand   _____ _____

21. Patient is draped without contamination:

a. abdomen   _____ _____

b. perineum (lithotomy)   _____ _____

c. extremity   _____ _____

d. *(Other)*_____   _____ _____

22. Patient is draped from the operative site to the periphery.   _____ _____

23. A cuff is formed from drape to protect gloved hand.   _____ _____

24. Drapes are not repositioned once placed.   _____ _____

Aseptic Practices

25. Gloved hands are kept in sight at or above the level of the sterile field.   _____ _____

26. (Circulating role) Items are checked for sterility prior to being dispensed to the sterile field (package integrity, chemical indicator, evidence of strike-through, expiration date if applicable).   _____ _____

27. (Scrub role) Sterility of items is checked prior to accepting for delivery to sterile field (packaging, chemical indicator, expiration date).   _____ _____

28. Items of questionable sterility and unsterile items are not entered into the sterile field.   _____ _____

29. Items are dispensed to the sterile field without contamination.   _____ _____

30. Ungloved hands and arms are not extended over the sterile field.   _____ _____

31. Fluids

    a. are dispensed to receptacle placed at the edge of the sterile field   _____ _____

    b. are poured carefully to prevent splashing   _____ _____

32. Sterile field:

    a. is set up as close to time of surgery as possible   _____ _____

    b. is not left unattended   _____ _____

    c. is not covered   _____ _____

33. Scrubbed nurse touches only sterile items.   _____ _____

34. Scrubbed nurse remains close to sterile field.   _____ _____

35. Movement around sterile field is back to back and front (sterile) to front (sterile).   _____ _____

36. Circulating nurse maintains safe distance from sterile field.   _____ _____

37. Circulating nurse approaches sterile field by facing sterile field.   _____ _____

Sanitation

38. Spills or splashes of blood and body fluids that occur in the immediate vicinity of the sterile field are promptly absorbed and cleaned with a germicide.   _____ _____

39. Soiled sponges are deposited into a plastic-lined bucket, counted, and sealed in an impervious receptacle.   _____ _____

40. Specimen containers are wiped as needed with EPA-registered hospital germicide.   _____ _____

OBSERVER'S SIGNATURE   INITIALS   DATE

_____

ORIENTEE'S SIGNATURE

_____

Chapter 5—Section Question Answers

Q1. False

Q2. Superficial incisional, deep incisional, organ/space

Q3. a, b, d, e

Q4. True

Q5. Extremes of age, nutritional status, obesity, preexisting disease, preexisting infection, use of nicotine, length of surgery, type of surgery, surgeon technique, extended preoperative hospital stay

Q6. True

Q7. False

Q8. True

Q9. False

Q10. 3

Q11. a, b, c, d, e, f

Q12. An inner commitment to strictly adhere to aseptic practice, to report any break in aseptic practice and to correct any violation, whether or not anyone is present or observes the violation

Q13. b, c

Q14. e

Q15. Cleanses effectively, reduces microbial count rapidly, has a broad spectrum of activity, is easy to apply, is nonirritating and nontoxic, provides residual protection

Q16. False

Q17. b

Q18. a, b, c

Q19. To prevent shedding from bare arms

Q20. a, b, c

Q21. False

Q22. b

Q23. b, c, d, e

Q24. a, c

Q25. False

Q26. True

Q27. a

Q28. True

Q29. Powders or talc on gloves can incite an inflammatory response and delay healing

Q30. a, c, d

Q31. Drapes serve as a barrier to prevent the passage of microorganisms between sterile and nonsterile areas

Q32. To reduce airborne contamination into the operative site (microorganisms are carried on dust particles)

Q33. False

Q34. The tips are contaminated

Q35. False

(continues)

Chapter 5—Section Question Answers (*continued*)

Q36. c
Q37. When liquids soak through a barrier from a sterile to an unsterile area and vice versa
Q38. b, c
Q39. False
Q40. True
Q41. Outside shipping cartons may harbor insects and dirt
Q42. a, b, c, d
Q43. False
Q44. Absorb first with a soft cloth, then clean with an EPA registered hospital-grade germicide
Q45. False
Q46. False
Q47. Disposal costs for infectious waste are higher than for noninfected waste
Q48. True
Q49. a. OR bed, kick buckets, visibly soiled area of the floor, patient transport vehicle
     b. floor, scrub sinks, ceiling mounted equipment, surgical lights
     c. locker areas, walls, ceiling, sterilizer

Chapter 5—Post Test Answers

1. True
2. False
3. *Staphylococcus aureas, Staphylococcus epidermidis,* coagulase-negative staphylococci, *Enterococcus* sp.
4. False
5. The integrity of the skin, the first line of defense, is broken
6. True
7. A susceptible host, a portal of entry, a mode of transmission
8. b, c; a; a; a, b, c, d
9. True
10. c, d
11. True
12. True
13. False
14. False
15. False
16. a, b, c, e, f, g
17. a
18. False
19. b

(continues)

Chapter 5—Post Test Answers (*continued*)
20. False
21. True
22. b
23. b
24. True
25. a, b, c
26. Because the back cannot be under constant observation and the cuffs may become contaminated by perspiration
27. True
28. False
29. False
30. a, c
31. a, b, c
32. The higher the number of personnel in the operating room, the higher the number of microorganisms present
33. 68°F, 73°F (20°C to 23°C); 30%, 60%
34. c
35. False
36. True

6

Prevention of Injury—Positioning the Patient for Surgery

LEARNER OBJECTIVES

After reading and completing "Prevention of Injury—Positioning the Patient for Surgery," the learner will:

- describe five common surgical positions
- list three factors that in combination create the potential for tissue damage
- describe the impact of surgical position upon the respiratory, circulatory, neuromuscular, and integumentary systems
- discuss body structures at risk in supine, prone, lateral, lithotomy, Trendelenburg, and sitting positions
- identify potential injuries related to improper and prolonged positioning
- list five positioning devices and their appropriate use
- describe nursing interventions to prevent patient injury in supine, prone, lateral, lithotomy, Trendelenburg, and sitting positions
- list the desired patient outcomes relative to positioning
- discuss the responsibilities of the perioperative nurse in patient positioning

. . . .
Lesson Outline

I.   OVERVIEW
II. DESIRED PATIENT OUTCOMES
III. IMPACT OF SURGICAL POSITIONING
     A. Overview of Injuries
     B. Respiratory and Circulatory System Compromise

C. Neuromuscular—Injury
1. Facial Nerves
2. Brachial Plexus
3. Lower Extremity Nerves
D. Integumentary System Injury
IV. RESPONSIBILITIES OF THE PERIOPERATIVE NURSE
A. Patient Advocate
B. Nursing Considerations
1. Patient Assessment
2. Planning Care
V. ADDITIONAL CONSIDERATIONS FOR POSITIONING
A. Surgical Procedure
B. Anesthesia
C. Patient Dignity
VI. POSITIONING DEVICES
VII. IMPLEMENTATION OF PATIENT CARE
A. Transportation and Transfer
B. Initial Position Techniques
VIII. BASIC SURGICAL POSITIONS
A. Supine (Dorsal Recumbent)
B. Trendelenburg
C. Reverse Trendelenburg
D. Lithotomy
E. Sitting (Semi-sitting; Semi-Fowler's; Lawnchair)
F. Prone
G. Jackknife (Kraske's)
H. Lateral
IX. EVALUATING IMPLEMENTATION OF POSITIONING
X. POSTOPERATIVE TRANSFER
XI. DOCUMENTATION OF NURSING ACTIONS

OVERVIEW

1. Many factors combine to create the potential for patient injury related to positioning. The degree of risk for injury is relative to whether or not the patient receives general or regional anesthesia, the type and length of the procedure, the required position, the patient's overall condition at the time of surgery, and whether or not the patient is positioned correctly and safely.

2. Impaired skin integrity, compromised respiratory effort, altered tissue perfusion, and neuromuscular and musculoskeletal injury are all possible consequences related to positioning.

3. When the patient is properly positioned, the surgeon will have optimal access to the surgical site, and the patient will not suffer injury. Improper positioning can result in severe and permanent patient injury and, at the least, can hinder the surgeon's ability to perform surgery.

4. Safe patient positioning in preparation for surgery is a critical component of perioperative nursing practice. Although patient positioning is a team responsibility, it is most often the perioperative nurse who coordinates the activities related to positioning.

DESIRED PATIENT OUTCOMES

5. Desired patient outcomes related to positioning are:
   a. skin—intact, smooth, free of ecchymosis, cuts, abrasions, shear injury, or blistering
   b. cardiovascular status—heart rate and blood pressure within expected ranges; peripheral pulses present and equal bilaterally; skin warm to touch
   c. neuromuscular status—flexes and extends extremities without assistance or pain, denies numbness or tingling of extremities (AORN, 2004, p. 199).

6. To achieve these outcomes, the perioperative nurse must have knowledge of

   - principles of anatomy and physiology
   - anatomical and physiological changes related to anesthesia and surgical position
   - the surgical procedure to be performed
   - proper positioning technique
   - appropriate positioning equipment
   - proper use of equipment

7. In addition to absence of injury related to positioning, maintenance of dignity and comfort are also desired outcomes.

IMPACT OF SURGICAL POSITIONING

Overview of Injuries

8. The basic positions used for surgery are supine, lithotomy, sitting, prone, and lateral. Injury can occur in any of these positions. Each is described later on in this chapter. Some of the complications that can arise from improper positioning are postoperative musculoskeletal pain, joint dislocation, peripheral nerve damage, skin breakdown including necrosis, and cardiovascular and respiratory compromise.

9. The anesthetized patient is at increased risk of positioning injury. General anesthetic and regional blocks prevent the body's normal defense of pain from warning of exaggerated stretching, twisting, and compression of body parts. Subsequent damage to nerves and vascular structures and compromise to respiratory and circulatory functions occur without patient awareness.

Respiratory and Circulatory System Compromise

10. Extreme or unnatural positions such as Trendelenburg, where the head and upper body are lower than the feet and lower body, affect circulation and oxygen–carbon dioxide exchange. Pulmonary capillary blood volume, and therefore the amount of blood available for oxygenation, is altered by gravity. When the lung becomes engorged with blood, the amount of space for alveolar expansion is decreased, thus reducing the amount of oxygenated blood. In addition, the air inspired in the lungs is redistributed and affects the amount of air that is available to oxygenate the blood.

11. Unfavorable positions can also decrease compliance or stretchability of the lung and the ability of the thoracic cage to expand. The amount of air that may be taken in for gas exchange can be reduced, and hypoventilation can result. In positions that compromise respiratory mechanics, muscles become fatigued as the patient attempts to compensate, and hypoventilation may occur. Even where respiratory function is supported through mechanical assistance, hypoxia and hypercarbia can still occur.

12. Lung expansion may be decreased by mechanical restriction of the ribs or sternum. Lung expansion may also be decreased by the diaphragm's reduced ability to push down against abdominal contents or retractors that are used during surgery.

13. General and regional anesthetics disrupt normal vasodilatation and constriction and frequently cause dilation of peripheral blood vessels and result in a drop in blood pressure. Dilated vessels allow venous blood to pool in areas that are dependent. This reduces the amount of blood returned to the heart and lungs for oxygenation and redistribution. In some operations, certain body parts may be placed in a dependent position for an extended period of time, causing a significant amount of pooling to occur.

14. The ability of the heart to contract is impacted by some positions and anesthetic agents. The result is a relaxation of skeletal muscles that normally support vein walls and help to propel blood. This in turn can cause a decrease in cardiac output.

15. Position or pressure that obstructs the flow of blood in the legs also has the potential to result in phlebothrombosis. Venous thrombosis can result when superficial veins are occluded by pressure, straps, or other positioning devices. Safety straps should be tight enough to secure the patient but not so tight as to impair superficial venous return.

Neuromuscular—Injury

16. In the awake patient, normal pain and pressure receptors of muscle groups warn against unnatural stretching and twisting of tendons, ligaments, and muscles. Opposing muscle groups also prevent strain on muscle fibers. The anesthetized patient, subjected to an exaggerated range of motion, is unable to indicate pain. Anesthetic agents and muscle relaxants further exacerbate the potential for injury by inducing loss of muscle tone and exaggerated muscle relaxation, which interferes with normal defense mechanisms against unnatural or excessive range of motion.

17. Evidence of hyperextension injury can range from mild postoperative joint pain to dislocation.

18. Musculoskeletal injury is minimized with adequate support of the extremities while being positioned and adequate padding at final positioning. Extremities should not be allowed to hang unsupported over the edge of an armboard or the operating table. Lower extremities should be moved slowly and in unison to prevent sacroiliac joint dislocation.

19. Crushing and pressure injuries to fingers, toes, ears, and nose are possible whenever the operating table, instrument table, or Mayo stands are adjusted. Team members are cautioned to visualize these body parts when positioning and repositioning. Equipment must not be allowed to rest or exert pressure contact against the patient. Surgical team members must not lean on the patient.

Facial Nerves

20. Injury to the facial nerve (buccal branch), resulting in motor injury to the mouth, can occur if the nerve is compressed from an improperly fitting face mask.

21. Injury to the suborbital nerve, resulting in numbness of the forehead, can occur from pressure on the nerve by endotracheal tube connectors.

22. Prolonged stretching or compression of nerves may result in postoperative numbness, tingling, or pain. Severe injury can result in permanent loss of sensation and paralysis in the affected area.

Brachial Plexus

23. Because of its superficial position and close proximity to bony structures, brachial plexus nerve injury is one of the more common positioning injuries.

24. Brachial plexus injury may result from improper positioning of the arm and/or armboard. The supine position, with one or both arms extended on armboards, is the most common surgical position. Brachial plexus nerve injury can occur in this position if the armboard is positioned so as to cause hyperextension of the arm. Unintentional movement of an armboard, causing the arm to be hyperabducted, may not be noticed because the arm is hidden by surgical drapes.

25. When the arm is positioned on an armboard, pronated, and extended more than 90 degrees, damage to the plexus can occur. To minimize pressure on the brachial plexus, the patient's head may be turned toward the extended arm and the palm supinated.

26. Injury to the brachial plexus may occur when shoulder braces are improperly applied. In Trendelenburg position, shoulder braces, used to prevent the patient from slipping from the table, can cause compression of the brachial plexus. If the brace is placed too far laterally and the arm is abducted, the head of the humerus can be pushed into the axilla, causing compression of the plexus. If the brace is positioned too far medially and the arm is abducted, the plexus can be compressed between the clavicle and the first rib. Shoulder braces should not be used unless absolutely necessary and, if used, must be adequately padded.

27. Motor and sensory loss to the arm and shoulder may be evidenced postoperatively if damage has occurred to the brachial plexus.

28. The radial or ulnar nerve may be injured if the elbow slips off the mattress onto the metal edge of the operating table and the nerve is compressed between the table and the medial epicondyle. Such an injury can occur when the surgical team leans against the table and is unaware that the patient's arm has slipped and is being compressed against the table.

29. The possibility of damage to the radial or ulnar nerve caused by compression against the table can be minimized by securing the arm with a draw sheet. The draw sheet begins from under the patient and is brought up over the arm and then tucked back under the patient, not under the mattress.

30. Ulnar nerve injury can also occur during anesthesia if the upper extremity of a supine patient is allowed to rest on a flexed elbow with the forearm pronated across the ventral trunk. Supination of the arm on an armboard is preferable because this shifts the elbow pressure away from the cubital tunnel onto the olecranon process of the ulnar and relieves compression from the ulnar nerve. Padding around the elbow can also help to protect the nerve (Martin, 1991, p. 70).

31. A malfunctioning automatic blood pressure cuff that recycles without allowing sufficient time between compressions can also cause ulnar nerve damage (Martin, 1991, p. 70).

32. Symptoms of ulnar nerve injury include tingling, pain, and numbness in the fourth and fifth fingers. Severe injury can result in a weak grip or contractures, leading to a "claw hand."

33. Radial nerve damage may be evidenced by wrist drop.

Lower Extremity Nerves

34. Improper placement in stirrups or improper movement of the legs can result in extension,

flexion, compression, or stretching that can cause injury to lower extremity nerves.

35. The peroneal, posterior tibial, femoral obturator, and sciatic nerves are at risk for injury in lithotomy position.

36. Injury to the peroneal nerve on the lateral aspect of the knee can occur if the nerve is compressed between the fibula and a laterally positioned stirrup bar. This injury can result in foot drop.

37. Injury to the posterior tibial nerve, resulting in numbness of the foot, can occur if the nerve is compressed. Popliteal knee supports should be padded to prevent compression injury of the tibial and femoral obturator nerves.

38. Injury to the femoral obturator nerve, resulting in paralysis and numbness of the calf muscles, can occur if the nerve is compressed between a metal popliteal knee support stirrup and the medial tibial condyle.

39. Padding at these potential compression sites can prevent injury.

40. Injury to the sciatic nerve, resulting in foot drop, can occur if the nerve is compressed or stretched. Compression and stretching can occur if the legs are fully extended in high lithotomy position and the thighs are flexed more than 90 degrees on the trunk.

Integumentary System Injury

41. Integumentary injuries are cause by friction, shearing, and pressure. Friction injuries occur when the skin moves or rubs across coarse surfaces such as bed linens or blankets. Friction injury can also be caused from excessive rubbing. Friction injuries are usually superficial and result in an abrasion or blister. These, however, can contribute to the more serious injury of a pressure ulcer.

42. Shearing injuries occur when the skin remains stationary while the tissue beneath is shifted. This can occur when linen or blankets underneath the patient are pulled or when the patient is pulled rather than lifted. Examples of when this can happen are when the anesthetized patient is repositioned or slides down or up when the table is adjusted. Shearing injuries result in the stretching or tearing of subcutaneous capillaries and can lead to ischemia and contribute to the development of a pressure ulcer.

43. External pressure can restrict blood flow and result in tissue ischemia that can lead to tissue breakdown. Lesions caused by unrelieved pressure are referred to as *pressure ulcers*. These occur most commonly over bony prominences where tissue tends to be thin. The anesthetized patient is immobile and subjected to uninterrupted pressure during a surgical procedure. The result may be an injury caused by tissue hypoxia that leads to eventual necrosis. The potential for tissue damage due to localized pressure increases markedly with procedures that last more than 2 to 2½ hours (Goodman, 2003, p. 21). Additionally, some patients are immobile in the pre- or postoperative periods, which further contributes to the possibility of pressure ulcer formation. It is estimated that the average incidence of pressure ulcer formation in surgical patients is 8% (Aronovitch, 2002, p. 1). The duration of unrelieved pressure impacts the extent of the injury. One study found that surgeries lasting from 2½ to 4 hours double the risk of skin changes and quadruple the risk of pressure ulcer formation (Shultz et al., 1999, p. 438). (Surgeries lasting longer than 8 hours put the patient at increased risk of pressure ulcers leading to necrosis [Hoyman & Gruber, 1992, p. 15]).

44. A pressure ulcer can develop during surgery and go unnoticed for hours or days because actual skin breakdown is not immediately visible postoperatively. The majority usually present 1 to 3 days after surgery (Schultz et al., 1999, p. 434). During pressure ulcer formation, the muscle closest to the bone is impacted first, so that tissue damage may occur in the deeper layers of tissue while the skin remains intact. Operating room–acquired pressure ulcers typically appear as a bruise and rapidly progress to a pressure ulcer. The damage originates from deep within the tissue and progresses to subcutaneous tissue damage and eventual skin rupture.

45. An area on the patient's skin that appears reddened after surgery may be an indication of the beginning of pressure ulcer formation, or it may be an indication of a self-healing transient reaction to pressure. In either case, the area should not be massaged. Massage may in fact compromise circulation to the affected area (Goodman, 2003, p. 23).

46. Areas most at risk for pressure ulcer formation are heels, elbows, scapula, sacrum, and coccyx. Risk factors include: age—older patients have less elastic, smaller blood vessels that hinder blood flow; weight—obesity causes additional weight and pressure on bony prominences; nutritional status—malnourished patients; presence of diabetes or hypertension—these conditions are associated with diminished circulation. Prevention of pressure ulcer formation is achieved through adequate padding and relief of pressure after 2 hours. (Figure 6-1, 6-2, 6-3, 6-4)

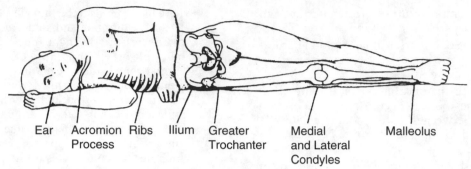

FIGURE 6-1 Potential Pressure Points in Lateral Position.
Source: Reprinted from *Operating Room Nursing: The Perioperative Role,* by L.K. Groah, p. 273, Reston Publishing Company, Inc., © 1983. Reprinted with permission of Appleton & Lange.

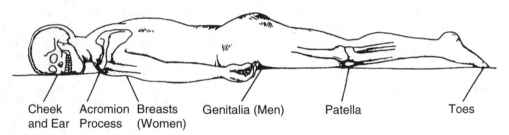

FIGURE 6-2 Potential Pressure Points in Prone Position.
Source: Reprinted from *Operating Room Nursing: The Perioperative Role,* by L.K. Groah, p. 265, Reston Publishing Company, Inc., © 1983. Reprinted with permission of Appleton & Lange.

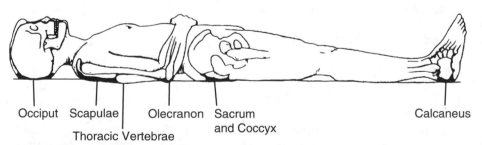

FIGURE 6-3 Potential Pressure Points in Supine Position.
Source: Reprinted from *Operating Room Nursing: The Perioperative Role,* by L.K. Groah, p. 271, Reston Publishing Company, Inc., © 1983. Reprinted with permission of Appleton & Lange.

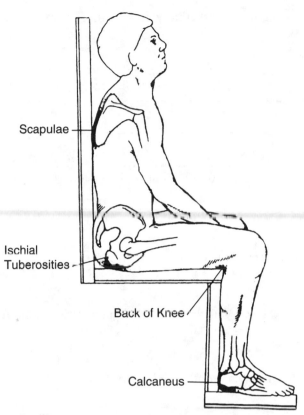

Scapulae

Ischial
Tuberosities

Back of Knee

Calcaneus

FIGURE 6-4 Potential Pressure Points in Sitting Position.
Source: Reprinted from *Operating Room Nursing: The Perioperative Role,* by L.K. Groah, p. 268, Reston Publishing Company, Inc., © 1983. Reprinted with permission of Appleton & Lange.

• •

SECTION QUESTIONS

Q1. List 3 possible consequences related to positioning. (Ref. 2)

_____

_____

_____

Q2. List three desired patient outcomes related to the integumentary system and two desired outcomes related to the neuromusculoskeletal system (Ref. 5):

Skin— _____

_____

Neuromusculoskeletal— _____

_____

Q3. List three respiratory system changes that occur with extreme or unnatural positions such as Trendelenburg. (Ref. 10, 11, 12)

_____

_____

_____

Q4. General anesthetics frequently cause _____ of peripheral blood vessels and also a(n) _____ in blood pressure. (Ref. 13)

    a. dilation/drop

    b. constriction/increase

Q5. An improperly positioned safety strap can result in venous thrombosis. (Ref. 15)

    True   False

Q6. What severe musculoskeletal injury may result from hyperextension? (Ref. 17)

_____

Q7. An improperly fitting face mask can result in injury to the (Ref. 20):

    a. suborbital nerve

    b. buccal branch of the facial nerve

    c. hypoglossal nerve

Q8. Why is brachial plexus injury one of the more common positioning injuries? (Ref. 23)

_____

_____

Q9. Hyperabduction of the arms on armboards is a common cause of brachial plexus injury. (Ref. 24)

    True   False

Q10. To minimize pressure on the brachial plexus, the patient's head may be turned _____ the extended arm and the palm_____ . (Ref. 25)

    a. toward/pronated

    b. away from/supinated

    c. toward/supinated

    d. away from/pronated

Q11. List two possible causes of ulnar nerve compression. (Ref. 28, 29, 30, 31)

_____

_____

Q12. Ulnar nerve injury is evidenced by tingling, pain, and numbness in the fourth and fifth fingers. (Ref. 32)

True   False

Q13. The following nerves may be injured by improper positioning with stirrups (Ref. 35):

a. peroneal

b. posterior tibial

c. radial

d. saphenous

Q14. Foot drop may occur as a result of peroneal nerve damage caused by pressure on the nerve from a laterally positioned stirrup bar. (Ref. 36)

True   False

Q15. An anesthetized surgical patient who remains on the table for an hour is at high risk for development of a pressure ulcer. (Ref. 43)

True   False

Q16. A pressure ulcer that develops during surgery will be immediately noticeable following surgery. (Ref. 44)

True   False

• •

RESPONSIBILITIES OF THE PERIOPERATIVE NURSE

Patient Advocate

47. The patient undergoing surgery is vulnerable to positioning injury, particularly when the procedure is performed under general anesthesia. Neuromuscular, musculoskeletal, integumentary, and physiologic systems can be severely compromised at a time when the patient is unable to indicate that there is a problem.

48. Although it is most frequently the perioperative nurse who positions the patient, the surgeon, surgical assistants, anesthesia personnel, and other members of the nursing team may all participate in patient positioning.

49. Every team member must serve as a patient advocate. The perioperative nurse is a crucial patient advocate, and at no time should the responsibility to ensure proper positioning be assumed to belong to another team member. The unconscious surgical patient is unable to self-advocate, and the responsibility for advocacy becomes a perioperative nursing responsibility for which the nurse is accountable.

Nursing Considerations

Patient Assessment

50. Planning for positioning begins with a nursing assessment of the patient. Assessment relative to positioning should include surgical procedure, age, height, weight, activity level, muscle tone, nutritional status, skin condition, and respiratory and cardiac status. Any physical limitations, injuries, or previous operations should also be noted.

51. The surgical procedure will determine the desired patient position. Lengthy procedures under general anesthesia require extended periods of immobility and increase the risk for injury. Surgeries performed on areas where access is difficult may result in unnatural positions that increase the risk for injury.

52. Elderly patients have decreased muscle tone, poor skin turgor, and less subcutaneous fat and muscle to cushion bony prominences. These

factors place the elderly patient at increased risk for impaired skin integrity.

53. Height and weight data are useful to determine appropriate positioning aids. Activity level and muscle tone data provide information about how well the patient moves and the degree to which the patient may participate in transfer to and from the operating room bed. Drugs and anesthetic agents can alter the patient's ability to move. Baseline data provide information that is useful for evaluating the impact of drugs and anesthesia on movement and muscle tone.

54. Patients with poor nutritional status are at increased risk for tissue injury. Malnourished patients lack protein reserves necessary to maintain healthy skin cells and are at increased risk for skin impairment. Obese patients may trap moisture and fluids from skin prep solutions in tissue folds, which may lead to skin breakdown. Adipose tissue is not well perfused, and the pressure resulting from positioning can cause a decrease in circulation to peripheral body areas. Excess body weight increases the strain on joints and ligaments. Respiratory function is compromised in obese patients because of increased weight on the chest. Anesthetic agents and positioning for surgery place additional strain on respiratory function. Obesity places an increased workload on the heart and circulatory system. Positioning that increases venous blood return to the heart can further compromise circulation.

55. Underweight patients experience greater than normal pressure on bony prominences and are therefore at greater risk for impaired skin integrity.

56. Patients with existing integumentary damage are at increased risk for further skin impairment. Diminished body fat provides little protection for peripheral nerves, and the underweight patient is at high risk for nerve damage.

57. Certain preexisting injuries or conditions and certain surgical procedures may require additional planning to prevent injury.

58. Preexisting conditions requiring additional considerations include:

   • demineralized bone conditions such as osteoporosis and malignant metastasis—increased risk of fracture
   • diabetes, anemia, and paralysis—increased risk for skin breakdown
   • arthritis and joint prosthesis—limited joint movement

   • edema, infection, obstructive pulmonary disease, and other conditions that reduce respiratory and cardiac reserves
   • immunocompromise—increased risk of skin breakdown

59. Surgical procedures requiring additional considerations include:

   • surgeries lasting 2 hours or longer—increased risk for skin breakdown
   • vascular surgery compromises blood perfusion to tissues—increased risk for skin breakdown
   • surgeries where prolonged traction or sustained pressure is required—increased risk for skin breakdown and nerve damage

Planning Care

60. The perioperative nurse should communicate with surgical and anesthesia personnel to determine any specific needs. This information, the procedure, assessment data, and nursing diagnoses serve as the basis for planning the care necessary to correctly position the patient. Appropriate positioning equipment is selected, and decisions are made regarding the number of persons needed to implement positioning and whether aspects of positioning can be assigned to ancillary personnel.

ADDITIONAL CONSIDERATIONS FOR POSITIONING

Surgical Procedure

61. The procedure being performed determines the necessary position. The surgical site should be readily accessible by the surgeon and assistants. Surgeon preference may also be a factor in positioning.

Anesthesia

62. Patients who are awake or lightly sedated are able to state objection to a particular position or a sensation of pain. Patients under general anesthesia are totally dependent on the surgical team to prevent injury from incorrect positioning. Patients who receive regional anesthesia will not feel or report pain and are at risk for injury to anesthetized regions that are improperly positioned.

63. When anesthesia personnel (anesthesiologist or nurse anesthetist) consider positioning, they are concerned with airway access, respiratory

and circulatory functions, and monitoring lines. Anesthesia has a profound effect on cardiac and respiratory function.

64. The anesthesiologist or nurse anesthetist will perform a patient assessment prior to delivering anesthesia. The assessment data coupled with the specialized body of knowledge of anesthesia will determine the limitations to positioning with regard to anesthesia.

Patient Dignity

65. Patient dignity should be a major consideration during positioning. The patient should not be exposed unnecessarily, and once positioning is complete, a final check should be made to ensure that the patient is appropriately covered. The patient should be made to feel that even when he or she is anesthetized, dignity will be maintained with adequate covers.

66. For some patients, the response to entering the operating room is to turn all control over to the personnel providing care. Even an awake patient who feels a loss of dignity while being exposed during positioning may not feel confident enough to cover an area inadvertently left exposed. The perioperative nurse, as patient advocate, must preserve the patient's dignity whether the patient is awake or asleep.

POSITIONING DEVICES

67. Each operating room facility has its own routine supplies and devices to be used for positioning. These should be clean, in good repair, and used only by staff who are knowledgeable in the mechanics of the equipment.

68. Every operating room must have some type of operating bed or table. A table may be designed specifically for general, urologic, ophthalmic, dental, neurological, orthopedic, or minor surgery. Tables have multiple parts and specific functions. Table attachments are designed to hold a body part stationary and to facilitate exposure during surgery. Persons who operate tables and utilize attachments should have demonstrated competency to do so.

69. Typical table attachments may include the following:

- head rest
- anesthesia screen
- padded armboards
- shoulder braces
- kidney brace
- table strap
- leg stirrups
- table extensions
- table attachment holders

Specialized tables, such as those designed for major orthopedic procedures, have dedicated attachments necessary to achieve the desired patient position.

70. In addition to attachments for the table, there are a number of positioning accessories that are needed to achieve certain positions and to provide patient safety and comfort:

- Blankets and sheets are for patient warmth. They are also used to form rolls and bolsters. A draw sheet under the patient's body can serve as a lift sheet. A draw sheet may be used to secure the patient's arms at the sides.

- A donut that is made of foam, contoured silicone gel, or fashioned from towels is used as a head rest and to protect the ears and nerves of the head and face. If sized properly, donuts can be used to protect knees and heels.

- Pillows are used to support and elevate body parts.

- Sandbags are used for immobilization.

- Beanbags—A beanbag is a waterproof pillow filled with small plastic beads. The patient is positioned with the beanbag molded to the position. The beanbag is then attached to suction, the air from inside the pillow is withdrawn, and the beanbag becomes rigid and holds the shape to which it was molded.

- Padding made of sheepskin, foam, felt, cotton, or contoured silicone gel can be used to protect bony prominences and pressure areas such as elbows, knees, and heels. Disposable foam and reusable contoured silicone gel pads are available in a variety of sizes and shapes.

- Tape is sometimes used to secure the patient or an extremity in a flexed position. A patient assessment for tape allergy should precede the use of tape as a positioning aid.

- A laminectomy frame, or body rolls made from sheets that extend from the acromioclavicular joint to the iliac crest, are used to support the body off the chest while in a prone position.

- Eye pads may be used to protect the eyes and maintain them in a closed position.

- Pneumatic sequential compression devices, elastic bandages, or antiembolectomy stockings are all appropriate for reducing venous pooling in certain positions, for certain conditions, and for lengthy surgeries. A pneumatic sequential compression device consists of a sleeve that is wrapped around the leg and is automatically inflated and deflated in sequential progression along the extremity.

Surgical procedures in general increase the risk of deep vein thrombosis (DVT), with 50% of all DVTs in surgical patients beginning in the operating room. The risk is highest in orthopedic procedures (Carroll, 1993, p. 856). General anesthesia causes dilation of peripheral vessels, which can result in endothelial damage that may serve as a site for formation of a thrombus. Sequential compression devices should be applied and activated before induction of general anesthesia. Patients should be assessed for DVT risk and sequential compression devices applied accordingly. Any patient with a history of previous DVT should be considered high risk for DVT formation. Prolonged hospitalization, malignancy, immobility, heart failure, varicose veins, leg ulcers, and stroke are additional risk factors. Others include age (over 40) and length of procedure. Patients undergoing total joint replacement or revision are also at risk. (Figure 6-5)

IMPLEMENTATION OF PATIENT CARE

Transportation and Transfer

71. Verification of the patient's identity and of the surgical procedure is completed before the patient is transported to the operating room.

72. The patient's condition, the presence of invasive lines, the planned procedure, and institutional policy determine whether the patient may ambulate to the operating room or whether a wheelchair or stretcher is used.

73. Stretchers used for transportation should have side rails, a safety strap, a locking mechanism, and the capability to alter the patient's position. Pediatric transport cribs should have rails on all four sides, bumper pads, and a canopy that prevents escape.

74. During transport, stretcher side rails are up and the safety strap is secured. The patient is covered to maintain body temperature and to preserve dignity.

75. The patient's condition, as determined from the nursing assessment, will aid in determining

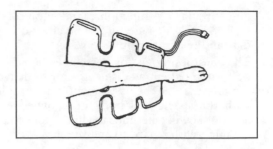

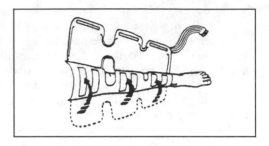

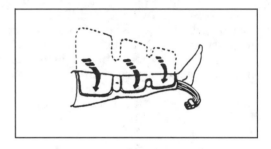

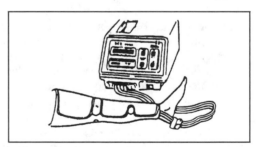

FIGURE 6-5   Application of Sequential Compression Device.
Source: Courtesy of Kendall Healthcare Products, Mansfield, Massachusetts.

whether special equipment is necessary for transport to the operating room and whether additional personnel are required. (For example, patients on ventilators are transported to the operating room in a bed rather than on a stretcher, and additional personnel are required to wheel the bed and maintain the patient's respirations during transport.) Institutional policy may require the presence of nursing and/or medical personnel during transport of critically ill or ventilator-dependent patients.

76. Verification of patient identity and the incision site is made before the patient is transferred to the operating table. Patient transfer from the stretcher to the operating table begins only when sufficient personnel are in attendance. Before transfer, the stretcher is brought adjacent to the operating table and the side rail that is proximal to the table is lowered. Both the stretcher and the table are locked in place and raised or lowered to equal height. All patient intravenous lines and catheters need to be visible and free from entanglement. All team members must be ready for patient transfer.

77. During transfer to the operating table, one team member stands at the far side of the table to receive the patient. Another team member stands at the near side of the stretcher to assist the patient to transfer and to ensure that the stretcher does not move away from the table should the lock fail. Operating room personnel must use good body mechanics to prevent injury to themselves.

78. If the patient is unable to move unaided, he or she is lifted or may be transferred with the assistance of a roller. The patient is not pushed or pulled. Pushing and pulling create a shearing effect that stretches blood vessels and obstructs blood flow, thus promoting the potential for a pressure ulcer.

79. Intravenous lines, monitoring devices, and endotracheal tubes are supported during transfer. The anesthesiologist supports the head and indicates readiness for any move.

Initial Position Techniques

80. Prior to being anesthetized, the patient is positioned supine with careful attention to proper body alignment. Legs are secured with the table strap applied 2 inches above the knees. The arms may be initially secured at the patient's side with a draw sheet drawn over the arm and tucked under the patient.

81. The patient is never left unattended while on the operating table.

82. If the patient is awake, all actions should be explained. The patient should be asked if he or she is comfortable, and if not, appropriate adjustments should be made.

83. Because the temperature in the operating room is generally cool, a warm blanket may be applied to the patient. This can prevent hypothermia and contributes to prevention of infection ("Preventing surgical infections," 2004, p. 1). Many patients are uncomfortable lying flat on their back, and when possible, a pillow is placed under the patient's head until anesthesia preparations necessitate removal.

84. To reduce the potential for compression injury and/or electrical burn, no part of the patient is allowed to contact a metal surface.

85. Extremities do not extend beyond the table. All body parts are supported and not allowed to hang free where they may be compressed or stretched and thus injured.

86. To prevent compression and trauma to blood vessels, skin, and the tibial nerve, legs must not be crossed at the ankles.

• •

SECTION QUESTIONS

Q17. The perioperative nurse is accountable for providing safety during positioning. (Ref. 49)

   True   False

Q18. In preparation to position a patient scheduled for a thoracotomy, the perioperative nurse should assess (Ref. 50, 51, 53, 70):

   a. bowel habits

   b. nutritional status

   c. height

   d. cardiac status

   e. respiratory status

    f. skin condition

    g. anticipated length of surgery

    h. tape allergy

Q19. Conditions that increase risk for skin breakdown include (Ref. 52, 54, 55, 56, 58):

    a. diabetes

    b. elderly

    c. underweight

    d. immunocompromised

Q20. What type of positioning device may be used to protect the patient's ears and nerves of the face? (Ref. 70)

_____

Q21. All patients should be transported to the operating room in either a wheelchair or a stretcher and should not be allowed to ambulate. (Ref. 72)

    True   False

Q22. If the patient is unable to move, the safest way to transfer the patient is to use a draw sheet to pull the patient. (Ref. 78)

    True   False

Q23. It is appropriate to secure the patient's arm at the side with a draw sheet drawn over the arm and tucked under the patient. (Ref. 29, 70)

    True   False

• •

BASIC SURGICAL POSITIONS

Supine (Dorsal Recumbent)

87. The supine position is the most common surgical position. (Figure 6-6) Procedures in this position include abdominal surgeries and those that require an anterior approach. Head, neck, and most extremity surgery is performed in the supine position. It is also the most common position for a wide variety of minimally invasive surgeries.

88. In the supine position, the patient is positioned flat on the back with the head and spine in a horizontal line. Hips are parallel to each other and the legs are positioned in a straight line, uncrossed, and not touching each other.

89. The head may be supported by a small donut, head rest, or pillow to prevent stretching of neck muscles that support the head. A donut may also help to prevent loss of hair that can occur as a result of prolonged pressure on the occiput.

90. Arms may be placed on padded armboards or at the patient's side. If the arm is extended on an armboard, it must be positioned at less than a 90 degree angle from the body and palms are supinated (palms up) to prevent ulnar nerve compression. If the arm is positioned next to the body, the elbows must not be flexed or extend beyond the mattress. The arm is secured with a draw sheet.

91. A small pillow may be placed under the lumbar curvature to prevent back strain that occurs when paraspinal muscles are relaxed from anesthetic and muscle relaxant agents. An anesthetized patient lying on the back for hours will likely experience temporary lumbar pain without a small pillow for support.

92. The table strap is applied loosely over the waist or mid thighs. The strap should be at

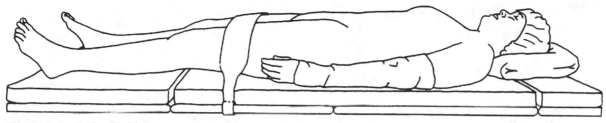

FIGURE 6-6 Supine Position.
Source: Courtesy of Reichart Consulting, Olmstead Falls, Ohio.

least 2 inches above the knees to prevent hyperextension of the knees. It should be secure but not constricting and should not be applied over a bony prominence.

93. If surgery is anticipated to extend beyond 2 hours, or if the patient's condition indicates an increased risk of skin injury, protective padding is placed at pressure points. To prevent plantar flexion and crushing injuries to the toes, the foot board must extend beyond the toes.

94. Pressure points at risk for skin injury in the supine position include skin over bony prominences, occiput, spinous processes, scapulae, styloid process of the ulnar and radius, olecranon process, sacrum, and calcaneus. Skin breakdown from pressure is most common on the styloid process of the ulnar and radius (elbows), the sacrum, and the calcaneus (heels). (Figure 6-3)

95. Nerves or nerve groups at risk include the brachial plexus, radial, ulnar, median, common peroneal, and tibial nerves.

96. Vital capacity can be reduced because of restriction of posterior chest expansion.

Trendelenburg

97. Trendelenburg is a supine position with the table tilted head down so that the head is lower than the feet. This position is used for surgery on the lower abdomen and pelvis. It is also indicated for patients who develop hypovolemic shock. (Figure 6-7)

98. The patient is positioned supine with knees over the lower break in the table. All safety measures are applied before the table is tilted. To help maintain this position, the lower part of the table may be adjusted so that the patient's legs are parallel with the floor.

99. Padded shoulder braces may be positioned against the acromion and spinous process of the scapula. Care is taken to ensure that they are not placed incorrectly over soft tissue of the shoulder where they can cause brachial plexus injury. Because of the high risk of injury, shoulder braces are used very infrequently and should not be used unless absolutely necessary.

100. The position of the arm and hand is checked to make certain that the elbow does not extend beyond the table and that the fingers are not at

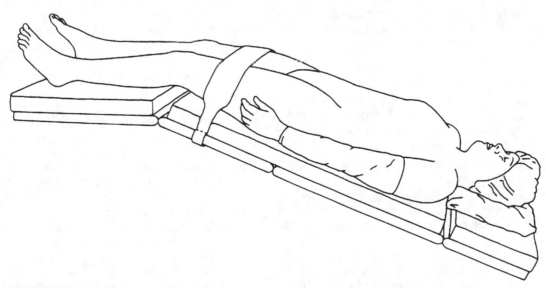

FIGURE 6-7 Trendelenburg.
Source: Courtesy of Reichart Consulting, Olmstead Falls, Ohio.

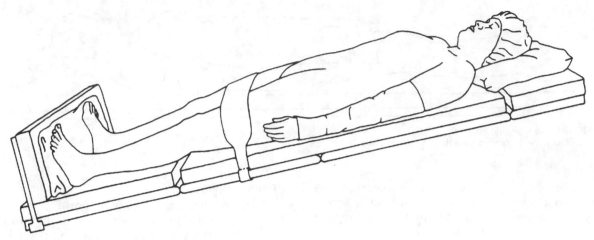

FIGURE 6-8 Reverse Trendelenburg.
Source: Courtesy of Reichart Consulting, Olmstead Falls, Ohio.

the lower break in the table where they can be crushed when the table is adjusted.

101. Before the patient is placed in Trendelenburg position, Mayo stands, tables, and other equipment are adjusted. When the position is attained, the toes are checked to ensure that the Mayo stand or other equipment is not pressing on them.

102. All movements are done slowly to allow the body enough time to adjust to the change in blood volume, respiratory exchange, and displacement of abdominal contents.

103. Respiratory and circulatory changes occur as a result of redistribution of body mass that limits diaphragm expansion and decreases ventilation-perfusion ratio. Trendelenburg position increases intrathoracic and intracranial pressure. Because of these changes, the patient should remain in Trendelenburg position for as short a time as possible.

Reverse Trendelenburg

104. Reverse Trendelenburg is a variation of the supine position in which the table is tilted feet down. This position is used for head and neck procedures. (Figure 6-8)

105. A padded foot board may be used to support the patient's body.

106. A pneumatic sequential compression device, elastic bandages, or antiembolectomy stockings are used to prevent pooling of blood in the legs.

107. Movement in and out of reverse Trendelenburg is performed slowly to allow sufficient time for the heart to adjust to change in blood volume.

Lithotomy

108. The lithotomy position is an extreme modification of the supine position in which the legs are elevated, abducted, and supported in stirrups. This position is used for procedures involving the perineum region, pelvic organs, and genitalia. (Figure 6-9)

109. The patient is positioned supine with buttocks even with the lower break in the table. For lengthy procedures, a sequential compression device or antiembolectomy stockings are applied to decrease pooling of blood in the lower legs.

110. Arms are secured on padded armboards to prevent injury to fingers and hands that can be compressed in the mechanism of the table when the bottom section of the table is lowered or raised.

111. Stirrups are securely attached to the table, positioned at equal height, and adjusted to the length of the patient's legs. This adjustment prevents pressure at the knee and lumbar region of the spine.

112. Three types of stirrups are available, and their selection should be made carefully. At-risk pressure points vary according to the type of stirrups that are used. Particular attention should be paid to the femoral epicondyle, tibial condyles, and lateral and medial malleolus. (Figure 6-10)

113. Padding on portions of the stirrups that contact the legs is appropriate to prevent external compression of nerves. Some stirrups come with a gel pad lining that provides an excellent cushion. Gel pads are made from oil-based chemical compounds or polymers. The poly-

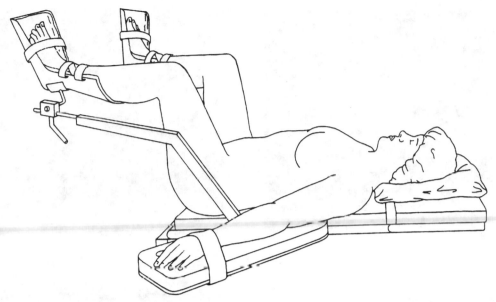

FIGURE 6-9 Lithotomy.
Source: Courtesy of Reichart Consulting, Olmstead Falls, Ohio.

mer is sealed in a sturdy membrane-like water-repellent covering. To prevent injury from pressure on the peroneal nerve, the lower part of the leg should be free from pressure against the stirrup. To prevent injury to the femoral and obturator nerve, the inner thigh should be free of pressure from the stirrup.

114. Although rare, compartment syndrome, characterized by pain, muscle weakness, and loss of sensation, can result if calf muscles remain in prolonged contact with leg supports (Walsh, 1993, p. 56).

115. To prevent hip dislocation or muscle strain from an exaggerated range of motion, the legs are raised or lowered simultaneously by two members of the surgical team. During leg elevation, the foot is held in one hand and the lower part of the leg in the other. The legs are flexed slowly, and the padded foot is secured in the stirrup.

116. After the legs are safely secured, the bottom section of the table is lowered or removed.

117. Padding may be placed under the sacrum to prevent lumbosacral strain.

118. Following the procedure, the lower section of the table is raised to align with the rest of the table, the legs are removed from the stirrups, extended fully to prevent abduction of the hips, and lowered slowly onto the table. The table strap is then applied.

119. When the legs are lowered, 500 to 800 ml of blood is diverted from the visceral area to the extremities, which can result in hypotension. To prevent severe sudden hypotension, the legs must be lowered very slowly.

120. Lithotomy position reduces respiratory efficiency because pressure from the thighs on the abdomen and pressure on the diaphragm from the abdominal viscera restrict thoracic expansion. Lung tissue becomes engorged with blood, and vital capacity and tidal volume are decreased.

121. If nursing assessment suggests a limited range of hip motion because of contractures, arthritis, prosthesis, or another condition, the patient may be placed in lithotomy position while awake to permit vocalization of pain or discomfort so that appropriate modifications can be made.

Sitting (Semi-sitting; Semi-Fowlers; Lawnchair)

122. The sitting position is used for certain cranial procedures.

123. The patient is initially positioned supine. The foot of the table is slowly lowered, flexing the knees and pelvis. The upper portion of the table is raised to become the back rest and the torso is in an either a semi-sitting or upright position. The head is supported in a cranial head rest. The feet are supported on a padded foot rest.

124. The torso and shoulders should be supported with a loose body strap. The arms may be flexed at the elbows and rest on a pillow on the

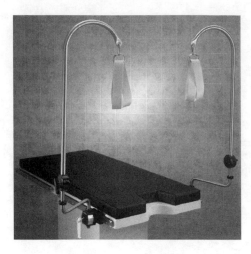
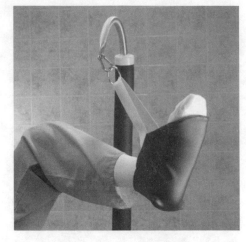
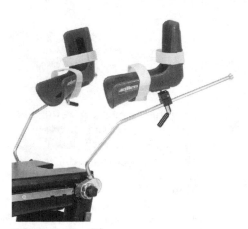
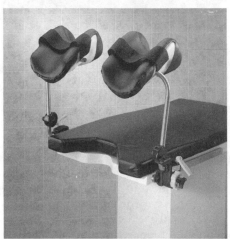

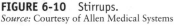
FIGURE 6-10 Stirrups.
Source: Courtesy of Allen Medical Systems

patient's lap or on an adjustable pillow in front of the patient. The arms should not fall into a dependent position.

125. Pressure points at increased risk for skin impairment include the scalp, scapulae, olecranon process, back of the knees, sacrum, ischial tuberosities, and calcaneus.

126. Padding at these pressure points is essential. Ischial tuberosities and the sacral nerve are especially at risk because most of the patient's body weight rests here. For this reason, it is critical that the operating table be well padded.

127. Antiembolism stockings or a sequential compression device is used to prevent postural hypotension and pooling of blood in lower extremities.

128. Because the sitting position causes negative venous pressure in the head and neck, the patient undergoing a craniotomy procedure in the sit-

ting position is at risk for air embolism. A central venous catheter with a Doppler ultrasound flowmeter is used to monitor the patient in this position. The Doppler is used to detect an air embolism, and the central venous pressure line is used to extract the air in this event.

129. In the semi-sitting position the patient's body is flexed at the pelvis and knees. The back of the table is not fully upright and the patient is in a reclining position. This position is used for nasopharyngeal, facial, breast reconstruction, and neck surgery. A roll may be placed under the patient's neck to hyperextend the neck and provide better access to the surgical site.

Prone

130. In the prone position, the patient is positioned on the abdomen. This exposure of the posterior body is used for procedures of the spine,

back, rectum, and the posterior aspects of extremities. (Figure 6-11)

131. The patient is initially positioned supine on the stretcher. The side rail closest to the operating table is lowered, and the stretcher is positioned adjacent to the operating table and locked. The other side rail is lowered, and anesthesia is administered prior to placing the patient in a prone position. Following induction, the anesthesiologist will secure the endotracheal tube to prevent dislocation and apply ointment to the eyes and tape them shut to prevent corneal abrasion. The anesthesiologist will indicate readiness of any movement of the patient.

132. A minimum of four persons is necessary to safely turn the patient from supine position on the stretcher to prone position on the operating table; one person supports and moves the head, one supports and moves the torso, one supports and moves the lower body, and one controls the body as it is rolled onto the operating table. All necessary equipment must be available. This includes padded armboards, a donut, body rolls or laminectomy frame, pillows, and padding.

133. All movement of the patient is done slowly and gently to allow the body time to adjust to the change in position. The anesthesiologist supports the head and neck and protects the patient's airway. A second person turns the patient from the stretcher onto the operating table into the waiting arms of a third person who supports the patient's chest and lower abdomen. A fourth person supports and turns the patient's legs. During turning, the patient's arms and hands are placed at the sides. The body is maintained in alignment, and all team members work in concert to turn the patient in a single motion.

134. After the patient is turned, the arms are brought down and forward in a normal range of motion and then placed on armboards positioned next to the head. The arms are flexed at the elbows with the hands pronated. When the patient's arms are in place, the person receiving the patient may then remove his or her arms from under the patient. Elbows should be padded.

135. The patient's head is turned to one side and supported on a small pillow or donut, and the airway is secured. The eyes are checked to ensure that they are closed in order to prevent corneal abrasion and free them from pressure, which can cause permanent eye injury. The ears are checked to ensure that they are not folded unnaturally. Neck and spine must be in good alignment.

136. The chest is supported by rolls or a laminectomy frame, such as the Wilson frame, which is positioned lengthwise from the acromioclavicular joint to the iliac crest. This facilitates respiratory expansion because the chest is lifted off the operating table and the weight of the abdomen is removed from the diaphragm. This is important because female breasts and male genitalia must be free of crushing pressure.

137. A pillow is placed under the ankles to prevent stretching of the anterior tibial nerve and to prevent pressure on the toes and feet that can cause plantar flexion and foot drop.

138. In the prone position, the table strap is placed over the mid thighs, which are covered with a sheet and/or a blanket. The strap should be at least 2 inches above the knees so as not to impede superficial venous return.

139. A small donut under the knees prevents pressure on the patellas.

140. If the patient has a stoma, precautions must be taken to prevent ischemic compression of the stoma against the frame or body rolls. Such pressure can lead to tissue necrosis and sloughing.

Jackknife (Kraske's)

141. In the jackknife position, the patient is positioned prone with the table flexed at the center

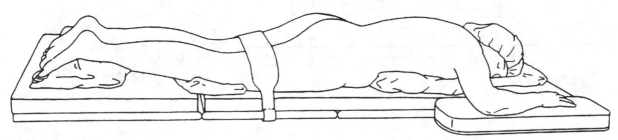

FIGURE 6-11 Prone.
Source: Courtesy of Reichart Consulting, Olmstead Falls, Ohio.

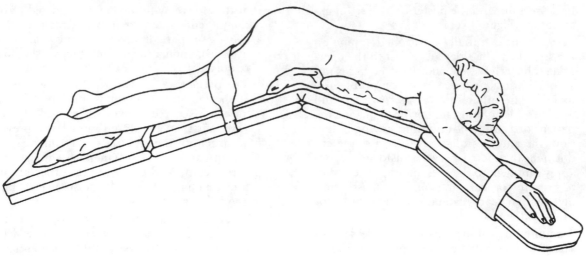

FIGURE 6-12 Kraske.
Source: Courtesy of Reichart Consulting, Olmstead Falls, Ohio.

break in the table. This position is often used for proctological procedures. (Figure 6-12)

142. Venous pooling in the chest and feet can cause a decrease in mean arterial blood pressure. Restriction of diaphragm movement combined with increased blood volume in the lungs can cause a decrease in ventilation and cardiac output. Because of its adverse effect on the respiratory and circulatory systems, the jackknife position is considered one of the most precarious surgical positions.

143. In the jackknife position, the patient is positioned as for prone, with the hips placed over the center table joint. Arms are positioned on padded angled armboards placed next to the head. Elbows are flexed, and palms are pronated. Chest rolls are placed to raise the patient's chest, and the head is turned to one side. (Chest rolls are not necessary if the patient is awake.) A pil-

low is placed under the ankles, and the table strap is applied to the thighs. The table is then flexed to a 90 degree angle, causing the hips to be raised and the head and legs to be lowered.

144. All precautions that are taken with the prone position are also taken with the jackknife position.

Lateral

145. In the lateral position, the patient lies on one side. In the right lateral position, the patient is placed on the right side for surgeries on structures on the left side of the body. The reverse is true for the left lateral position. (Figure 6-13)

146. The lateral position is used for access to the thorax, kidney, retroperitoneal space, and hip.

147. The patient is initially positioned supine on the operating table and anesthetized. A team of four persons will then lift and turn the patient

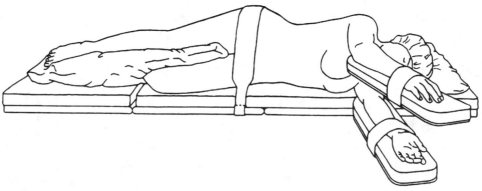

FIGURE 6-13 Lateral.
Source: Courtesy of Reichart Consulting, Olmstead Falls, Ohio.

onto the nonoperative side. The anesthesiologist's responsibility is to support the head and neck, guard the airway, and initiate any movement. A second person will lift and support the chest and shoulders, while a third will lift and support the hips. A fourth person is needed to support and turn the legs.

148. The patient is lifted in supine position to the edge of the operative side of the table and then turned on the side toward the center of the table. For kidney procedures, it is important that the patient's flank be positioned over the kidney rest with the iliac crest just below the table break. The patient's head is supported with a pillow or donut, and the body is checked for proper alignment. The head must be placed in cervical alignment with the spine. The lower leg is flexed. The lateral aspect of the lower knee is well padded to prevent peroneal nerve damage resulting in foot drop caused by pressure from the fibula on the nerve. A pillow is placed between the legs, and the upper leg is extended out straight. Feet and ankles are padded and supported to prevent foot drop and pressure injuries of the malleolus. The patient is secured with the table strap or with wide tape applied across the upper hip and fastened to the table.

149. A small roll or padding is placed under the patient's lower axilla to relieve pressure on the chest and axilla, to allow sufficient chest expansion, and to prevent compression of the brachial plexus by the humeral head. The lower arm is slightly flexed and placed on a padded armboard. The upper arm may rest on a padded elevated armboard or other padded support. Care must be taken not to abduct the arm more than 90 degrees, which can cause brachial plexus injury.

150. For kidney procedures, the patient is supported on the operating table with well-padded braces, rolls, or sandbags. Extra padding is applied to bony prominence areas of the ankles, knees, greater trochanter, iliac crest, shoulders, elbows, and wrists.

151. The table is flexed at the center break in the table. The kidney elevator (kidney rest) portion of the table is raised to provide greater exposure of the area from the twelfth rib to the iliac crest. Kidney braces that fit over the kidney elevator may be used to support and maintain the patient in this position. Kidney braces must always be well padded.

152. Respiratory efficiency is affected by pressure from the weight of the body on the lower chest. The lower lung receives more blood from the right side of the heart, so it has increased perfusion but less residual air because of mediastinal compression and weight from abdominal contents.

153. Circulation is compromised by pressure on abdominal vessels and pooling of blood in the lower extremities. In the right lateral position, compression on the vena cava impairs venous return. If the kidney elevator is raised, additional pressure on abdominal vessels can further compromise circulation.

154. Injury of the eye or ear is a special concern with the patient in the lateral position. The ear must be laid flat against the operating table and the eyelid must be closed.

• •

SECTION QUESTIONS

Q24. In the supine position, the arms may be positioned at the patient's side, flexed, and secured with a draw sheet. (Ref. 90)

True   False

Q25. In the supine position, what intervention may be taken to prevent back strain and lumbar pain? (Ref. 91)

_____

_____

Q26. List five bony prominence areas that are susceptible to pressure injury in the supine position. (Ref. 94)

_____

_____

_____

_____

_____

Q27. Explain why all movement of the patient into Trendelenburg position should be done slowly. (Ref. 102)

_____

_____

_____

Q28. In lithotomy position the patient's buttocks are positioned even with the lower break in the table. (Ref. 109)

True   False

Q29. One person is sufficient to place an anesthetized patient in stirrups, provided the legs are raised slowly. (Ref. 115)

True   False

Q30. Explain why sudden hypotension can occur when a patient's legs are lowered from stirrups. (Ref. 119)

_____

_____

_____

Q31. Explain why lithotomy position reduces respiratory efficiency. (Ref. 120)

_____

_____

Q32. Explain why a central venous pressure line with a Doppler ultrasound is used to monitor a patient in a sitting position. (Ref. 128)

_____

_____

_____

Q33. Which member of the team initiates readiness to move the patient from supine to prone position? (Ref. 131)

    a. perioperative nurse

    b. anesthesiologist

    c. surgeon

    d. scrub person

Q34. In the prone position, the patient's arms will be brought down and forward, placed on armboards with the elbows flexed, and the hands pronated. (Ref. 134)

True   False

Q35. When the prone position is used in surgery, the perioperative nurse facilitates diaphragmatic expansion by (Ref. 136):

    a. repositioning the patient several times during surgery

    b. pressing down on the OR table mattress periodically throughout the procedure

    c. placing supporting rolls from the acromioclavicular joint to the iliac crest under the patient

    d. placing the patient's head on a neck roll

Q36. Describe an intervention for the patient in the prone position to prevent stretching of the anterior tibial nerve and pressure on the toes that can cause plantar flexion and foot drop. (Ref. 137)

_____

_____

Q37. A patient who is having a hemorrhoidectomy may be placed in which position for surgery? (Ref. 141)

    a. right lateral

    b. jackknife

    c. prone

Q38. A team of four persons is necessary to safely position the patient in the lateral position. (Ref. 147)

True   False

Q39. In the lateral position, the patient's lower leg is positioned straight and the upper leg is flexed with a pillow between them. (Ref. 148)

True   False

Q40. In the lateral position, it is appropriate to place a small roll under the patient's upper axilla to relieve pressure on the chest and promote chest expansion. (Ref. 149)

True   False

· ·

EVALUATING IMPLEMENTATION OF POSITIONING

155. The anesthetized patient cannot report discomfort or pain related to positioning, and the effects of improper positioning are not generally known until the patient recovers from anesthesia and is able to report pain and injury. The patient relies on the surgical team to ensure that positioning injuries do not occur.

156. Once the patient is in position for the surgery, the perioperative nurse should do a thorough, once-over check to ensure that the patient's body is in alignment, extremities are not extended beyond their natural range of motion, bony prominences are padded, pressure is removed from nerves where injury can occur, respiratory and circulatory efforts are restricted as little as possible, and positioning devices are appropriately positioned and padded and hold securely without excessive restriction on body structures. Intermittent reevaluation of the patient's position throughout the procedure is important. If the patient is repositioned during the procedure, a thorough reevaluation is critical, with adjustments made as necessary.

POSTOPERATIVE TRANSFER

157. When surgery is completed and the anesthesiologist indicates that the patient is stable and can be moved, the postoperative bed or stretcher is brought adjacent to the operating table. It is raised or lowered to the level of the operating table and locked into place.

158. Ideally four staff should be available to transfer the anesthetized patient in a slow and smooth manner to the bed or stretcher. The airway and proper body alignment must be maintained. Lines and catheters must be transferred intact and free from entanglement.

159. The patient is lifted or rolled onto the bed or stretcher. Pushing and pulling is avoided. Side rails are raised and locked for safe patient transfer and recovery.

DOCUMENTATION OF NURSING ACTIONS

160. Nursing documentation related to positioning should include but not be limited to the following:

- assessment, considerations for positioning—desired outcomes
- overall skin condition on arrival and discharge from the perioperative suite
- position
- placement of extremities
- placement of positioning devices such as rolls, padding, and restraints
- precautions to protect eyes
- any changes made in positioning during the procedure
- who positioned patient
- presence and placement of safety strap or equivalent
- patient condition following surgery—whether desired outcomes were met
- signature

SECTION QUESTIONS

Q41. Once the patient is in final position, the perioperative nurse should do an overall check to ensure that positioning will not cause injury. Describe what the perioperative nurse should assess. (Identify at least four implementations to check for.) (Ref. 156)

_____

_____

_____

_____

Q42. Assessment of the patient's position should be performed (Ref. 156):

a. just prior to surgery

b. intermittently throughout the procedure

c. whenever the patient is repositioned

d. following the procedure

Q43. Information that should be included in nursing documentation relative to positioning should include at least five items (Ref. 160):

_____

_____

_____

_____

_____

• •

• • • References

Association of periOperative Registered Nurses (AORN). (2004). Standards: Patient outcomes. In *Standards, recommended practices and guidelines* (pp. 197–206). Denver, CO: Author.

Aronovitch, S. A. (2002). How to prevent pressure ulcers. *Outpatient Surgery Magazine, 111*(5), 61–66.

Goodman, T. (2003). *Positioning: A patient safety initiative, study guide for nurses.* ConMed Corporation. Denver, CO: Healthstream.

Hoyman, K., & Gruber, N. (1992). A case study of interdepartmental cooperation: Operating room acquired pressure ulcers. *Journal of Nursing Care Quality: Special Report, 15,* 12–17.

Peterson, C. (2004). Clinical issues. Deep vein thrombosis. *AORN Journal, 79*(4), 856–861.

Preventing surgical infections by keeping patients warmed. (2004). *OR Manager, 20*(4), 1, 9–15.

Martin, J. (1991). Updating the concepts of patient positioning during anesthesia and surgery. *Current Reviews for Nurse Anesthetists, 14,* 67–76.

Schultz, A., Bien, M., Dumond, K., Brown, K., Myers, A. (1999). Etiology and incidence of pressure ulcers in surgical patients. *AORN Journal, 70*(3), 434–449.

Stewart, T. P., & Magnano, S. J. (1988). Burns or pressure ulcers in the surgical patient. *Decubitus, 1*(1), 36–40.

Walsh, J. (1993). Postop effects of OR positioning. *RN, 56*(2), 50–57.

• • • Suggested Reading

Goodman, T. (2003). *Positioning: A patient safety initiative: Study guide for nurses.* ConMed Corporation. Denver, CO: Healthstream.

Phillips, N. (2004). Positioning, prepping, and draping the patient. In *Operating Room Technique* (10th ed., pp. 470–511). St. Louis, MO: Mosby.

Appendix 6-A

• •

Chapter 6 Post Test

Instructions: Fill in the blank(s), mark the correct answer(s), or answer the question as appropriate.

1. The patient undergoing surgery for a thoracotomy is at high risk for (Ref. 2):

   a. impaired skin integrity

   b. compromised respiratory effort

   c. altered tissue perfusion

   d. musculoskeletal injury

2. A desired patient outcome related to positioning is skin is free of ecchymosis. (Ref. 5)

   True   False

3. List four things necessary for the perioperative nurse to know for safe positioning of the patient. (Ref. 6)

   _____

   _____

   _____

   _____

4. Maintenance of patient dignity is a desired patient outcome relative to positioning. (Ref. 7, 65, 66)

   True   False

5. Complications that can occur as a result of improper positioning include (Ref. 8):

   a. pain

   b. joint dislocation

   c. fracture

   d. cardiovascular compromise

   e. paralysis and paresis

   f. necrosis

6. Trendelenburg position can result in hypoventilation. (Ref. 10, 11)

   True   False

7. Muscle relaxants decrease risk of hyperextension injury. (Ref. 16)

   True   False

8. When the Mayo stand or operating room table is repositioned during surgery, what should the perioperative nurse check for to prevent injury to the patient? (Ref. 19)

   _____

   _____

9. Select the correct statement(s) concerning prevention of brachial plexus nerve injury. (Ref. 25, 26, 27, 90)

   a. The arm is positioned on an armboard at a greater than 90 degree angle and the palm pronated.

   b. The arm is positioned on an armboard at a less than 90 degree angle to the body and the palm supinated.

c. Injury can occur if a shoulder brace is positioned too far medially with the arm abducted.

d. Motor and sensory loss to the arm and shoulder may occur as a result of brachial plexus injury.

10. Ulnar nerve injury (Ref. 31, 32):

a. may occur as a result of a malfunctioning blood pressure cuff

b. may result in symptoms of numbness in the fourth and fifth fingers

c. may result in a weak grip

11. The position most likely to lead to injury of the peroneal nerve is (Ref. 35, 36):

a. prone

b. supine

c. lithotomy

d. jackknife

12. Shearing injury can contribute to the development of a pressure ulcer. (Ref. 41, 42)

True   False

13. An anesthetized patient is at risk for pressure ulcer after (Ref. 43):

a. 30 minutes

b. 1 hour

c. 2 hours

14. The elderly are at greater risk for skin breakdown during surgery because (Ref. 52):

a. surgery on the elderly generally lasts longer than on young people

b. they have less subcutaneous fat and muscle tissue

c. they are usually malnourished

15. Immunocompromised patients are at increased risk of (Ref. 58):

a. joint dislocation

b. skin breakdown

c. circulatory insufficiency

16. List three safety features that should be present in a pediatric transport crib. (Ref. 73)

_____

_____

_____

17. Explain why two persons should be present when a patient transfers from a stretcher to the operating room bed. (Ref. 77)

_____

18. The longer that pressure is applied, the more severe is the tissue damage. (Ref. 43, 59, 93)

True   False

19. Concerning positioning (Ref. 18, 80, 82, 84, 85, 86):

a. All actions are explained to the awake patient.

b. The safety strap is applied 2 inches below the knee.

c. No part of the patient is touching metal.

d. No extremity is allowed to hang free.

e. Legs are not crossed at the ankles.

20. Match the position to the pressure areas. (Ref. 94, 135, 136, 148, 150)

    a. Supine   _____ occiput, scapulae, spinous processes, medial epicondyle of the humerus, sacrum, olecra-
    non process, calcaneus

    b. Prone   _____ ear, patella, breasts, genitalia, cornea, toes

    c. Lateral   _____ malleolus, greater trochanter, iliac crest, lateral aspect of the knee

21. In which position are the ischial tuberosities and sacral nerve are at high risk of injury? (Ref. 125, 126)

    a. supine

    b. lateral

    c. lithotomy

    d. sitting

22. Another name for the dorsal recumbent position is _____. (Ref. 87)

23. Although rare, compartment syndrome injury can occur when calf muscles remain in prolonged contact with
    leg stirrups. (Ref. 114)

    True   False

24. Explain why in the lithotomy position it is safer to position the patient's arms on armboards than next to the
    body. (Ref. 110)

    _____

    _____

25. The sitting position is used most often for (Ref. 122):

    a. perineal procedures

    b. cranial surgeries

    c. neck surgery

    d. gastrointestinal surgery

26. Describe the position of the patient in reverse Trendelenburg. (Ref. 104)

    _____

    _____

27. What intervention may be undertaken to prevent pooling of blood in lower extremities during a procedure?
    (Ref. 109, 127)

    _____

    _____

28. List three positioning devices that are necessary when positioning the patient in prone position.
    (Ref. 135, 136)

    _____

    _____

    _____

29. Explain the purpose of placing a pillow under the feet and ankles in the prone position. (Ref. 137)

_____

_____

30. In which position is the female at greatest risk for injury to breasts? (Ref. 136)

_____

_____

31. Because of its adverse effects on the respiratory and circulatory systems, the jackknife position is considered one of the most dangerous positions. (Ref. 142)

    True   False

32. Venous thrombosis can result from an improperly placed safety strap. (Ref. 15, 138)

    True   False

33. When positioning a patient in the lateral position (Ref. 147, 148):

    a. a team of three people is needed for positioning

    b. a pillow is placed between the patient's legs

    c. the lateral aspect of the lower knee is well padded

    d. the lower leg is flexed and the upper leg is straight

    e. feet and ankles are supported and padded

34. For surgery on the left side, the patient is positioned in the _____ lateral position. (Ref. 145)

    a. right

    b. left

35. In the right lateral position, circulation is compromised from pressure on the vena cava. (Ref. 153)

    True   False

36. Which statement(s) concerning patient transfer from the operating room table are correct? (Ref. 158, 159)

    a. Four persons should be available to transfer the anesthetized patient.

    b. The surgeon initiates transfer of the patient.

    c. The stretcher is positioned lower than the operating table.

    d. The patient may be lifted or rolled onto the stretcher.

37. List five items of information that should be included in nursing documentation relative to positioning. (Ref. 160)

_____

_____

_____

_____

_____

Appendix 6-B

• •

Competency Checklist: Positioning the Patient for Surgery

Under "Observer's Initials," enter initials upon successful achievement of competency.
Enter N/A if competency is not appropriate for institution.

NAME _____

	OBSERVER'S INITIALS	DATE
1. Table Operation		
a. armboards—attach, remove, adjust	_____	_____
b. rotation—right, left, Trendelenburg, reverse Trendelenburg, flex	_____	_____
c. lower leg portion of table and remove section (lithotomy position)	_____	_____
d. attach/remove side rail stirrup holders	_____	_____
e. other	_____	_____
2. Patient Transfer		
a. side rails up and secure during transport	_____	_____
b. patient covered	_____	_____
c. stretcher adjacent to table with proximal side rail lowered	_____	_____
d. stretcher and table locked	_____	_____
e. stretcher and table are equal height	_____	_____
f. two team members present during transfer	_____	_____
g. patient lifted or rolled, not pulled	_____	_____
3. Supine		
a. patient is flat on back with head and spine in a straight, horizontal line	_____	_____
b. hips are parallel and legs are in a straight line and uncrossed	_____	_____
c. safety strap is placed at least 2 inches above the knees (secure but nonconstricting)	_____	_____
d. small pillow is placed beneath the patient's head	_____	_____
e. arms extended on armboards are at less than a 90 degree angle from the body and supinated	_____	_____
f. arms at patient's side are not flexed and do not extend beyond the mattress; arms are secured with a draw sheet	_____	_____
g. protective padding is placed at pressure points	_____	_____
4. Trendelenburg		
a. patient is positioned supine	_____	_____
b. knees are over lower break of the table	_____	_____

    c. table is tilted head down   _____   _____

    d. following table tilt, patient's toes are checked   _____   _____

5. Reverse Trendelenburg

    a. patient is positioned supine   _____   _____

    b. table is tilted feet down   _____   _____

6. Lithotomy

    a. equipment assembled

      • appropriate stirrups   _____   _____

      • OR table stirrup holders   _____   _____

      • padding   _____   _____

    b. patient is initially positioned supine   _____   _____

    c. buttocks are positioned directly above the break in the table   _____   _____

    d. both legs are simultaneously and slowly raised and positioned in stirrups by two people   _____   _____

    e. both stirrups are at even height   _____   _____

    f. fibular head free of pressure from stirrups   _____   _____

    g. stirrups are not exerting pressure against the upper inner aspect of the calf   _____   _____

    h. padded stirrups do not compress vascular structures in the popliteal space   _____   _____

    i. padding is placed beneath the sacrum   _____   _____

    j. both legs are slowly and simultaneously lowered to the bed by two people   _____   _____

7. Sitting

    a. patient is initially positioned supine   _____   _____

    b. foot of table is slowly lowered   _____   _____

    c. upper portion of table is raised   _____   _____

    d. feet are supported on a padded foot rest   _____   _____

    e. torso and shoulders are secured with table strap   _____   _____

    f. arms are flexed and positioned on a pillow on the patient's lap   _____   _____

    g. pressure points are padded   _____   _____

8. Prone

    a. equipment assembled

      • chest roll or laminectomy frame   _____   _____

      • donut   _____   _____

      • pillows and padding   _____   _____

    b. patient is logrolled from the stretcher to the OR table onto chest rolls or laminectomy frame by four people   _____   _____

    c. arms are rotated through their normal range of motion and positioned on padded armboards next to the patient's head   _____ _____

    d. arms are not abducted beyond 90 degrees   _____ _____

    e. elbows are padded   _____ _____

    f. patient's head is positioned to one side and supported on a donut   _____ _____

    g. eyes and ears are checked for pressure points   _____ _____

    h. male genitalia are checked for pressure points   _____ _____

    i. female breasts are checked for pressure points   _____ _____

    j. knees and toes are protected with padding   _____ _____

9. Jackknife (Kraske's)

    a. patient is positioned prone   _____ _____

    b. hips are placed over the center table break   _____ _____

    c. arms are positioned on padded armboards next to the patient's head   _____ _____

    d. elbows are flexed; palms are pronated   _____ _____

    e. pillow is placed beneath the ankles   _____ _____

    f. table strap is placed across thighs   _____ _____

    g. table is flexed to a 90 degree angle   _____ _____

10. Lateral

    a. equipment assembled

      • tape   _____ _____

      • pillows/padding/donut   _____ _____

      • axillary roll   _____ _____

    b. patient is initially positioned supine   _____ _____

    c. patient is turned onto the nonoperative side by four people   _____ _____

    d. patient's head is in cervical alignment with the spine   _____ _____

    e. bottom leg is flexed   _____ _____

    f. lateral aspect of lower knee is padded   _____ _____

    g. upper leg is extended   _____ _____

    h. pillow is placed between the legs   _____ _____

    i. patient is secured with table strap or tape across hips   _____ _____

    j. axillary roll is placed at the lower axilla   _____ _____

    k. lower arm is flexed on a padded armboard   _____ _____

    l. upper arm is supported on a padded elevated armboard/pillow/padded support   _____ _____

    m. arms are not abducted more than 90 degrees   _____ _____

    n. lower ear is flat and eyes are closed   _____ _____

11. Documentation

   a. documentation includes:

      • preoperative assessment of skin   _____   _____

      • assessment—considerations for positioning   _____   _____

      • position   _____   _____

      • placement of padding   _____   _____

      • who positioned patient   _____   _____

      • intraoperative changes made to position   _____   _____

      • safety strap   _____   _____

      • outcome   _____   _____

      • signature   _____   _____

OBSERVER'S SIGNATURE   INITIALS   DATE

_____

ORIENTEE'S SIGNATURE

_____

CHAPTER 6—Section Question Answers

Q1. Impaired skin integrity, compromised respiratory effort, altered tissue perfusion, neuromuscular and musculoskeletal injury

Q2. Skin—intact, free of ecchymosis, cuts, abrasions, shear injury, blisters
Neuromuscular—flexes and extends extremities without assistance or pain, no numbness or tingling of extremities

Q3. The lung can become engorged with blood and decrease space for alveoli expansion; amount of oxygenated blood is reduced; lung compliance and expansion is decreased and amount of air taken in is reduced, which can lead to hypoventilation, hypoxia, hypercarbia; diaphragm is less able to work against pressure from abdominal contents

Q4. a

Q5. True

Q6. Joint dislocation

Q7. b

Q8. Because of its superficial position and close proximity to bony structures

Q9. True

Q10. c

Q11. If the elbow slips off the mattress onto the metal edge of the table and is compressed between the table and the medial epicondyle, if the arm is allowed to rest on a fixed elbow with the forearm pronated across the ventral trunk, a malfunctioning blood-pressure cuff that does not allow sufficient time between compressions

Q12. True

Q13. a, b

Q14. True

Q15. False

Q16. False

Q17. True

Q18. b, c, d, e, f, g, h

Q19. a, b, c, d

Q20. Donut

Q21. False

Q22. False

Q23. True

Q24. False

Q25. A small pillow may be placed under the lumbar curvature

Q26. Occiput, spinous processes, scapulae, styloid process of the radius and ulnar, olecranon process, sacrum, calcaneus

Q27. To allow the body enough time to adjust to the change in blood volume, respiratory exchange, and displacement of abdominal contents

Q28. True

Q29. False

Q30. 500 to 800 ml of blood is rapidly diverted from the visceral area to the extremities, which can result in sudden hypotension

(continues)

CHAPTER 6—Section Question Answers (*continued*)

Q31. Pressure from the thighs on the abdomen and pressure on the diaphragm from the abdominal viscera restrict thoracic expansion. Lung tissue becomes engorged with blood; vital capacity and tidal volume are decreased.

Q32. The sitting position causes negative venous pressure in the head and neck, and the patient is at risk for air embolism. The central venous pressure line with a Doppler ultrasound flowmeter will detect an air embolism.

Q33. b

Q34. True

Q35. c

Q36. A pillow is placed under the ankles

Q37. b (b and c are also correct)

Q38. True

Q39. False

Q40. False

Q41. Alignment, extremities not hyperextended, bony prominences padded, pressure relieved from nerves, respiratory and circulatory efforts restricted as little as possible, positioning devices appropriately positioned and padded as needed, no excessive restriction

Q42. a, b, c

Q43. Assessment considerations for positioning; preoperative and postoperative skin condition; position; placement of extremities; placement of positioning devices, rolls, and padding; restraints; precautions to protect eyes; changes in positioning; presence of safety strap; who positioned patient; outcome of positioning; signature

---

Chapter 6—Post Test Answers

1. a, b, c, d
2. True
3. Principles of anatomy and physiology, anatomical changes and physiologic changes related to anesthesia and surgical positions, surgical procedure to be performed, proper positioning techniques, appropriate positioning equipment and its use
4. True
5. a, b, d, e, f
6. True
7. False
8. That equipment is not resting or exerting pressure on the patient
9. b, c, d
10. a, b, c
11. c
12. True

(continues)

Chapter 6—Post Test Answers (*continued*)

13. c
14. b
15. b
16. Side rails, bumper pads, canopy
17. One team member to receive the patient, another to assist in transfer and prevent stretcher from moving away from operating table during transfer
18. True
19. a, c, d, e
20. a, b, c
21. d
22. Supine
23. True
24. To prevent fingers and hands from being crushed in table mechanism
25. b
26. Supine position, table tilted with head higher than feet
27. Application of antiembolectomy stockings, elastic bandage, or sequential compression device
28. Padded armboards, donut, body rolls or laminectomy frame, pillows, padding
29. To prevent stretching of anterior tibial nerve and prevent pressure on the toes that can cause plantar flexion and foot drop
30. Prone
31. True
32. True
33. b, c, d, e
34. a
35. True
36. a, d
37. Assessment considerations for positioning; pre- and postoperative skin condition; position, placement of extremities; placement of positioning devices, rolls, padding; restraints; precautions to protect the eyes; changes made in positioning during the procedure; presence and position of safety strap; who positioned patient; outcome; signature

CHAPTER

7

Prevention of Injury—Counts in Surgery

LEARNER OBJECTIVES

After reading and completing "Prevention of Injury—Counts in Surgery," the learner will:

- identify the desired patient outcome relative to counts in surgery
- discuss nursing responsibilities related to counts in surgery
- describe the procedure for sponge, sharp, and instrument counts
- list what should be documented with regard to counts

• • • • • • • • • • • •
Lesson Outline

I.   DESCRIPTION
II. NURSING DIAGNOSIS—DESIRED PATIENT OUTCOME
III. OVERVIEW
IV. NURSING RESPONSIBILITIES
V.   COUNT PROCEDURES
    A. Sponge Counts
    B. Sharps Counts
    C. Instrument Counts
VI. DOCUMENTATION

DESCRIPTION

1. Surgical counts refers to the counting of sponges, sharps such as blades and needles, and instruments that are opened and delivered to the field for use during surgery. The purpose is to reconcile what was delivered to the sterile field before an incision is made and during the surgery with what remains at the end of surgery. For example, if 20 sponges are delivered to the sterile field before the incision and 10 more are added during the procedure, there should be 30 sponges accounted for at the end of surgery. Counts are performed for sponges, sharps, instruments, and any other items, such as vessel loops and vein introducers, that could be retained.

NURSING DIAGNOSIS—DESIRED PATIENT OUTCOME

2. Patients undergoing surgery are at risk for injury related to an unintentionally retained foreign body. Although the occurrence of a retained foreign body is not common, it does happen. Extraneous objects such as sponges, sharps, or instruments, if unintentionally retained inside the patient, constitute serious patient injury. Patients suffer unnecessary pain, possible readmission to the hospital or extended stay, additional surgery, and delayed healing.

3. Cramping, fever, pain, or cavity abscess of unknown origin are possible signs of a retained foreign body. Often these symptoms do not occur until well after the patient has returned home.

4. A desired outcome at the end of surgery is that the patient is free from signs and symptoms of injury caused by extraneous objects (AORN, 2004b, p. 198).

OVERVIEW

5. In addition to the harm incurred by the patient, malpractice litigation frequently results when foreign objects are retained. Because a retained foreign body in a patient is almost always indefensible, such cases usually do not come before a jury. Any or all members of the surgical team may be held liable.

6. One mechanism to reduce the potential for a retained foreign body is surgical counts.

7. Counts are usually performed by the scrub person and the circulating nurse. Legal accountability for counts is a primary responsibility of the perioperative nurse; however, the entire surgical team has a responsibility to protect the patient from foreign body injury.

8. The Association of Perioperative Registered Nurses recommends counting sharps and related miscellaneous items on all procedures, and sponge and instrument counts on procedures where the likelihood exists that a sponge or instrument could be retained (AORN, 2004b, p. 231).

9. Many healthcare facilities have established count policies that reflect the AORN Recommended Practice for Sponge, Sharp and Instrument Counts; however, there are many facilities where count policies differ from the AORN Recommended Practice. With the advent of minimally invasive surgery, the opportunity for a retained foreign body has been reduced and count policies have often been developed that do not mandate instrument counts unless an open procedure is performed. All policies, however, should specify when counts are to be taken, by whom, and what is counted.

10. Policies determining what is counted are often based on the nature of the procedure and the probability of a retained item, the anticipated size of the incision, and the supplies required for the procedure. Some healthcare facilities have policies that identify specific procedures or specialties, such as ophthalmology, for which a count may be omitted.

11. Some institutions use a count sheet to record count results. Others employ a wallboard where counts are recorded during the procedure and only the final results are documented as a permanent record.

NURSING RESPONSIBILITIES

12. Counts in surgery provide a mechanism to provide for patient safety during surgery. As patient advocates, perioperative nurses have a responsibility to ensure that count procedures are carried out according to institutional policy.

13. Surgical counts are not a guarantee that items will not be retained in a patient. Existence of a documented "*correct count*" usually accompanies a lawsuit for a retained item. The item was not intentionally retained, nor does the documentation intentionally misrepresent the count.

An error in the count process accounts for this phenomenon. Over time, counting becomes a routine task, which contributes to the potential for error. Other factors that can contribute to error are excessive talking during counts, sponges placed in cavities for packing during the case, circulating nurse out of the room when sponges are added to the field, and signing for counts that were not performed (Beyea, 2003, p. 291). All counts must be performed carefully, and the scrub person and the circulating nurse must share the responsibility equally. Counts must be done together, concurrently, and aloud. Items being counted must be visible to both persons.

14. When an incorrect count occurs, it is the responsibility of the nurse to inform the surgeon and for all team members to assist in locating the missing item before the surgery is completed.

15. In an extreme emergency situation, such as multiple trauma, a count before the procedure may not be possible. In such an instance, the omission and the rationale should be documented and institutional policy for this occurrence should be followed.

16. As a general procedure, counts are performed and documented prior to the beginning of the surgery, during surgery when items are added to the field, before closure of a body cavity or deep incision, before closure of a cavity within a cavity (cesarean section), and at skin closure. Additional counts may be performed as needed to verify accuracy. In fact, during long procedures where many sutures and sponges are used it is wise, if possible, to verify sponges and needles from time to time.

17. All counted items should be removed from the room at the end of surgery. Items left in the room may cause an incorrect count in a subsequent procedure in that room.

18. Counts should be verified when either the scrub person or the circulating nurse is relieved by a new team member.

19. The nurse is responsible for documenting the information related to counts and for notifying the surgeon of count results.

. . . .

SECTION QUESTIONS

Q1. List three categories of items that surgical counts refer to. (Ref. 1)

_____

Q2. A patient undergoing an invasive surgical procedure such as a total joint replacement is at high risk for an unintentionally retained foreign body. (Ref. 2)

   True   False

Q3. The Association of periOperative Registered Nurses (AORN) recommends counting all sponges, sharps, and instruments on all surgical procedures. (Ref. 8)

   True   False

Q4. Perioperative nurses have a responsibility to ensure that count procedures are carried out according to (Ref. 12):

   a. institutional policy

   b. the AORN recommendations

   c. the surgeon's recommendation

Q5. Counts are performed (Ref. 16, 18):

    a. prior to the procedure

    b. when items are added to the sterile field

    c. following all X-rays

    d. when either scrub person or circulator is relieved

    e. as needed to verify accuracy

COUNT PROCEDURES

Sponge Counts

20. The word *sponges* refers to materials designed to absorb blood and fluids. All sponges placed on the sterile field should incorporate a radiopaque strip or thread that makes them X-ray detectable. An X-ray-detectable strip facilitates location of sponges presumed to be retained in the patient should a count discrepancy occur. Sponges include:

    - Lap pads (also referred to as tapes and lap packs)—square or rectangular gauze pads with an X-ray-detectable tape sewn in the corner of the pad. These are used where moderate to large amounts of blood or fluid are encountered.

    - Gauze sponges (also referred to as raytec and swabs)—approximately 4×4 inch squares of gauze used where a small amount of blood or fluid is anticipated. They may also be folded and clamped to forceps to be used for swabbing an area.

    - Peanuts—very small sponges approximately the size of a peanut. They are clamped to forceps and used for dissection or to absorb a small amount of fluid or blood on delicate tissue.

    - Kitner dissectors—a small roll of heavy cotton tape that is clamped to forceps and used for dissection or absorption.

    - Tonsil sponges—cotton-filled gauze in the shape of a ball. They have a long tape attached to them and are used in tonsil surgery, where they are inserted into the mouth to absorb blood and stop bleeding. The tape extends outside the mouth and is used for retrieval.

    - Cottonoid patties (also referred to as neuro sponges)—small sponges made of compressed cotton and supplied in a variety of sizes. They are used for surgeries on delicate structures such as the brain and spinal cord. Small patties include a long radiopaque thread. When these patties become saturated with blood they are difficult to see. The thread facilitates location.

    - Pledgets—small pieces of felt used as a support under sutures in friable tissues.

21. Before surgery begins, the scrub person and the circulating nurse count all sponges on the field and document the count. The count is performed aloud and together. Sponges must be handled so that both persons can visually verify the count.

22. Sponges are generally supplied from the manufacturer in packs of five and ten and are held together with a paper strip. It must never be assumed that the amount indicated on the package label is accurate. The paper strip must be removed and all sponges must be separated and individually counted. If a commercially prepared package of sponges is found to be incorrect, it should be removed from the field, bagged, labeled as such, and isolated from the rest of the sponges in the room.

23. If additional sponges are needed during the procedure, they are delivered to the sterile field, counted together and aloud, and the addition is recorded.

24. During surgery, the scrub person discards used sponges into a plastic-lined kick bucket provided for this purpose.

25. When a unit of five or ten sponges accumulates, the circulating nurse counts them aloud together with the scrub person and places them in an impervious bag. Soiled sponges are handled with an instrument or with gloved hands and never with bare hands. At the end of the procedure, the bags containing sponges are disposed of in a manner that reduces the risk of bloodborne pathogen dis-

ease transmission. Sponges contaminated with blood, which if compressed would release blood, are placed in leak-proof containers/bags that are color coded, labeled, or tagged as infectious waste (AORN, 2004a, p. 275). Individual healthcare facility policy and the United States Department of Labor, Occupational Safety and Health Administration, Bloodborne Pathogen Standard 1910-1030 (2001) should be consulted for guidelines related to personal protective equipment and disposal of infectious waste. In some states, the regulations for definition and disposal of regulated waste may be more stringent than federal regulations. As a result, policies for managing soiled sponges will vary with the institution.

26. All sponges that were opened for the procedure should remain in the room until the procedure is completed and the patient has left the room. Trash and linen containers should also remain in the room. This will assist in locating a missing sponge in the event that the count cannot be immediately reconciled.

27. As wound closure begins, the scrub person and the circulating nurse count aloud and together all sponges on the sterile field and any in the bucket. This number is added to the number of bagged sponges. The total should equal the number supplied for the surgery.

28. The procedure for counting sponges should be consistent, that is, follow the same sequence each time. Typically the count starts at the surgical site, continues to the Mayo stand, then the back table, and finally to the discarded sponges. Consistency promotes efficiency and continuity.

29. The surgical team is informed of the results of the count. If the count is accurate, closure will continue. As skin closure begins, a final count of sponges is conducted in the same manner. The results are reported to the surgical team and are documented.

30. If a count is found to be incorrect at the time of wound closure, the surgical team is notified and a thorough search, beginning within the wound and including the operative field, the room, and the trash, is initiated for any missing sponge.

31. Common institutional policy is that if the count remains incorrect after skin closure, an incident report is filed and an X-ray taken before the patient leaves the operating room. If an X-ray reveals a retained sponge, appropriate measures are taken to retrieve it and complete the surgery.

32. Steps to minimize the possibility of an incorrect sponge count include keeping to a minimum the amount, size, and types of sponges opened for a procedure, and containing all sponges in the room by not removing any linen, trash, or supplies from the operating room until after the patient leaves the room.

33. If the surgeon chooses to pack the surgical wound, the packaging should not be with X-ray-detectable sponges. X-ray-detectable sponges should not be used as a dressing for the wound. Should an X-ray be required, any X-ray-detectable sponge in or on the patient could appear to be a retained sponge.

· ·

SECTION QUESTIONS

Q6. Only sponges that contain a(n) _____ strip should be used on the surgical field. (Ref. 20)

Q7. List five types of sponges that should be counted. (Ref. 20)

_____   _____

_____   _____

_____

Q8.   Sponge counts should be (Ref. 21):

   a. performed silently

   b. performed by the scrub person and the circulating nurse

   c. visually verified

Q9. Sponges are generally supplied by the manufacturer in packs of five and ten and are held together by a strip. It is acceptable practice to accept the amount on the package label as accurate. (Ref. 22)

True   False

Q10. As sponges are discarded during surgery they should be counted in units of five and ten and placed on a sheet until wound closure, when they are placed in an impervious bag. (Ref. 24, 25)

True   False

Q11. Steps to minimize the possibility of an incorrect sponge count include (Ref. 32):

a. keeping the type of sponges used for a procedure to a minimum

b. containing all sponges in the room until the patient leaves the room

c. counting together each time a sponge is discarded from the sterile field during the procedure

• •

Sharps Counts

34. Sharps include but are not limited to scalpel blades, suture needles, hypodermic needles, cautery blades and needles, and safety pins.

35. The procedure for counting sharps is essentially the same as for counting sponges. Counting must be done concurrently, visibly, and aloud by the scrub person and the circulating nurse. Sharps counts are documented.

36. Atraumatic sutures may be supplied in packages containing multiple sutures. When counting these sutures, it is acceptable practice to count needles according to the number indicated on the packet label. Once the scrub person opens a suture package, both the scrub person and the nurse must verify the number of needles inside (Fogg, 1994, p. 848). To prevent an excess of needles on the field, it is good practice to keep the packet unopened until needed.

37. Occasionally a needle or blade will break during a surgical procedure. When this occurs, the sharp(s) in question must be accounted for in their entirety. On occasion, the risk of injury to a patient may be greater if a needle or piece of a needle is retrieved than if it is left to encapsulate in tissue. The decision not to retrieve a needle rests with the surgeon. Individual institutional policy dictates documentation of such an occurrence.

38. If a sharp is removed from the sterile field for any reason during a procedure, the circulating nurse should isolate it and keep it in a designated place in the operating room until the final count is performed and the procedure is complete. As with sponges, the procedure for counting sharps should be consistent.

39. Some surgical procedures require the use of a large number of suture needles. Frequent needle counts can help reduce the risk of an incorrect count.

40. Sharps should be contained on a magnetic needle mat or other device designed for this purpose. Sharps pose a risk of inflicting injury and permitting transmission of infectious disease to patients and personnel. Loose sharps should never be permitted on the sterile field.

41. Following the procedure, sharps must be disposed of in containers that are leak proof, puncture resistant, and color coded, or labeled as biohazardous waste (OSHA, 2001, [d][2][vii][A]).

Instrument Counts

42. Although the risk of a retained instrument is small, there are documented cases where it has occurred. Instrument counts are a means to reduce this risk. Instrument counts are most appropriate for procedures where a body cavity is entered or where an incision is large enough to permit an instrument to be accidentally retained (Gawande et al., 2003, p. 229).

43. In addition to being a means of providing safe patient care, instrument counts are a means of inventory control and cost containment. Instruments are less likely to be lost if they must be accounted for.

44. The procedure for counting instruments is essentially the same as for counting sponges and sharps; however, instruments are generally counted two times: once just prior to the procedure and again at wound closure. Instrument counts must be done concurrently, visibly, and aloud by the scrub person and the circulating nurse. Instrument counts are documented.

45. With the proliferation of minimally invasive surgery, many institutions have instituted a policy whereby instruments set up in the event that the surgery becomes an open procedure are counted prior to the procedure. If the case does not convert to an open procedure, a second instrument count is not taken.

46. Instruments that are removed from the sterile field should be retained in the operating room until the final count is performed and the patient leaves the room. Removal of an instrument from the room increases the potential for an incorrect count.

47. It is helpful when instrument sets are standardized and when the number of instruments in sets is kept to a minimum.

DOCUMENTATION

48. Count sheets, used for documentation of counts, may be either generic, specialty specific, or set specific. When sets are standardized, count sheets can be preprinted so that what is listed on the count sheet is identical to the contents of the set. Preprinted count sheets may list only the names of instruments contained within the sets, or they may list both the names and the amounts. Preprinted count sheets are helpful for those who are responsible for set assembly.

49. Counts should be documented. Some institutions require that the documentation be placed in the patient's intraoperative record. Other facilities maintain the documentation elsewhere. Regardless of where the documentation is maintained, it must be retrievable and should included the following information:

- what was counted, e.g., types of sponges, instruments, etc.
- results of the count
- surgeon who was notified of count results
- names, titles, and signatures of those who performed the count
- any item intentionally retained
- actions taken when a count is incorrect
- reason counts that would normally be performed were omitted, e.g, emergency, insufficient time
- action taken as a result of omitted count (Exhibit 7-1, 7-2, 7-3)

Exhibit 7–1 Instrument/Sponges/Needle Count Record

ST. VINCENT'S MEDICAL CENTER OF RICHMOND
INSTRUMENT/SPONGE/NEEDLE COUNT RECORD

OPERATION   DATE

SECTION A	COUNT BEFORE SURGERY	ADDED DURING SURGERY	COUNT BEFORE PERITONEUM	FINAL COUNT (BEFORE SKIN CLOSE)
Raytec Sponges (4x4)				
Laparotomy Sponges				
Cottonoid				
Peanuts				
Tonsil Sponges				
Umbilical Tapes				
Vessel Loops				
Scalpel Blades				
Reel Ties				
Retention Sutures				
Free Needles				
Atraumatic Needles				

SECTION B	BEFORE SURGERY	ADDED	BEFORE PERITONEUM	FINAL COUNT INSTS. AFTER PERITONEUM	SECTION B CONTINUED	BEFORE SURGERY	ADDED	BEFORE PERITONEUM	FINAL COUNT INSTS. AFTER PERITONEUM
Mosquitos (curv)					Richardson Retractors				
Criles					Deaver Retractors				
Kelly (med)					Ribbon Retractors				
Allis					Balfour, Blade, Screw				
Babcock					Self-Retaining				
Kelly (lg)					McBurney Retractors				
Allis (lg)					Vein Retractors				
Babcock (lg)					Allen (anastomosis)				
Kochers					Bowel (rt) Angle				
Adson					DeMartel Applier				
Mixters					DeMartel Clamps				
Metzenbaum Scissors					Mayo Robson Clamps				
Mayo Scissors (curv)					Payr Pylorus Clamps				
Mayo Scissors (str)					Bakes (dilators)				
Metzenbaum (lg)					Randall Stone				
Mayo (lg str)					Trocar				
Potts Scissors					Heaney				
Needle Holders					Kochers (curv)				
Sponge Sticks					Phaneuf				
Adson Forceps (plain)					Tenaculum				
Adson Forceps (mt)					Uterine Packing				
Forceps (plain)					Pedicle				
Forceps (mt)					Bronchus				
Forceps (plain/long)					Lung Clamps				
Forceps (mt/long)					Bulldog Clamps			'	
Arterial Forceps					Vascular Clamps				
Rings					Baby Mosquitos				
Suction					Baby Rt. Angles				
Towel Clips					Skin Hooks				
Scalpel Handle #3					Lahey				
Scalpel Handle #7					Hemoclip appliers				
Scalpel Handle #3L					Other				
Rakes									
Army/Navy									
Parker Retractors					COUNTS ARE:				

SCRUB NURSE   RELIEF-SCRUB NURSE   CIRC. NURSE   RELIEF CIRC. NURSE

FORM 996 (9/86) MADISON BUSINESS FORMS

Source: Courtesy of St. Vincent's Medical Center of Richmond, Staten Island, New York.

Exhibit 7–2 Instrument/Sponge/Needle Count Record

GENERAL INSTRUCTIONS:

1. Instruments will be counted on all procedures which include invasion of peritoneum and an anticipated incision of more than three inches.
2. Instruments will be counted on all other procedures which do not invade the peritoneum but where incision is anticipated to be greater than three inches.
3. Sponges and needles will be counted on all procedures.
4. Incorrectly numbered packaged sponges must be isolated and not used during the procedure.
5. Instruments, counted sponges, and needles should never be taken from the O.R. for any reason during a procedure.
6. Instruments or needles broken or disassembled during a procedure must be accounted for in their entirety.
7. Used needles should be kept on a needle pad to insure their containment on the table.

PROCEDURE:

1. Before surgery begins, the scrub nurse and circulating nurse count instruments, sponges, and needles together and out loud as each item is separated in the counting procedure.
2. This original count is recorded immediately after being taken by the circulating nurse, on the Instrument/Sponge/Needle Count Record Form #998A.
3. All instruments/sponges and needles added to the operative field during surgery are counted together and out loud by the scrub and circulating nurses and recorded immediately by the circulating nurse on Form #998A in the column marked "Added".
4. During the operative procedure, the circulating nurse:
   a) counts all sponges that are discarded from the operative field together and out loud with the scrub nurse.
   b) separates sponges into units.
   c) places counted sponges by units into plastic bags.
5. Before closure of peritoneum begins, the scrub nurse and the circulating nurse count together and out loud:
   a) all instruments/sponges/needles contained within the operative field which were counted before surgery and which were added during surgery.
   b) all instruments/sponges/needles which have been discarded from the operative field which were counted before surgery and which were added during surgery.
   c) the circulating nurse records the tally in the column marked "Before Peritoneum Closure".
   d) the circulating nurse reports to the surgeon, out loud, the results of this count.
6. Before skin closure begins the scrub and circulating nurses count out loud and together all instruments which were used after the peritoneum closure and all items included in Section A of the Instrument/Sponge/Needle Count Record Form #998A.
   a) This final count is recorded by the circulating nurse in the column marked "Final Count" on Form #988A.
   b) Result of this count, e.g. correct or incorrect, is recorded on Form #998A in the appropriate space.
   c) The scrub nurse and circulating nurse write their name and status in the appropriate space on Form #998A.

Source: Courtesy of F. Zarnick, Director of Nursing Services, St. Vincent's Medical Center of Richmond, Staten Island, New York.

Exhibit 7–3 Instrument Count Sheet

Minor Set SMC

Setcode ID/SN: GEN01 / 00010
Department/Speciality:
Packaging: 3/4 Size Container
Remarks:
Comments:

Production No.: 20040513000001
Printed On: 5/13/2004 8:28 PM
User: Joan Spear

Act	Min	Tgt	Catalog	Instrument Name	1st	2nd	Add	Final
				PUT ON STRINGER				
2		2	BH648R	Kocher Forceps Str 1×2 9"				
4		4	BH201R	Adson Delicate Forceps Cvd 7 1/4"				
4		4	BH443R	Rochester-pean Forceps Cvd 6 1/4"				
8		8	BH167R	Crile Forceps Cvd 6 1/4"				
4		4	EA030R	Babcock Tissue Forceps 6"				
4		4	EA016R	Allis Forceps 5×6 6"				
2		2	BH144R	Crile Forceps Str 5 1/2"				
4		4	BF463R	Lorna Towel Clamp Non-perf 5 1/8"				
1		1	BM065R	Tc Mayo-hegar Needle Holder Hvy Serr 6"				
2		2	BM066R	Tc Mayo-hegar Needle Holder Hvy Serr 7"				
1		1	BC242R	Tc Mayo Disect Scis Rnd Bld Str L-6 3/4"				
1		1	BC243R	Tc Mayo Disec Scis Rnd Blds Cvd L-6 3/4"				
1		1	BC261R	Tc Metzenbaum Scissors Cvd 5 3/4"				
1		1	BC263R	Tc Metzenbaum Scissors Cvd 7"				
				LAY IN PAN				
1		1	BF122R	Foerster Sponge Fcps Serr Str 9 1/2"				
2		2	SU3472	Richardson Retractor 9-1/4 32×29mm				
2		2	SU3474	Richardson Retractor 10 38×38mm				
2		2	SU3470	Richardson Retractor 9-1/4 25×19mm				
2		2	BT041R	Usa-army Retractors 8 3/4" 2/set				
1		1	BV200R	Self-retaining Retr 3×4 Sharp 7 3/4"				
1		1	GF862R	Pool Suction Cannula Charr. 30				
2		2	BD512R	Adson Tissue Fcps Fine Serr 4 3/4"				
1		1	BD579R	Tissue Forceps 2×3 6 1/4"				
2		2	BB074R	Scalpel Handle #3 With Measure				
2		2	BD701R	Brown Atraumatic Tissue Forceps 6"				
1		1	US061R	Metal Sponge Bowl 1 Qt				
1		1	US066R	Metal Medicine Cup 2 Oz				
2		2	FB414R	Debakey Atra Fcps 2.8mm Str 6"				
1		1	00107	Cautery Holder				
2		2	BV996R	Gelpi Vaginal Retractor 5 1/4"				

Actual: 64   Target: 64   Assembled By: Joan Spear

instacount PLUS   Aesculap 3773 Corporate Parkway; Center Valley PA 18034 800258-1946

Source: Adapted from Aesculap, Inc. Used with permission.

SECTION QUESTIONS

Q12. If a sharp is removed from the sterile field for any reason during the surgical procedure, the circulating nurse should immediately dispose of it in a proper sharps container. (Ref. 38, 41)

True   False

Q13. Instrument counts (Ref. 42, 43, 44):

a. do not require documentation

b. are a means of inventory control

c. reduce risk of patient injury

Q14. Contaminated instruments removed from the sterile field should be retained in the operating room until the patient leaves the room. (Ref. 46)

True   False

Q15. List 5 things regarding counts that should be documented. (Ref. 49)

• • • References

Association of periOperative Registered Nurses (AORN). (2004a). Recommended practices for environmental cleaning. In *Standards, recommended practices and guidelines* (pp. 273–279). Denver, CO: Author.

AORN. (2004b). Standards: Patient outcomes. In *Standards, recommended practices and guidelines* (pp. 197–206). Denver, CO: Author.

Beyea, S. (2003). Counting instruments and sponges. *AORN Journal, 78*(2), 291.

Fogg, D. (1994). Clinical issues: Counting multipack suture. *AORN Journal, 60*(5) 854–859.

Gawande, A. A., Studdert, D. M., Orav, E. J., Brennan, T. A., Zinner, M. (2003). Risk factors for retained instruments and sponges after surgery. *New England Journal of Medicine, 348*(3), 229–235.

U.S. Department of Labor, Occupational Safety & Health Administration (OSHA). Jan 18, 2001. (Regulations—Standards-29CFR), Bloodborne pathogens. 1910-1030. Retrieved February 25, 2004, from www.osha.gov/pls/oshaweb/owadisp.show_document?p_table=STADARDS&p_id=10051

Appendix 7-A

. . . .

Chapter 7 Post Test

Instructions: Fill in the blank(s), mark the correct answer(s), or answer the question as appropriate.

1. Surgical counts guarantee that unintended items will not be retained in the patient. (Ref. 6, 13)

   True   False

2. Indicate three consequences for a patient who experiences an unintended retained foreign body. (Ref. 2)

   _____

3. List three symptoms of a retained foreign body. (Ref. 3)

   _____

4. Surgical counts (Ref. 5, 6, 7, 9, 12, 16, 19)

   a. are a means to reduce the patient's risk of injury

   b. are a shared responsibility

   c. should be documented

   d. should be performed according to institutional policy

   e. that are incorrect may incur liability for any or all members of the surgical team

5. A correct count at the end of a procedure is a guarantee that no unintended foreign body has been retained. (Ref. 13)

   True   False

6. Explain why all counted items should be removed from the room at the end of surgery. (Ref. 17)

   _____

7. The count procedure should start at the back table, progress to the Mayo stand, and then to the surgical site. (Ref. 28)

   True   False

8. If a count is found to be incorrect during the procedure, the _____ is notified immediately so that a search may be initiated. (Ref. 30)

   a. surgical team

   b. supervisor

   c. OR director

9. Suture needles (Ref. 36, 37):

   a. should be accounted for in their entirety

   b. should always be retrieved in their entirety

   c. should be counted according to the amount indicated on the package and confirmed when the package is opened

   d. should be stored in a medicine cup to keep them together

10. Instruments removed from the sterile field during a surgical procedure requiring an instrument count should be immediately sent to the instrument processing room for decontamination. (Ref. 46)

    True   False

11. Circle the correct statement(s). (Ref. 8, 9, 10, 13, 19, 48)

    a. According to the AORN Recommended Practice on Counts, instruments should be counted on all procedures.

    b. Policies determining what is counted may be based on the anticipated size of the incision.

    c. A documented "correct count" is a guarantee that nothing has been retained unintentionally.

    d. The nurse is responsible for documenting information related to counts.

    e. Counts must be performed together, concurrently and aloud and counted items must be visible to both persons counting.

    f. Preprinted instrument count sheets with instrument names and amounts may be used for performing counts.

12. The following should be documented and saved as a permanent record (Ref. 49):

    a. results of the count

    b. whether a count was omitted as a result of an emergency

    c. names and amounts of sponges, sharps and miscellaneous items

    d. intentionally retained items

    e. name, title and signature of those who performed count

    f. that an X-ray was taken because of an incorrect count

Appendix 7-B

• •

Competency Checklist: Counts in Surgery

Under "Observer's Initials," enter initials upon successful achievement of competency.
Enter N/A if competency is not appropriate for institution.

NAME _____

	OBSERVER'S INITIALS	DATE
1. Counts are performed and documented:		
a. prior to procedure	_____	_____
b. during procedure when items are added	_____	_____
c. before closure of a body cavity	_____	_____
d. prior to skin closure	_____	_____
e. at time of relief	_____	_____
2. Count is performed together, concurrently, and aloud by scrub person and circulating nurse.	_____	_____
3. Items being counted are visible to scrub person and circulating nurse.	_____	_____
a. sponges are separated for visibility	_____	_____
4. Sharps are maintained on a needle mat (or other device designed for this purpose).	_____	_____
5. Counts are verified when personnel are relieved.	_____	_____
6. Contents of multipack sutures are verified when package opened	_____	_____
7. Sponges that are discarded are counted in units of five or ten and bagged.	_____	_____
8. All sponges, sharps or instruments opened for the procedure are retained in the room until the procedure is completed.	_____	_____
9. Count begins at the surgical site and progresses to the Mayo tray and the back table.	_____	_____
10. Sponges are handled according to OSHA guidelines.	_____	_____
11. Surgeon is notified of count results.	_____	_____
12. Names of all persons who performed counts during procedure are documented.	_____	_____
13. Documentation is complete.	_____	_____

OBSERVER'S SIGNATURE   INITIALS   DATE

_____

ORIENTEE'S SIGNATURE

_____

Chapter 7—Section Question Answers

Q1. Sponges, sharps, instruments
Q2. True
Q3. False
Q4. a
Q5. a, b, d, e
Q6. X-ray-detectable
Q7. Gauze, laps, peanuts, cottonoid, kitner dissectors, tonsil sponges, pledgets
Q8. b, c
Q9. False
Q10. False
Q11. a, b
Q12. False
Q13. b, c
Q14. True
Q15. What was counted; results of the count; name and signature of those who performed the count; surgeon notified of count results; items intentionally retained; action taken when count is not correct; reasons counts that would ordinarily be taken were omitted; action taken as a result of omitted count

Chapter 7—Post Test Answers

1. False
2. Pain, readmission, additional surgery, extended hospital stay, delayed healing
3. Cramping, fever, pain, cavity abscess
4. a, b, c, d, e
5. False
6. May cause an incorrect count in a subsequent surgical procedure in that room
7. False
8. a
9. a, c
10. False
11. b, d, e, f
12. a, b, c, d, e, f

Prevention of Injury—Hemostasis, Tourniquet, and Electrosurgical Equipment

---

LEARNER OBJECTIVES

After reading and completing "Prevention of Injury—Hemostasis, Tourniquet, and Electrosurgical Equipment," the learner will:

- describe the natural process of hemostasis
- list five means of artificial hemostasis
- identify three potential patient injuries related to use of tourniquet
- list two criteria for evaluating achievement of desired patient outcome relative to use of tourniquet
- describe nursing interventions to prevent patient injury when tourniquet is used
- identify three potential patient injuries related to the use of electro-surgical equipment
- identify and define general electrosurgical terms
- describe potential injury related to capacitive coupling
- identify the desired patient outcome relative to use of electrosurgical equipment
- list four criteria for evaluating achievement of desired patient outcome relative to electrosurgical equipment
- describe nursing interventions to prevent patient injury when electro-surgical equipment is used
- list information that should be documented when tourniquet or electro-surgical equipment is used
- discuss use of an ultrasonic energy device (scalpel) and an argon beam coagulator

. . . .
Lesson Outline

I. HEMOSTASIS
  A. Natural Methods of Hemostasis
  B. Artificial Methods of Hemostasis
    1. Chemical Hemostasis
      a. Thrombin
      b. Absorbable Gelatin
      c. Oxidized Cellulose
      d. Microfibrillar Collagen
      e. Styptic
    2. Mechanical Hemostasis
      a. Instruments, Ties, Suture Ligatures, Ligating Clips
      b. Bonewax
      c. Pressure
II. TOURNIQUET
  A. Overview
  B. Nursing Diagnosis—Desired Patient Outcome
  C. Nursing Interventions
III. ELECTRICAL HEMOSTASIS—ELECTROSURGERY
  A. Overview
  B. Electrosurgical Components
    1. The Generator
    2. The Active Electrode
    3. The Dispersive Electrode
  C. Application
  D. Nursing Diagnosis—Desired Patient Outcomes
    1. Desired Patient Outcome/Criteria
  E. Nursing Interventions—Patient and Staff Safety
    1. Electrosurgical Use During Endoscopic Surgery—Special Precautions
IV. ULTRASONIC ENERGY DEVICES
  A. Overview
  B. System Components
  C. Tissue Effects
  D. Technology Characteristics
  E. Applications
V. ARGON BEAM–ENHANCED ELECTROSURGERY
  A. Overview
  B. System Components
  C. Application/Characteristics

HEMOSTASIS

1. *Hemostasis* is the arrest or control of bleeding. Historically, attempts to achieve hemostasis have included applications of egg yolk, dust, cobwebs, hot oil, cautery with hot irons, and use of crude sutures made from materials such as cotton or harp strings derived from sheep intestine. Until the advent of modern hemostatic methods, blood loss made surgery difficult and was a serious surgical complication.

2. Modern hemostatic methods, including electrosurgery and tourniquet application, have greatly enhanced the surgeon's ability to perform slow, deliberate surgery and to operate in a field where control of bleeding permits excellent visualization of anatomical structures.

3. Hemostasis may be achieved by natural or artificial methods.

Natural Methods of Hemostasis

4. When an injury occurs to a blood vessel, a roughened surface is created. Platelets are attracted to and adhere to this surface. Several layers accumulate, and a platelet plug is formed. A platelet plug is often sufficient to seal small injuries. As the platelets break down, they release thromboplastin into the blood. Thromboplastin is necessary for coagulation to occur.

5. Platelet plug formation is not the same as coagulation. In coagulation, a fibrin clot is formed. Coagulation is a complex mechanism involving multiple clotting factors and a series of reactions. During coagulation, prothrombin, which is present in blood, reacts with thromboplastin, which is released when tissues are injured and platelets break down. Prothrombin, thromboplastin, and calcium ions in the blood form thrombin. In the final step, thrombin unites with fibrinogen, a blood plasma, to form fibrin. Fibrin is the basic structure of the clot and reinforces the platelet plug. Initially this fibrin is white. As platelets, white cells, and red cells become entangled in the fibrin, the clot becomes red, taking on the appearance of a blood clot. The process of coagulation is regulated so that, as blood loss is controlled, coagulation ceases.

6. In spite of the complexity of the coagulation process, it is rapid and sufficient to prevent blood loss from most small wounds.

Artificial Methods of Hemostasis

7. Natural hemostasis is not sufficient to control bleeding during surgery. Gross bleeding and oozing occur during surgery, and both are controlled through artificial hemostatic methods. Chemical, mechanical, or thermal methods may be used and can include the use of thrombin, absorbable gelatin, oxidized cellulose, microfibrillar collagen, collagen pads, styptics, pressure, instruments, ties, suture ligatures, ligating clips, staples, bonewax, tourniquet, and electrosurgery. Tourniquet and electrosurgery have significant patient safety implications and are addressed in depth in this chapter.

Chemical Hemostasis

THROMBIN

8. Thrombin is an enzyme made from dried beef blood. It combines with fibrinogen and accelerates the coagulation process. Thrombin is useful in controlling capillary bleeding. It is supplied as a dry white powder that may be sprinkled on an oozing site. More often, it is mixed with water or saline to form a solution and is used in conjunction with a gelatin sponge. Thrombin is for topical use only and must never be injected. Thrombin will lose its potency within 3 hours and should be mixed just prior to use. Thrombin in combination with gelatin sponge is particularly useful in vascular surgery for controlling capillary bleeding at the site of a vascular graft.

ABSORBABLE GELATIN

9. Absorbable gelatin is made from a purified gelatin solution. It is available as a powder or a compressed pad (Gelfoam). In the compressed form it resembles Styrofoam. When placed on an area of capillary bleeding, fibrin will be deposited in the interstices of the pad, the pad will swell, and clot formation will progress. Gelfoam pads are available in a variety of sizes and may be cut to desired size. Gelfoam may be used alone, but is frequently dipped in a thrombin solution. Gelfoam may also be soaked in epinephrine before application. Gelfoam absorbs 45 times its weight in blood. It is not soluble; however, when left in the body it will be absorbed in 20 to 40 days. In the powder form, gelatin is mixed with sterile saline to form a paste. Once hemostasis has been achieved, it is common to remove gelatin to prevent compression of adjacent anatomic structures.

OXIDIZED CELLULOSE

10. Oxidized regenerated cellulose (Oxycel, Surgicel, and Surgicel Nu-Knit) is a specially treated knitted gauze or cotton applied directly to an oozing surface to control bleeding. It absorbs seven to eight times its own weight. When oxidized cellulose contacts whole blood, it increases its size, forms a gel, and causes clot formation. The pressure of the swollen cellulose also encourages hemostasis. Oxidized cellulose is used to control bleeding in areas that are difficult to control by other means of hemostasis. Oxidized cellulose may be applied in layers, in tufts, or in a roll. It may be left on an oozing surface and will be absorbed by the body in 7 to 14 days. It must, however, be removed when used around the optic nerve or spinal cord, where swelling of the cellulose can exert harmful pressure on these structures.

MICROFIBRILLAR COLLAGEN

11. Microfibrillar collagen (Avitene, Instat) is a fluffy, white, absorbable material made from purified bovine dermis. It is applied dry and directly over the source of bleeding. Its form allows it to be placed in crevices and areas of irregular contour. Hemostasis is achieved when platelets and fibrin adhere to the collagen and clot formation pro-

gresses. Microfibrillar collagen is useful where tissue is friable. Collagen pads, sponges, and felt are also available and are applied directly to a bleeding surface. Microfibrillar collagen is absorbable; however, excess material should be removed once hemostasis has been achieved.

Styptic

12. Styptics are agents that cause blood vessel constriction. Epinephrine is a frequently used styptic. It is often added to a local anesthetic, such as lidocaine, to constrict blood vessels and decrease bleeding at the site of the surgery.

13. Silver nitrate, in the form of a stick or pencil with a silver nitrate crystal head, is another form of styptic. It is applied topically to small vessels.

14. Tannic acid, silver nitrate, and 95% phenol in combination with 95% alcohol are three less frequently used topical agents. Tannic acid may be used on mucous membranes in the nose. Silver nitrate mixed with silver chloride and formed into an applicator stick is used as a topical hemostatic agent. A phenol and alcohol combination is sometimes used to seal the site where the appendix was removed.

Mechanical Hemostasis

Instruments, Ties, Suture Ligatures, Ligating Clips

15. A hemostatic clamp may be used to occlude the end of a bleeding vessel. As long as the clamp is in place, bleeding will not occur. Clamping is a temporary means of hemostasis and is followed by the application of a tie, a suture ligature, a ligating clip, or electrocautery. A tie is a strand of material tied around the vessel to occlude the lumen. A suture ligature is a tie with an attached needle that is used to anchor the tie through the vessel. A ligating clip (Hemoclip, Ligaclip, Surgiclip) is a stainless steel, tantalum, or titanium clip used to permanently close off a vessel. Except for clips made from synthetic absorbable suture, ligating clips remain permanently within the patient.

Bonewax

16. Bonewax is made from beeswax and is used to stop bleeding from bone. It is rolled into a ball and rubbed over a cut bone surface to control bleeding. Bonewax is used most often in neurosurgery and orthopedic surgery.

Pressure

17. Pressure is applied when sponges are used to blot areas of bleeding. When a sponge is removed, it is possible to identify the area of bleeding and to employ additional methods of hemostasis. Manual pressure applied directly to small vessels may delay bleeding long enough for clot formation to begin.

• •

SECTION QUESTIONS

Q1. Coagulation (Ref. 4, 5, 6):

   a. is a natural process

   b. is the same as a platelet plug formation

   c. is a complex process that involves multiple clotting factors

   d. is a slow deliberate process

   e. ceases as blood loss is controlled

   f. is a process that is sufficient to prevent blood loss from most small wounds

Q2. Artificial means of hemostasis include (Ref. 7):

   a. gelatin sponge

   b. suture ligatures

   c. blood transfusion

   d. ligating clips

   e. electrosurgery

Q3. Match the method of hemostasis with its description. (Ref. 8–15)

a. absorbable gelatin   _____ epinephrine

b. thrombin   _____ stainless steel clip used to clamp a vessel

c. oxidized cellulose   _____ specially treated gauze or cotton used to control bleeding

d. styptic   _____ enzyme made from dried beef blood used to control capillary bleeding

e. hemoclip   _____ resembles Styrofoam, used to control capillary bleeding, may be dipped in thrombin

Q4. _____ is used in orthopedic surgery to control bleeding from bone. (Ref. 16)

• •

TOURNIQUET

Overview

18. Application of a tourniquet prior to surgery provides a bloodless surgical field. A pneumatic tourniquet is often used for surgery on an extremity. The resultant bloodless field enhances the surgeon's ability to complete the surgery and prevents blood loss for the patient. Once the tourniquet is released the severed vessels will bleed, and cauterization or ligation will be necessary to stop bleeding.

19. Tourniquets of various types are available. The simplest tourniquet is a piece of rubber tubing, such as a Penrose drain, that is used around an extremity in preparation for a venipuncture.

20. An Esmarch bandage is a long piece of rolled latex that is wrapped tightly around an extremity from the distal end toward the proximal end. Before application of a tourniquet, the extremity is raised to permit gravity to drain blood from the extremity. The Esmarch compresses superficial blood vessels and further forces the blood from the extremity. The Esmarch is removed, and while the limb is raised a pneumatic tourniquet is then applied.

21. Pneumatic tourniquets are inflated and maintained at a specified pressure required for the surgery and requested by the surgeon. Pneumatic tourniquets contain an internal bladder housed in a pressure cuff. The bladder is inflated with either ambient air or compressed gas from a cartridge, tank, or compressed-air line.

Nursing Diagnosis—Desired Patient Outcome

22. The nursing diagnosis of high risk for injury related to use of tourniquet is appropriate for the patient on whom a tourniquet is used.

Tourniquet injury can include skin injury, such as chemical burn from prep solutions; abrasion, bruise or blister formation; swelling, pain or nerve injury, including paralysis.

23. The Association of periOperative Registered Room Nurses (AORN) outcome standard states, "The patient is free from signs and symptoms of injury caused by extraneous objects (AORN, 2004b, p. 198). The patient should not experience an injury as a result of tourniquet use.

Nursing Interventions

24. Nursing interventions to prevent injury from tourniquet application require knowledge of equipment use and appropriate safety precautions. Institutional policy and practice may dictate who has responsibility for tourniquet application. Regardless of who actually applies the tourniquet, patient safety with regard to its use is a responsibility shared by nursing, surgeon, and anesthesia personnel. The perioperative nurse must be able to select a tourniquet of the appropriate size and in good working condition; and the nurse must be knowledgeable regarding the principles of application.

25. Prior to tourniquet application, the patient's skin should be assessed for integrity and turgor; and the extremity size should be evaluated in order to select an appropriately sized tourniquet cuff.

26. The pneumatic tourniquet should be tested and inspected for integrity, cleanliness, and function prior to use. Testing should be performed according to the manufacturer's written instructions and healthcare facility policy. Most policies for tourniquet testing require periodic testing to ensure that the pressures are accurate and that the tourniquet functions properly. Most automated systems contain a microprocessor that performs self-calibration.

27. The cuff and tubing should be free of cracks. Cracks can result in unintentional pressure loss. Connections should be secure, and electrical cords should be intact. Inspection should also include a check of the last inspection by biomedical engineering. A sticker indicating inspection by biomedical engineering within the last 12 months should be present. When nitrogen gas is used to inflate the cuff, the level of gas in the tank should be checked before each use to ensure that there is an adequate amount for the duration of the intended surgery. Close inspection of the cuff for cleanliness is important. Velcro fasteners are areas where microorganisms and other debris can collect. Water left in a tourniquet cuff port can cause microbial growth with the potential for entry of microorganisms into the tourniquet-regulating mechanism when the cuff is deflated (AORN, 2004d, p. 336). Tourniquet cuffs and bladders should be cleaned and dried between patient uses. An Environmental Protection Agency (EPA) registered tuberculocidal germicide should be used to clean, and manufacturer's instructions for use strictly followed. The gauges and pressure source should also be inspected for cleanliness and cleaned as needed.

28. The selection of a tourniquet cuff should take into consideration the size of the patient's extremity. As wide a cuff as possible should be selected because a wider cuff occludes blood flow at a lower pressure. The length of the cuff should permit an overlap that is adequate to provide even pressure on the circumference of the extremity. Overlap should be approximately 3 to 6 inches. Too much overlap can cause increased pressure in the area of the overlap (AORN, 2004d, p. 336).

29. Except where the manufacturer specifies in writing that padding is not required, the tourniquet should not be applied to unprotected skin. A Webril or stockinette material should be wrapped around the extremity where the tourniquet will be applied. Care must be taken to prevent bunching or wrinkling the material, which can result in uneven pressure against the skin and create the potential for the impairment of skin integrity. When a patient is extremely obese, an assistant should apply traction of the excess skin until the tourniquet is applied to prevent overlapping of skin and possible shearing injury.

30. The tourniquet should be placed on the limb at the point most proximal to the surgery and at the point of maximum circumference, according to the manufacturer's written instructions for use. This area provides the greatest amount of soft tissue and therefore protection of underlying nerves and blood vessels (AORN, 2004b, p. 336). Care should be taken when a tourniquet is applied to the calf not to compromise the head of the fibula, which can result in damage to superficial nerves in the area.

31. The area of tourniquet application should be protected from any potential or actual pooling or collection of fluids, which can irritate the skin. Prepping agents, if allowed to pool under the cuff, have the potential to cause a chemical burn to the skin. The nurse should remove excess liquid resulting from the prep and should protect the area from subsequent pooling of fluids during surgery by applying a protective fluid barrier. Such a barrier may be included as part of the extremity drape and will be applied during the draping procedure.

32. Exact tourniquet inflation pressures have not been determined. The lowest pressure needed to create a bloodless field should be used. Patient age, extremity size, systolic blood pressure, and tourniquet cuff size are factors that determine inflation pressures. Excessive inflation pressure can cause muscle weakness or paralysis, and insufficient pressure can result in passive congestion of the limb and hemorrhagic infiltration of a nerve (AORN, 2004d, p. 338). Newer tourniquet systems automatically measure the minimum cuff pressure needed to occlude arterial blood flow distal to the cuff and will maintain the cuff at this pressure.

33. The exact length of time for tourniquet inflation has not been determined; however, inflation times should be kept to a minimum. Excessive inflation times can damage underlying tissue and cause injury as severe as permanent paralysis. For an adult, 1 hour for an upper extremity and $1\frac{1}{2}$ to 2 hours for a lower extremity are usual inflation times. A lower pressure is used for children and for patients in whom blood supply to the extremity is diminished. Insufficient pressure and subsequent prolonged venous congestion can also result in nerve injury.

34. During the surgery, the nurse should periodically report to the surgeon the length of time that the tourniquet has been inflated. Most tourniquet systems automatically display pressure readings and inflation time and will sound an alarm when a predetermined time is reached. Intervals for reporting inflation times should be agreed upon between the surgeon and the nurse and may be indicated in the facility policy for tourniquet application. Anesthesia personnel also monitor inflation times. All team members must work in concert to ensure adequate and appropriate communication.

35. Throughout the surgery the nurse should refer to the tourniquet gauge to determine fluctuations in pressure that may indicate a tourniquet failure.

36. In the case of inadvertent loss of pressure, the tourniquet should be totally deflated, the extremity allowed to reperfuse, and an elastic bandage or the action of gravity should be used to force the blood out of the extremity before the tourniquet is reinflated. The tourniquet should not be reinflated over an area already engorged with blood. To do so creates a risk for intravascular thrombosis (AORN, 1995a, p. 229)

37. The tourniquet should be deflated upon instructions from the surgeon. When bilateral tourniquets are used, as in the case of bilateral arthroscopies, the cuffs should be deflated individually, with a 30-minute minimum time frame between extremities. This action will prevent excessive metabolites from rapidly entering the blood stream.

38. AORN Recommended Practices for use of the pneumatic tourniquet state that the perioperative nurse should document:

    - the assessment of skin and tissue integrity under the cuff before and after tourniquet use
    - the location of the cuff
    - the material used under the cuff to protect the skin
    - the cuff pressure
    - the time of inflation and deflation
    - the identification/serial number and model of the equipment used
    - the identification of the person who applied the cuff (AORN, 2004d, p. 339)

39. Documentation should also include an evaluation of the achievement of desired outcome.

• •

SECTION QUESTIONS

Q5. What is the purpose of an Esmarch bandage? (Ref. 20)

_____

_____

Q6. The patient on whom a tourniquet is used is at high risk for injury. List three potential injuries that can result from pneumatic tourniquet use. (Ref. 22)

_____

_____

_____

Q7. Prior to the application of a tourniquet the patient's extremity should be assessed for (Ref. 25):

    a. size

    b. skin turgor

    c. skin integrity

    d. capillary fill

Q8. Explain why a cuff as wide as possible should be selected for use with a pneumatic tourniquet. (Ref. 28)

_____

_____

Q9. Tourniquet pressure is determined by (Ref. 32):

    a. patient age

    b. size of extremity

    c. make of tourniquet

    d. tourniquet cuff size

Q10. Monitoring of inflation time and pressure is not the responsibility of the perioperative nurse. (Ref. 34, 35)

    True   False

Q11. Documentation regarding tourniquet application and use should include (Ref. 38, 39):

    a. skin assessment before and after cuff application

    b. location of cuff

    c. tourniquet cuff pressure

    d. inflation time

    e. evaluation of achievement of desired patient outcome

●●

ELECTRICAL HEMOSTASIS— ELECTROSURGERY

Overview

40. Electrosurgery is used routinely in most surgical procedures. Radio-frequency electrical current is passed through the patient's body for the purpose of cutting tissue or coagulating bleeding points.

41. As the current passes through the tissue, heat is generated in sufficient amounts to produce cutting and/or coagulation.

42. There are two different types of electrosurgery: bipolar and monopolar.

Electrosurgical Components

43. Three components necessary to perform monopolar electrosurgery are: (1) an electrosurgical unit (ESU) or generator, (2) an active electrode, and (3) a dispersive electrode. Bipolar electrosurgery requires only a generator and an active electrode handpiece that delivers current to the patient and also returns current back to the generator.

The Generator

44. The unit that supplies the current is referred to as an electrosurgical unit or generator. (Figure 8-1)

45. In the 1920s, Dr. William Bovie was instrumental in the development of the first spark-gap vacuum tube generator that produced cutting with hemostasis. This was the basis of electrosurgical units until the 1970s, when solid-state electrosurgical units were introduced. Solid-state units with small printed circuit boards and transistors have replaced the vacuum tube. However, many persons still

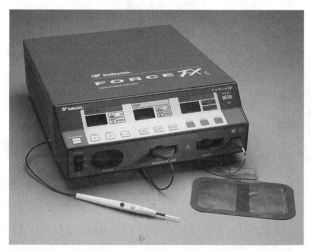

FIGURE 8-1 Electrosurgical generator, active and dispersive electrodes.
Source: Copyright © 2002, 2003, 2004 Valleylab, a division of Tyco Healthcare Group LP: Force FX?, REM?. All rights reserved.

refer to the solid-state electrosurgical units as "Bovie" machines.

46. Current is provided by the generator to the active electrode accessory that is used to introduce current into the patient. The dispersive electrode is an accessory that is in contact with the patient and returns the current from the patient back to the electrosurgical generator.

47. Early electrosurgical units presented significant risk for a burn or shock injury. Generators manufactured today are both solid-state and isolated systems and have dramatically reduced the risk of injury.

48. Early generators were the ground-referenced type. In a ground-referenced system, the generator acts as a ground to earth. If the circuit whereby the current returns to the machine is broken, the current may seek an alternate pathway and cause a burn at the site of contact. Alternate sites might include electrocardiogram electrodes and sites where the patient is touching a grounded metal item. If there is not proper contact between the patient and the dispersive electrode, there will be an interruption in the current. Use of ground-referenced generators in the United States is extremely rare. Ground-referenced systems have been replaced with isolated systems.

49. Isolated systems are a significant improvement over ground-referenced systems. In an isolated system there is a transformer within the generator that isolates the current from the ground. Current is restricted to pathways to and from the generator. In addition to isolated currents, systems used today include a patient-return electrode-monitoring system. The current that enters the patient is measured and compared with current returning to the dispersive electrode. If the currents are not sufficiently balanced, the unit will alarm and deactivate. These systems have virtually eliminated burns under the dispersive electrode.

50. Electrosurgical units are designed to deliver current that will cut, coagulate, or combine the two. The type of waveform that is selected determines whether cutting, coagulation, or a combination of the two will occur.

51. A continuous-frequency waveform will cause cutting to occur. In the cutting mode, tissue is severed as intense heat is delivered from the active electrode and focused at the intended site. The active electrode is held slightly above the tissue.

52. An interrupted-frequency waveform will cause coagulation to occur. In the coagulation mode, when the active electrode is in direct contact with the tissue, the ends of small- to moderate-sized vessels are seared and bleeding is controlled. When the active electrode is slightly above the tissue, a spark is produced and tissue is charred.

53. When a combination of the cut and coagulation waveform is selected, cutting and coagulation will occur simultaneously.

54. The amount of power and the type of current are regulated by controls on the electrosurgical unit and the accessories.

55. The selection of the type of current (waveform) and the amount of power is made by the surgeon and is determined by the procedure being performed and by surgeon preference.

The Active Electrode

56. The active electrode delivers current from the generator to the operative site. Active electrodes may be disposable or reusable. Most active electrodes are handheld devices with a cord that attaches to the electrosurgical generator. Active electrode tips may be shaped as a blade, ball, loop, hook, or needle that fits into a pencil-shaped handle or other device. (Figure 8-2) Active electrodes may also be combined with a suction catheter.

57. Active electrodes are activated by either a foot control or a control on the handpiece.

58. Active electrodes may be bipolar or monopolar. A monopolar electrode has one active pole or tip. This tip delivers concentrated current to the target tissue. The current is then dissipated through the patient's body, to the dispersive electrode, and then returned to the generator.

59. Bipolar electrodes are shaped as forceps with two poles or tips. One tip acts as the active electrode, and the other tip acts as the return or dispersive electrode. Current flows from the generator down one tine of the forceps, through the tissue between the forcep's tips, and is returned to the generator through the other tine of the forceps. Because the current flows only between the tips of the forceps, only low wattage is necessary. Precise hemostasis is provided, and current does not disperse

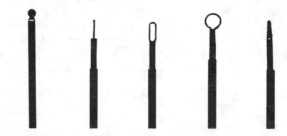

FIGURE 8-2   Examples of Active Electrode Tips.

throughout the patient. Because one tip of the forceps acts as a dispersive electrode, it is not necessary, as it is in monopolar electrosurgery, to attach a dispersive electrode to the patient.

The Dispersive Electrode

60. Dispersive electrodes are referred to by many names. These include grounding pad, inactive electrode, patient plate, "Bovie" pad, and return electrode.

61. Current enters the patient via the active electrode, where it is concentrated at the operative site and where tissue destruction is achieved. Current is then dissipated through the patient and returned to the generator via the dispersive electrode. Because the dispersive electrode is much larger than the active electrode, the current density is low at this site and therefore burns do not normally occur. (Figure 8-3)

62. Dispersive electrodes may be reusable or disposable.

63. Reusable dispersive electrodes made from metal have been replaced with products that incorporate a patient-return electrode with a pressure reduction pad and have current-limiting abilities to protect the patient from pad-site burns. One commonly used pad (MEGA 2000® Soft) measures 920 square inches. The pad is placed on the OR table to maximize contact with the pa-

tient. The patient lies directly on the pad, or a sheet can be placed between the patient and the pad. Unlike a disposable dispersive electrode, the pad does not adhere or stick to the patient. A cord connects the pad to the generator. Reusable dispersive electrodes may have patient weight minimums and requirements for placement. The pad must be used according to manufacturer's instructions. (Figure 8-4)

64. The most commonly used dispersive electrode is a disposable adhesive foil pad covered with a foam and impregnated with electrolyte gel. The dispersive electrode is in direct contact with the patient's skin. It has a cord that attaches to the generator. The dispersive electrode disperses the current released into the patient from the active electrode and provides the return path to the generator. The pad easily conforms to the patient's body contour and provides uniform contact with the patient. The adhesive promotes good conductivity. Newer electrosurgical systems employ a dispersive electrode that works with the generator to identify potential current concentration at the dispersive electrode site sufficient to cause a burn. When this occurs, the machine will alarm and deactivate. A scenario in which this might occur is if a dispersive electrode loosens from the patient and is only partially in contact with the patient's skin.

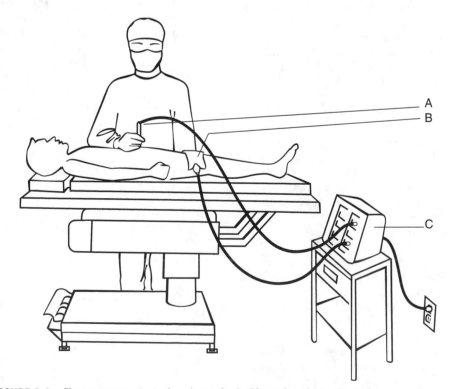

FIGURE 8-3　Electrosurgery. A. Active electrode. B. Dispersive electrode. C. Generator.

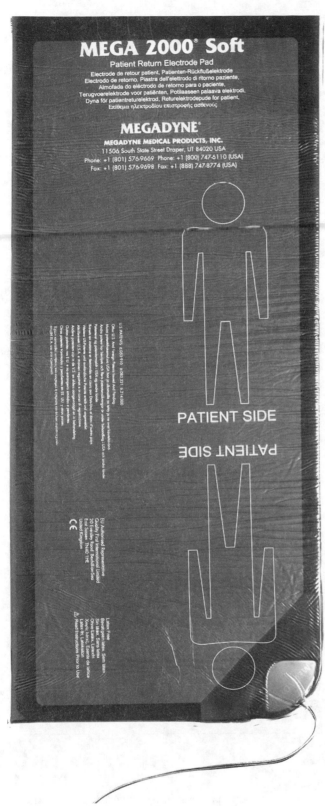

FIGURE 8-4 Patient Return Electrode Pad.
Source: Printed with permission from Megadyne Draper, Utah.

Application

65. Many surgeons prefer electrosurgery to other methods of hemostasis that involve cutting and tying tissue. Use of electrosurgery permits rapid achievement of cutting and coagulation and may reduce surgical time. However, coagulated tissue produces a foreign-body reaction and must be absorbed during the healing process. If there is an excessive amount of coagulated tissue in the wound, sloughing may occur and healing by first intention may not occur.

66. Electrosurgery is used in many types of surgery. A single power setting is not appropriate for all surgery. Differences in generator performance, surgical technique, and active electrode size determine power settings. Generally, low power is used in neurosurgery, dermatology procedures, and oral and plastic surgery.

67. Fulguration and desiccation are two types of coagulation. Fulguration is the use of sparking to coagulate large bleeders and to char tissue. In fulguration the active electrode does not actually contact the tissue. As sparks contact tissue, superficial coagulation initially results. As the sparking continues, this superficial coagulation is followed by necrosis. Fulguration is frequently used by urologists in transurethral resections where the intent is to cause necrosis and destroy tissue.

68. Coagulation in which the active electrode is in direct contact with the tissue is referred to as *desiccation* and is the type of coagulation used in most surgeries. Most surgeons will operate using a coagulation current, which actually cuts and coagulates tissue. Desiccation results in hemostasis but does not always result in necrosis. Desiccation slowly drives the water content out of the cell.

• •

SECTION QUESTIONS

Q12. Electrosurgery may be used to _____ tissue or _____ bleeding points. (Ref. 40)

Q13. An isolated electrosurgery system is _____ than a ground-referenced electrosurgery system. (Ref. 49)

    a. safer

    b. less safe

Q14. Explain the function of the active electrode. (Ref. 56)

_____

Q15. The active electrode (Ref. 56, 57, 58):

    a. may be a handheld device

    b. may be a foot-controlled device

    c. disperses current

    d. may be monopolar

    e. may be bipolar

Q16. The dispersive electrode provides a return path for electrical current from the patient to the electrosurgical generator. (Ref. 61)

True   False

Q17. Coagulated tissue causes a foreign-body reaction. Describe a complication of healing that can occur if there is an excessive amount of coagulated tissue in the wound. (Ref. 65)

_____

_____

Q18. Desiccation and fulguration are forms of coagulation. (Ref. 67)

True   False

Q19. Explain the difference between desiccation and fulguration. (Ref. 67, 68)

_____

_____

• •

Nursing Diagnosis—Desired Patient Outcomes

69. The nursing diagnosis of high risk for injury related to use of electrosurgery is appropriate for the patient on whom electrosurgery is used. Although improvements in electrosurgical equipment have minimized the risk of burn, the risk of patient injury, i.e., impaired skin integrity, remains. All operating rooms are not equipped with the most modern equipment, and even modern machines do not eliminate the potential

for injury. Older dispersive electrode pads can permit concentration of current and subsequent burn if there is poor contact, i.e., poor electrical connection between the patient and the dispersive electrode. Poor contact can be caused by the incorrect placement of the pad.

70. A patient burn can occur from inadvertent contact of an active electrode with the patient at an unintended site if the generator is accidentally activated and the active electrode is not housed in a protective receptacle.

71. The advent of minimally invasive endoscopic surgery has brought with it an increased risk of burn injury from electrosurgery. A 1999 study titled "Laparoscopic Bowel Injury: Incidence and Clinical Presentation" indicated a complication rate of 1.3 for every thousand cases. Fifty percent of the injuries were caused by electrosurgery, and of those 67% were not detected at the time of surgery (Bishoff, 1999, p. 887).

72. In laparoscopic surgery, the active electrode is introduced into the patient through the abdominal wall via a cannula. The internal view is limited and the shaft of the laparoscope and the cannula are not visualized. Unintended transfer of energy along the laparoscope or cannula shaft, or along the active electrode shaft, can result in an internal burn that may go unnoticed. Inadvertent activation of the active electrode outside the visible field can also cause an internal burn. The result may be an undiagnosed burn that perforates the bowel and results in postoperative peritonitis, which is then life threatening because of the time lapse between when a patient is discharged and when the infection is diagnosed.

73. Electrosurgical complications in laparoscopic surgery are caused by three mechanisms: (1) insulation failure on the active electrode, (2) direct coupling between the active electrode and other metal instruments or with tissue, and (3) capacitive coupling.

74. Insulation failure occurs when the insulation of an active electrode is not intact and causes current to flow to an unintended area where it may contact tissue and result in a burn injury to the abdominal viscera. Insulation failures occur in laparoscopic instruments such as a suction cautery where the tip of the suction cannula acts as an active electrode. The shaft of the instrument is insulated to prevent current from exiting other than at the active electrode end; however, if the insulation is not intact, current can flow unimpeded to tissue where it can burn through abdominal viscera and cause life-threatening injury. A less serious injury will occur if the current is directed to the cannula in which the electrode is housed. In this instance, the patient will experience a burn to the abdominal wall or skin where there is contact with the cannula.

75. Insulation defects may be so small as to go unnoticed during routine instrument examination.

76. In direct coupling, the tip of the active electrode touches another metal instrument. The current is transferred to that instrument, which in turn acts as an active electrode, causing a burn at the contact site.

77. This type of injury is within the surgeon's view, and repair can be attempted before the completion of surgery.

78. Capacitive coupling is the transfer of electrical current from the monopolar active electrode through the coupling of stray current into other conductive surgical equipment. When radio-frequency currents flow through an electrode, the flow induces stray currents onto other nearby conductors. Currents are induced onto the nearby conductors even though the insulation on the active electrode is intact. The current may be passed on to a metal cannula or working channel of a laparoscope or other metal instrument through which the electrode is passed. This creates the potential for a burn, most probably at the abdominal wall or on external skin. The current transfers to the second metal surface through intact insulation, creating a chrona that electrifies the entire instrument. This can result in an intra-abdominal burn, which in turn creates a risk of peritonitis for the patient.

79. Recent advances in endoscopic instrumentation include laparoscopic bipolar active electrodes and shielded monopolar active electrodes with monitors designed to detect insulation failure. Active Electrode Monitoring (AEM) detects for insulation failure and capacitive coupling and will deactivate the electrosurgical system from delivering current. Shielded monopolar monitoring systems detect insulation failure and will automatically deactivate in such an event. Bipolar electrodes localize current. These systems offer safety advantages.

80. The risk for capacitive coupling injury increases when high voltage and fulguration are used.

81. Two other risks associated with the use of electrosurgery are fire and plume inhalation.

82. The current from an active electrode is sufficient to initiate a fire. The National Fire Protection Association has identified electrosurgical units as high-risk equipment (AORN, 2004c, p. 246). An active electrode that has

been engaged and is in contact with a flammable item, such as a drape, a piece of gauze, or linen, has the potential to start a fire. The operating room is an oxygen-enriched environment that quickly helps to spread fire that can become intense in just a few minutes.

83. Fire in the operating room from electrosurgical equipment is not unknown. Patient injury and death have been reported. (See Chapter 12, "Workplace Safety.")

84. Plume or surgical smoke resulting from electrosurgical application is a concern. The National Institute for Occupational Safety and Health (NIOSH) has detected chemicals in surgical smoke that may be harmful and has identified electrosurgical smoke as a potential health hazard. A Japanese study has shown that electrosurgical smoke is mutagenic (Patterson, 1993, pp. 6–7). NIOSH, the American National Standards Institute, and the Association of periOperative Registered Nurses recommend smoke evacuation when there is electrosurgical smoke. In the absence of a dedicated smoke evacuator, suction should be used.

Desired Patient Outcome/Criteria

85. The desired patient outcome is that the patient will experience no injury as a result of the use of electrosurgery.

86. The criteria to evaluate successful achievement of the desired outcome are no evidence of:

- impaired skin integrity (burn) at dispersive electrode site or alternate current path such as electrocardiograph monitoring leads
- burn at an unintended site
- burn at the entrance site of laparoscopic instrumentation
- fever or abdominal pain associated with peritonitis

Nursing Interventions—Patient and Staff Safety

87. Although electrosurgery is performed by the surgeon and/or assistants, perioperative nursing interventions are critical to a safe patient outcome.

88. Prior to surgery the patient's skin should be assessed overall for the placement of the dispersive electrode. The presence of scar tissue, excessive adipose tissue, metal prosthetic implant, pacemaker, or automatic implantable cardioverter defibrillator (ICD) should be noted. This information is necessary for selecting a site for the dispersive electrode placement.

89. Implementation of the following guidelines and safety measures will minimize the risk of electrosurgical burn. The scrub person will implement some of the measures; the circulating nurse will implement others:

- Use only those dispersive and active electrodes that are compatible with the generator.
- Inspect the generator for frayed cords, loose connections, and an intact and activated alarm system.
- Use only equipment that has been inspected by biomedical engineering. Inspection sticker should be visible, and inspection must not have expired.
- Test the alarm and set it loud enough to be heard during surgery.
- Place the generator close enough to the patient to prevent cords from being pulled taut and thus creating tension at the connection sites. Electrical cords should be free of bends and kinks as well.
- Verbally confirm the power settings with the surgeon. Power settings should be kept as low as possible. If a request is made for an unusually high setting because the present setting is no longer adequate, check for loose connections and malfunction. In older equipment, this may signal that the current is seeking an alternate path. Replace the generator if a malfunction is discovered or suspected.
- Do not place liquids on the generator as these may spill, leak into the generator, and cause the equipment to malfunction. Foot pedals must also be kept dry. Placing the foot pedal into a plastic bag will keep it dry.
- Do not use electrosurgery in the presence of flammable agents. Prep solutions containing flammable agents should be permitted to dry before electrosurgical application. Open suture packages containing alcohol should be kept away from the area of the active electrode. Sponges are flammable, and those used in the area of the active electrode should be moistened. Extreme care must be taken when using electrosurgery in oxygen-enriched environments, such as around a nasal cannula. Methane gas, which occurs in the intestinal tract, is flammable. The active electrode should not be activated in the presence of this gas.

- In older generators in which two electrodes are attached to the generator, when one active electrode is activated the other is automatically activated. These generators should not be used when it is anticipated that two electrodes will be required.
- Prior to surgery, inspect the active electrodes for insulation defects. If a defect is noted, the device must not be used.
- Do not use single-use electrodes that have been reprocessed (unless reprocessed by a reprocessing company registered with the FDA and in compliance with FDA guidelines for reprocessing). Integrity and function of single-use devices that have been reprocessed cannot be guaranteed. For example, the insulation may not be designed to withstand reprocessing.
- Do not use reusable active electrodes beyond their intended life. Refer to manufacturer's guidelines for the permitted number of uses.
- Position the active electrode on the sterile field, close to the operative site, and in a protective container or holster so that accidental activation will not cause incidental burn to the patient or ignite drapes.
- Keep the active electrode clean during surgery by periodically removing charred tissue from the electrodes. Clean the tip with a moist sponge or a scratch pad intended for this purpose. Do not clean with a dry sponge. An active electrode inadvertently activated and in contact with a dry sponge (gauze pad) can start a fire.
- Select a dispersive electrode appropriate to the patient's size and in accordance with the manufacturer's guidelines. Do not cut the dispersive electrode to modify its size or shape.
- Check the dispersive electrode to ensure that there is adequate adhesive and gel, that cord connections are secure, and the expiration date has not been exceeded.
- Place the dispersive electrode on the patient over clean dry skin that covers a large muscle mass and as close to the operative site as possible. Such placement will help ensure good contact with the patient's skin, will ensure sufficient current dispersal, and will minimize current through the patient's body. Because bony prominences and scar tissue can concentrate current, these areas should not be selected as placement sites for the dispersive electrode. Areas of excessive hair and areas where fluids can accumulate and compromise the adhesive should be avoided. If necessary to ensure adherence, hair should be shaved at dispersive electrode site. Areas of excess adipose tissue should also be avoided. Fatty undervascularized tissue can impede conductivity of electrical current and dissipation of heat. Muscular areas generally have adequate blood circulation and promote conductivity of the electrical current. Suitable areas of placement include the anterior and posterior thigh, the calf, the upper arm, the buttock, the midback, and the abdomen. Areas close to electrocardiographic electrodes are avoided because current may be attracted to these electrodes and cause a patient burn at these sites.
- Avoid placement of the dispersive electrode between the patient and a warming device. The combination of heat at the dispersive electrode site and heat from a warming device can increase the risk of a thermal burn (Healthstream, 2003, p. 13).
- Position the patient free from contact with metal surfaces, such as the operating room table.
- Do not include metal implants in the circuit path from the active electrode to the dispersive electrode.
- During lengthy procedures, or when the patient is repositioned during surgery, verify patient contact with the dispersive electrode.
- Suction electrosurgical smoke from the field.
- In the event of the failure of any of the electrosurgical components, retain the defective items for follow-up with biomedical personnel and for reporting of medical instrumentation failure as required.

Electrosurgical Use During Endoscopic Surgery— Special Precautions

90. The following additional precautions are appropriate when using electrosurgery during endoscopic surgery:

- Prior to surgery, inspect the active electrodes for insulation defects. If a defect is noted, the electrode must not be used. If the defect is noted during the surgery or after the procedure, inform the surgeon that the patient may have sustained an inadvertent internal burn.

- Whenever available, use equipment designed to check insulation.
- Active electrode monitoring equipment is used to detect insulation failures and capacitive coupling on active electrode instrumentation in use during endoscopic surgery. Active electrode monitoring equipment should be used whenever available.
- Use all-metal trocar cannula systems. All-metal trocar systems reduce the risk of inadvertent direct coupling. Should the active electrode inadvertently come in contact with a metal surgical instrument, the metal cannula will direct current to the abdominal wall. A combination of plastic and metal trocar cannula systems should not be used. All-plastic trocar cannula systems are acceptable but are not preferable to all-metal systems.

91. The patient who has an internal cardioverter defibrillator (ICD) will need to have the device deactivated prior to surgery and reactivated after surgery. The presence of an ICD should be noted, and institutional procedures designed to implement deactivation and reactivation should be followed. Regardless of who has the responsibility for activation and deactivation, the perioperative nurse must ensure that the ICD has been noted and appropriate action has been taken. As an alternative, bipolar electrosurgery should be used when possible.

92. The use of electrosurgery in patients with a pacemaker represents a potential electrical hazard. Electrosurgery can interfere with the operation of some pacemakers. To prevent current from passing near the heart or pacemaker, the tip of the active electrode should be as far from the pacemaker as possible. The dispersive electrode should not be placed near the pacemaker. It should be placed as close as possible to where the active electrode will be used. Safety guidelines for patients with a pacemaker should be prepared in advance of surgery according to pacemaker manufacturer's instructions.

93. Patients with a pacemaker or ICD should have continuous electrocardiogram monitoring during procedures where electrosurgery is used, and a defibrillator should be readily available.

94. Following surgery, the dispersive electrode should be removed slowly and carefully to prevent denuding the skin. The placement area should be inspected for injury. The patient's skin should be checked for integrity and incidental burns, with particular attention given to electrocardiogram electrode sites and temperature probe entry sites.

95. Documentation of electrosurgical use should include the following:

- assessment of the skin preoperatively
- identification of electrosurgical equipment and settings
- site of dispersive electrode placement
- name of person who applied electrode
- assessment of skin postoperatively

ULTRASONIC ENERGY DEVICES

Overview

96. With an ultrasonic energy device, ultrasonic motion is used to cut and coagulate tissue. The ultrasonic scalpel generator is a microprocessor that uses controlled high-frequency power to drive an acoustic system within a handpiece. Electrical energy is converted into mechanical energy or ultrasonic waveforms. The energy is transmitted to a handpiece with a blade that then vibrates.

97. The mechanical vibrations move at a speed of 55,500 times per second. The mechanical vibrations are transferred to the blade that when in contact with tissue denatures protein and creates a sticky coagulum, thus sealing blood vessels. Cutting and coagulation occur simultaneously.

System Components

98. System components include a generator, a handpiece, and a foot pedal. The generator is a microprocessor that converts electrical energy into mechanical energy. A cable attaches the handpiece to the generator.

99. Various configured blades and accessories permit use of this technology in both open and endoscopic surgery.

Tissue Effects

100. Ultrasonic technology balances cutting and coagulation. It cuts and coagulates at temperatures lower than those used in electrosurgery. The cutting speed and the coagulation effects are inversely related. The following four factors control the effect upon tissue:

- Tissue tension—More tension, faster cutting, less hemostasis. Less tension, slower cutting, more hemostasis.
- Blade sharpness—The shear mode cuts faster than the blunt mode. The blunt mode

provides more coagulation when vascular structures are encountered.

- Power—Increasing the power on the generator increases the cutting speed and decreases the coagulation. Decreasing the power results in slower cutting and increased coagulation.
- Time—With shorter tissue application there is faster cutting and less hemostasis. The longer the tissue application, the slower the cutting and the more the hemostasis.

Technology Characteristics

101. The ultrasonic scalpel may be used as an adjunct to or a substitute for electrosurgery.

102. Because mechanical motion is the basis for this technology, no electrical energy is required nor transferred through the patient. Therefore, a dispersive electrode is not required.

103. Because there is minimal thermal damage, precise dissection near vital structures is possible.

104. The controlled coagulation effect results in minimal char and tissue desiccation. Ultrasonic energy coagulates at temperatures up to 100°C (212°F) versus electrosurgery temperatures of 150°C (302°F) or higher. This also results in less plume than electrosurgery.

Applications

105. The ultrasonic scalpel is intended for soft tissue where bleeding control and minimal thermal damage is desired.

ARGON BEAM–ENHANCED ELECTROSURGERY

Overview

106. Argon beam–enhanced electrosurgery technology uses a beam of ionized argon to achieve rapid hemostasis by coagulation. Argon gas combined with an electrosurgical pencil delivers radio-frequency energy to tissue in a white light beam of ionized argon. The flow of the argon gas clears the tissue of liquid blood and other fluid, and the energy from the ionized argon beam creates a superficial eschar directly on the tissue that causes coagulation and helps to prevent further bleeding. Coagulation does not occur from the argon gas. It occurs from the arcing effect of electrical energy.

System Components

107. System components include a generator, a multifunction handpiece that may be used for open or endoscopic surgery, and a dispersive electrode. Active electrodes include blade and needle electrodes for open procedures and a variety of electrode tips for endoscopic surgery. Flexible coagulation electrodes are available in a variety of lengths.

108. The dispersive electrode functions in the same manner as the dispersive electrode used with a monopolar electrosurgical system.

109. The clinical benefits of argon beam coagulation are rapid efficient coagulation, formation of a thin, flexible eschar, less charring, and less tissue damage than with traditional electrosurgical coagulation.

Application/Characteristics

110. Argon beam coagulation is used for open and endoscopic procedures in which coagulation and low tissue penetration is desired. It is used to control bleeding from vascular structures where large areas of coagulation are needed and to control surface bleeding of organs such as the liver.

111. Argon is an inert gas and is noncombustible. Plume, odor, and tissue damage are decreased.

SECTION QUESTIONS

Q20. The patient undergoing laparoscopic surgery in which electrosurgery is used is at risk of (Ref. 72):

a. internal burn from unintended transfer of energy along the laparoscope cannula

b. internal burn from inadvertent activation of the active electrode outside the field of vision

c. excessive tissue desiccation

Q21. When nonintact insulation on an active electrode results in patient injury during electrosurgery application, the injury can be life threatening. (Ref. 74)

True   False

Q22. If insulation is intact on an active electrode used in laparoscopic surgery, there is no risk of injury from capacitive coupling. (Ref. 78)

True   False

Q23. In addition to patient injury, such as burn, hazards associated with electrosurgery include (Ref. 81–84):

a. paralysis

b. fire

c. plume

Q24. List four criteria used to evaluate successful achievement of the desired patient outcome of no injury as a result of electrosurgery. (Ref. 86)

_____

_____

_____

_____

Q25. Suitable areas for placement of the dispersive electrode include (Ref. 89):

a. anterior thigh

b. posterior thigh

c. upper arm

d. buttock

e. over a bony prominence

f. abdomen

g. midback

Q26. A clean, dry sponge or a scratch pad should be used to periodically remove debris from the active electrode tip. (Ref. 89)

True   False

Q27. Combination plastic and metal trocar cannula systems are preferred when using electrosurgery during endoscopic surgery. (Ref. 90)

True   False

Q28. List four pieces of information relative to the use of electrosurgery that should be documented. (Ref. 95)

_____

_____

_____

_____

Q29. Two characteristics of argon gas are that it is _____ and _____. (Ref. 111)

• •

• • • References

AORN. (1995a). Recommended practices for use of the pneumatic tourniquet. In _Standards, recommended practices and guidelines_ (p. 126). Denver, CO: Author.

AORN. (2004b). Patient Outcomes. In _Standards, recommended practices and guidelines_ (pp. 197–206). Denver, CO: Author.

Association of periOperative Registered Nurses (AORN). (2004c). Recommended practices for electrosurgery. In _Standards, recommended practices and guidelines_ (pp. 245–259). Denver, CO: Author.

AORN. (2004d). Recommended practices for use of the pneumatic tourniquet. In _Standards, recommended practices and guidelines_ (pp. 335–339). Denver, CO: Author.

Bishoff, J. T., Allaf, M., Kirkels, W., Moore, R., Kavoussi, L., Schroder, F., et al. (1999). Laparoscopic bowel injury: Incidence and clinical presentation. _The Journal of Urology, 161_(3), 887–890.

Healthstream. (2003). Electrosurgery: Answers to the most frequently asked questions. _Study guide._ Denver, CO: Author.

Patterson, P. (1993, June). OR exposure to electrosurgery smoke a concern. _OR Manager, 9_(6), 6–7.

• • • Suggested Readings

Association for the Advancement of Medical Instrumentation (AAMI). (1993). _American national standard: Electrosurgical devices._ Arlington, VA: Author.

National Institute for Occupational Safety and Health (NIOSH). (1996, Sept.). Control of smoke from lasers/electric surgical procedures (NIOSH Publication No. 96-128). Cincinnati, OH: U.S. Department of Health and Human Services.

Tucker, R. D., & Voyles, C. R. (1995). Laparoscopic electrosurgical complications and their prevention. _AORN Journal, 62_(1), 58.

Ulmer, B. C. (1997). _Electrosurgery self study guide._ Boulder, CO: Valleylab.

Appendix 8-A

• •

Chapter 8 Post Test

Instructions: Fill in the blank(s), mark the correct answer(s), or answer the question as appropriate.

1. In natural hemostasis the protein fibrinogen is converted to _____, which forms the basic structure of a clot. (Ref. 5)

2. Thrombin, absorbable gelatin, and ties are examples of artificial methods of hemostasis. List four additional artificial methods. (Ref. 7)

   _____

   _____

   _____

   _____

3. It absorbs 45 times its weight in blood and is used to control capillary bleeding. (Ref. 9)

   a. absorbable gelatin

   b. thrombin

   c. oxidized cellulose

4. It is a specially treated gauze or cotton used to control oozing of blood in areas that are difficult to control by other methods of hemostasis. (Ref. 10)

   a. absorbable gelatin

   b. styptic

   c. oxidized cellulose

5. It is a fluffy white material made from purified bovine dermis. (Ref. 11)

   a. thrombin

   b. microfibrillar collagen

   c. absorbable gelatin

6. List two types of injury that a patient could sustain from improper tourniquet use. (Ref. 22)

   _____

   _____

7. The pneumatic tourniquet should be tested and inspected prior to use. What is tested? (Ref. 26, 27)

   _____

   _____

8. The length of the tourniquet cuff should (Ref. 28):

   a. wrap around the extremity so the ends of the cuff meet

   b. wrap around the extremity so there is overlap of 6 or more inches

   c. wrap around the extremity so there is an overlap of 3 to 6 inches

9. Before the tourniquet is applied, the extremity should be padded with _____. (Ref. 29)

10. The tourniquet should be applied (Ref. 30):

    a. at the point most proximal to the operative site

    b. at the point most distal from the operative site

11. What is the risk to the patient if prep solutions are allowed to pool under the tourniquet? (Ref. 31)

    _____

    _____

    _____

12. The maximum length of time for tourniquet inflation has not been determined; however, 2 hours for an arm and 2½ hours for a leg are usual inflation times. (Ref. 33)

    True   False

13. Reinflating a pneumatic tourniquet over an area already engorged with blood creates a risk for what type of injury? (Ref. 36)

    _____

    _____

    _____

14. The nurse should periodically report to the surgeon the length of time the tourniquet has been inflated. (Ref. 34)

    True   False

15. In addition to documentation as to whether the desired patient outcome was achieved, list four other pieces of information that should be documented regarding tourniquet use. (Ref. 38)

    _____

    _____

    _____

    _____

    _____

16. The purpose of electrosurgery is to _____ bleeding points or _____ body tissue using a high radio-frequency current. (Ref. 40)

17. Why are solid-state electrosurgery units sometimes referred to as "Bovie" machines? (Ref. 45)

    _____

    _____

18. What is the purpose of the active electrode? (Ref. 46)

    _____

    _____

19. In a ground-referenced generator, the dispersive electrode is connected or grounded to earth. If there is an interruption in the ground connection (Ref. 48):

    a. the current could seek an alternate path and cause the patient to sustain a severe burn

    b. the machine would automatically shut itself off

20. Explain why a return electrode-monitoring electrosurgery unit system is safer than the isolated electrosurgery unit system and the ground-referenced system. (Ref. 49)

_____

_____

_____

21. An advantage of bipolar surgery is (Ref. 59):

    a. the ability to perform electrosurgery with precise hemostasis

    b. current does not disperse throughout the patient

    c. the ability to perform electrosurgery without a separate dispersive electrode

    e. high-wattage current is provided

22. Dispersive electrodes are often referred to by many names. Give two other names for the dispersive electrode. (Ref. 60)

    _____

    _____

23. The active electrode (Ref. 56, 57, 67):

    a. delivers current to the operative site

    b. channels current back to the generator

    c. may be used to desiccate or fulgurate

24. The patient undergoing endoscopic surgery may sustain an injury from an active electrode (Ref. 72, 73, 75):

    a. that will not be detected until after discharge

    b. as a result of nonintact insulation on an active electrode instrument

    c. as a result of direct coupling

25. Capacitive coupling can occur in laparoscopic surgery (Ref. 78):

    a. when insulation on the active electrode is intact

    b. only if the dispersive electrode is not adequately adhered to the patient

    c. when stray current from the active electrode couples with other conductive surgical instrumentation

26. Fire is a hazard associated with use of electrosurgery. (Ref. 82, 83)

    True   False

27. The desired patient outcome is that the patient will experience no injury as a result of the use of electro-surgery. List two criteria that may be used to evaluate whether this outcome has been achieved. (Ref. 86)

    _____

    _____

28. Why should the active electrode be maintained in a holster when on the sterile field? (Ref. 89)

    _____

    _____

29. Identify two sites/areas where the dispersive should *not* be placed. (Ref. 89)

_____

_____

30. During a procedure where the patient is repositioned, what intervention should the nurse take to ensure patient safety? (Ref. 89)

_____

31. Describe an action that may be taken to reduce risk to personnel of the potential health hazards associated with plume. (Ref. 89)

_____

_____

32. The active electrode should not be operated very close to a pacemaker because it may interfere with the pacemaker's functioning. (Ref. 92)

True   False

33. A dispersive electrode is needed with: (Ref. 102, 108)

a. enhanced argon electrosurgery

b. an ultrasonic scalpel

34. In an ultrasonic scalpel, mechanical vibrations are transferred to an attached blade configuration that when in contact with tissue: (Ref. 97, 102, 104)

a. denatures protein in the tissue to form a sticky coagulum and seal blood vessels

b. vaporizes tissue through fulguration

c. creates large amounts of smoke

d. sends electrical current through the patient

35. The clinical benefits demonstrated by argon beam coagulation include rapid and efficient coagulation, a thinner more flexible eschar, less charring, and less tissue damage. (Ref. 109)

True   False

Appendix 8-B

• •

Competency Checklist: Hemostasis—Tourniquet

Under "Observer's Initials," enter initials upon successful achievement of competency.
Enter N/A if competency is not appropriate for institution.

NAME _____

	OBSERVER'S INITIALS	DATE
1. Assembles equipment:		
a. Webril	_____	_____
b. tourniquet	_____	_____
c. Esmarch	_____	_____
d. other	_____	_____
2. Assesses skin condition on extremity.	_____	_____
3. Appropriate size cuff selected.	_____	_____
4. Tourniquet inspected and tested:		
a. cuff	_____	_____
b. console	_____	_____
c. tubing	_____	_____
d. connections	_____	_____
e. electrical cords	_____	_____
f. power source/amount of gas in tank	_____	_____
g. cleanliness	_____	_____
5. Cuff applied:		
a. over padding	_____	_____
b. proximal point of limb selected (at maximum circumference)	_____	_____
c. tourniquet covers intended area only—nothing unintended under cuff	_____	_____
6. Tourniquet inflated and deflated upon surgeon instructions.	_____	_____
7. Length of inflation reported at agreed-upon intervals.	_____	_____
8. Pressure gauge checked during procedure for fluctuations in pressure.	_____	_____

9. Documentation of:

    a. skin assessment under cuff before and after tourniquet application   _____   _____

    b. location of cuff   _____   _____

    c. time of inflation and deflation   _____   _____

    d. tourniquet identification number   _____   _____

    e. identification of person who applied the cuff   _____   _____

OBSERVER'S SIGNATURE   INITIALS   DATE

_____

ORIENTEE'S SIGNATURE

_____

Appendix 8-C

· ·

Competency Checklist: Electrosurgical Equipment

Under "Observer's Initials," enter initials upon successful achievement of competency.
Enter N/A if competency is not appropriate for institution.

NAME _____

	OBSERVER'S INITIALS	DATE
1. Equipment assembled:		
a. electrosurgical generator	_____	_____
b. active and dispersive electrode	_____	_____
c. foot pedal	_____	_____
2. Generator:		
a. inspected for frayed cords and loose connections	_____	_____
b. alarm checked and setting is audible	_____	_____
c. inspected for biomedical inspection	_____	_____
d. no liquids placed on top of generator	_____	_____
3. Skin is assessed for integrity prior to application of dispersive electrode.	_____	_____
4. Dispersive electrode:		
a. appropriate size chosen	_____	_____
b. inspected for adequate adhesive/gel	_____	_____
c. positioned over large muscle mass (not positioned over bony prominence, excessively hairy site, large metal prosthetic implant, pacemaker)	_____	_____
d. contacts skin uniformly	_____	_____
e. areas close to electrocardiographic electrodes avoided	_____	_____
f. pad used/placed according to manufacturer's instructions for use	_____	_____
5. Active electrode:		
a. inspected for insulation defects (equipment for testing insulation used)	_____	_____
b. inspected for loose connections	_____	_____
c. housed in protective container/holster on the field	_____	_____
6. Power settings confirmed with surgeon.	_____	_____
7. Equipment positioned so as not to cause tension at connection sites (generator close to patient).	_____	_____

8. Troubleshooting:

    a. Surgeon repeatedly requests higher settings

       • All connections checked   _____   _____

       • Adherence of dispersive electrode checked   _____   _____

    b. Alarm sounds

       • All connections checked   _____   _____

       • Adherence of dispersive electrode checked   _____   _____

9. Dispersive pad removed slowly.   _____   _____

10. The following is documented:

    a. assessment of skin preoperatively and postoperatively   _____   _____

    b. identification of electrosurgical equipment and settings   _____   _____

    c. site of dispersive electrode placement and person who applied electrode   _____   _____

    d. assessment of skin   _____   _____

OBSERVER'S SIGNATURE   INITIALS   DATE

_____

ORIENTEE'S SIGNATURE

_____

Chapter 8—Section Question Answers

Q1. a, c, e, f

Q2. a, b, d, e

Q3. d, e, c, b, a

Q4. Bonewax

Q5. To force blood from an extremity by compressing superficial blood vessels

Q6. Chemical burn from prep solutions, abrasion, bruise, blister, swelling, pain, nerve damage

Q7. a, b, c

Q8. To occlude blood flow at a lower pressure

Q9. a, b, d

Q10. False

Q11. a, b, c, d, e

Q12. Cut, coagulate

Q13. a

Q14. Delivers current from the generator to the operative site

Q15. a, b, d, e

Q16. True

Q17. Tissue sloughing, healing by first intention may not occur

Q18. True

Q19. Fulgaration uses sparking to coagulate large bleeders. The active electrode does not contact the tissue. The intent is to cause tissue necrosis. Desiccation results in hemostasis without necrosis. In desiccation, the electrode is in contact with the tissue.

Q20. a, b

Q21. True

Q22. False

Q23. b, c

Q24. No evidence of burn at dispersive electrode site or alternate current path; no evidence of burn at unintended site; no evidence of burn at entrance site of endoscopic instrumentation; no evidence of fever or abdominal pain associated with peritonitis.

Q25. a, b, c, d, f, g

Q26. False

Q27. False

Q28. Preoperative skin assessment, identification of electrosurgery equipment, site of dispersive electrode, person who applied dispersive electrode, postoperative skin assessment

Q29. Inert, noncombustible

Chapter 8—Post Test Answers

1. Fibrin
2. Oxidized cellulose, microfibrillar collagen, styptic, pressure, instrument, suture ligature, ligating clip, bonewax, tourniquet, electrosurgery
3. a
4. c
5. b
6. Chemical burn from prep solutions, bruise, blister, pain, swelling, nerve damage
7. Accuracy of pressure, connection, amount of gas in tank, fasteners
8. c
9. Webril or stockinette material
10. a
11. Chemical burn
12. False
13. Intravascular thrombosis
14. True
15. Skin assessment prior to and following tourniquet use, location of cuff, cuff pressure, time of inflation and deflation, identification of equipment used, material used to protect skin, identification of person who applied cuff
16. Coagulate, cut
17. Dr. Bovie was instrumental in the development of the first spark-gap vacuum generator that produced cutting with hemostasis. This was the precursor for today's electrosurgery units.
18. Delivers current from the generator to the operative site
19. a
20. Current that enters the patient is measured and compared with current returning to the dispersive electrode. If they are not sufficiently balanced, the unit will alarm and deactivate. This allows less chance for burn injury.
21. a, b, c
22. Grounding pad, inactive electrode, patient plate, "Bovie pad," return electrode
23. a, c
24. a, b, c
25. a, c
26. True
27. No evidence of burn at dispersive electrode site or alternate current path, no burn at unintended site, no burn at entrance of laparoscopic instruments, no fever or abdominal pain associated with peritonitis
28. In the event of accidental activation, the active electrode will not cause an incidental fire or burn
29. Bony prominence, scar tissue, area of excessive hair, fatty undervascularized areas
30. Verify patient contact with dispersive electrode
31. Use a smoke evacuator or suction
32. True
33. a
34. a
35. True

9

Prevention of Injury—Use and Care of Basic Surgical Instrumentation

LEARNER OBJECTIVES

After reading and completing "Prevention of Injury—Use and Care of Basic Surgical Instrumentation," the learner will:

- identify potential patient injury that is related to failed surgical instrumentation
- discuss the relationship of proper care and use of surgical instruments to patient injury
- identify basic surgical instruments
- describe the basic categories and functions of surgical instrumentation
- list six conditions that should be checked during the inspection of instruments
- describe the process for the care and cleaning of basic surgical instrumentation
- describe the process for care and handling of rigid endoscopes, cameras, and fiberoptic light cables

• • • • • • • • • • • • •

Lesson Outline

I. NURSING DIAGNOSIS—DESIRED PATIENT OUTCOME
II. OVERVIEW
    A. Evolution of Surgical Instruments
    B. Proper Care and Handling—Departmental Impact
    C. Manufacture of Surgical Instruments
III. NURSING RESPONSIBILITIES RELATED TO SURGICAL INSTRUMENTATION

IV. CATEGORIES OF INSTRUMENTS
    A. Cutting and Dissecting Instruments
    B. Clamps
        1. Hemostatic Clamps
        2. Noncrushing Vascular Clamps
        3. Occluding Clamps
        4. Grasping/Holding Clamps
    C. Grasping Forceps
    D. Retractors
    E. Suction
    F. Other
V. CARE AND HANDLING
    A. Cleaning
    B. General Guidelines for Care and Cleaning
    C. Inspection

NURSING DIAGNOSIS—DESIRED PATIENT OUTCOME

1. The patient undergoing surgery is at risk for injury and infection related to use of surgical instrumentation.

2. Potential injury can include tearing of tissue caused by an instrument that does not perform as expected or the retention of a foreign body caused by a portion of an instrument that breaks off inside the patient and is not retrieved. A patient may also incur an infection or a foreign-body reaction from an improperly cleaned or sterilized instrument (Centers for Disease Control [CDC], 1999; pp. 1–3). An instrument that is inappropriately processed may have a retained toxic residue that can harm a patient (CDC, 1998, pp. 306–309). Finally, an instrument that is processed incorrectly or that malfunctions can be cause to delay a patient's surgery, which in turn can increase the patient's anxiety over pending surgery.

3. At the end of surgery the patient should be free from infection and free from injury related to improperly processed or malfunctioning instruments.

4. When a patient sustains an injury or an infection during surgery, it is sometimes difficult or impossible to trace the exact cause. For example, a postoperative infection may result from poor aseptic technique, poor surgical technique, inadequate skin preparation, improperly cleaned and processed instrumentation, the patient's state of health, or a combination of any of the above.

5. If an instrument was inadequately processed and a toxic residue results, the effect of that residue may not be measurable for some time, and a cause-and-effect relationship may never be established. This does not negate the necessity to take all requisite steps to protect the patient from injury that could possibly be related to instrumentation.

6. Meticulous aseptic technique coupled with proper use and care of surgical instruments provides the best insurance against an injury or infection related to surgical instrumentation. Absence of excessive swelling or discoloration at the surgical site, minimal pain (excluding the incision site), no sign of infection, and no evidence of retained instrument or instrument part upon instrument count or subsequent X-ray are several measures of appropriate use and care of surgical instruments.

OVERVIEW

Evolution of Surgical Instrumentation

7. Surgical instrumentation dates back to 10,000 B.C., when stone knives were used to perform surgery. Trephined skulls dating to the Neolithic era provide evidence that surgery was performed long before sophisticated surgical instrumentation was developed. Some early surgical implements included sharpened flints used for circumcision and sharpened animal teeth used for blood letting.

8. Until the 1700s, instruments were made by blacksmiths, cutlers, and armorers. In the eighteenth and nineteenth centuries, when surgery gained recognition as a scientific discipline, skilled craftsman—silversmiths, wood turners, coppersmiths, and steel workers—began to make surgical instruments.

9. Instruments were made to individual specifications and often incorporated ornate, finely carved wooden or ivory handles. They were often cased in velvet-lined boxes.

10. The advent of anesthesia in the 1840s permitted surgeons to work slowly and deliberately and also generated the need for more precise and varied surgical instrumentation. With the concurrent acceptance of instrument sterilization, wooden and ivory handles were replaced by all-metal instruments suitable for sterilization.

11. The development of stainless steel in the 1900s further enhanced the manufacturer's ability to make precise surgical instruments, and instrument making evolved into a highly skilled occupation. Many craftsmen from Europe, especially Germany, came to the United States to instruct apprentices. Germany is often considered the home of high-quality surgical instruments, and many instruments used in the United States today continue to be manufactured in Germany.

12. The majority of surgical instruments are manufactured from stainless steel, although titanium, vitallium, and other metals are also used.

13. Recent advances in surgery, especially in minimally invasive endoscopic surgery, combined with the discoveries of new materials, has led to the development of many precise, sophisticated, complex, delicate, and very expensive surgical instruments.

Proper Care and Handling—Departmental Impact

14. A large portion of the operating room budget is devoted to purchase and repair of surgical instruments. Proper instrument care and handling can preserve inventory and reduce expenditures for repair. Instruments that do not function properly, are out for repair, or are processed incorrectly can lead to a delay in surgery and can be a source of frustration for members of the surgical team. Proper care and handling of surgical instruments demands knowledgeable personnel with critical thinking skills who understand the processes necessary to prepare a variety of instruments for surgery and who have demonstrated competence in instrument care.

Manufacture of Surgical Instruments

15. The majority of basic instruments are made from stainless steel, which is composed of iron ore and varying amounts of carbon and chromium. Carbon provides the necessary hardness to the steel, and chromium provides a stainless, corrosion-resistant quality. Most stainless-steel instruments are made with alloys that are high in carbon and low in chromium.

16. There are more than 80 different types of stainless steel. The quality of stainless steel varies according to its composition. The American Iron and Steel Institute grades steel using a 3-digit number, based on various qualities and on the amount of carbon and chromium it contains. Stainless steel series 300 and 400 are commonly used for the manufacture of surgical instruments. The 300 series is used primarily for noncutting instruments, while the 400 series is used for both cutting and noncutting. High-quality stainless steel resists rust and corrosion, has good tensile strength, and maintains a keen edge. Both the 300 and 400 series resist rust and corrosion, have good tensile strength, and maintain a sharp edge. The stainless steel selected for instrument manufacture is determined by the intended use and desired flexibility and malleability of the instrument.

17. Stainless steel is not totally stainless. The chemical composition and the final heat and rinsing processes during manufacture determine the degree to which an instrument resists staining. Although stainless steel resists corrosion and staining, over time and with repeated use, some spotting and/or staining will occur. The degree of spotting, staining, or corrosion of stainless steel instruments also is dependent on how they are used, cleaned, processed, and cared for.

18. The initial step in instrument manufacture is the conversion of raw steel into sheets that are milled, ground, or lathed into instrument blanks that are forged, die-cast, molded, or machined into specific instrument pieces of various shape and size. Excess metal is trimmed, and the pieces are hand assembled, ground, and buffed. The instrument is then heat treated, or tempered, to achieve desired spring, temper, and balance. Balance and temper provide the flexibility that is necessary to withstand the stress of repeated use.

19. After an inspection that may include X-ray or fluoroscopy to expose any defects, the instrument is subjected to a finishing process to protect the surface and to minimize corrosion. In the finishing process, referred to as passivation, the instrument is immersed in a nitric-acid-bath solution that removes carbon steel particles and promotes the formation of a chromium oxide surface coating. Removal of the carbon particles may leave behind tiny pits that must be polished away. The final step is polishing, which creates a smooth surface on which a continuous layer of chromium oxide forms. Passivation and polishing essentially close the instrument pores and prevent corrosion. The chromium oxide layer continues to form when the instrument is exposed to the atmosphere and when it is subjected to the oxidizing agents contained in cleaning agents.

20. There are three types of instrument finish: bright, highly polished; satin or dull; and ebony. The highly polished finish resists surface corrosion. It is shiny and reflects light, which, on occasion, may distract the surgeon or obscure visibility. The majority of instruments have this finish.

21. The satin finish eliminates glare and is slightly more susceptible to corrosion.

22. The ebony finish is black and also eliminates glare. The black surface is useful in laser surgery to prevent reflection of the laser beam. Ebony is the least common finish.

23. Instruments made with titanium have a bluish finish. Titanium is stronger and lighter than stainless steel and more corrosion resistant. Titanium instruments are primarily manufactured for use in microsurgical procedures. They tend to be very delicate and are frequently used where extreme precision is necessary, such as in neurosurgery.

24. There are three types of joints used in the manufacture of instruments that are composed of two halves. These are the screw, the box lock, and the semibox joints. In the screw joint, a screw is used to secure the two halves of the instrument. This type of joint is not common and is sometimes seen in older instruments. In the box-lock joint, one arm of the instrument is passed through a slot in the other arm. In the semibox joint, the two halves can be separated.

25. Two very similar instruments may be known by two or more different names, depending upon the manufacturer or the facility in which they are used. Instrument catalogues from various manufacturers may identify instruments differently. Some instruments are spelled with a capital letter because the name is derived from the person responsible for its development.

NURSING RESPONSIBILITIES RELATED TO SURGICAL INSTRUMENTATION

26. Responsibility for the care and handling of instruments is shared by operating room and sterile processing personnel. Instruments are usually purchased upon operating room request and processed in the sterile processing department. Perioperative nurses who order and use surgical instruments have a responsibility to be knowledgeable about instrument care and handling, even if they are not responsible for implementation of the cleaning and sterilization process.

27. Perioperative nursing personnel responsible for setting up for a surgical procedure and nurses or technicians who function in the scrub role should be able to determine whether instruments are adequately prepared and functioning and ready for use in surgery. In addition to the inspection of instruments in the central service department prior to packaging and sterilization, instruments should be checked during setup for surgery, i.e., prior to surgery or before being handed to the surgeon.

28. The complexity of instrumentation, diversity of materials, high cost, and potential for patient injury require that the nurse know what special handling is required, what cleaning and sterilization methods are appropriate, and how to determine whether an instrument is functioning properly and therefore safe for use in surgery. In addition, urgent need for a particular instrument or instrument set may necessitate the nurse's implementing or directing the cleaning and sterilization process. Sterile processing personnel are the experts in instrument processing, and when a question arises about cleaning and or processing they should be consulted. The ultimate responsibility of the perioperative nurse is to provide for patient safety. Proper care and handling of instruments are deterrents to patient injury.

CATEGORIES OF INSTRUMENTS

Cutting and Dissecting Instruments

29. Dissecting instruments are used to cut or separate tissue. Such instruments may be sharp or blunt.

30. Scalpels and scissors are examples of sharp dissectors. Scalpels consist of a handle and a blade. The handle has a groove at the tip for attaching the blade. This makes it possible to change the blade as needed during the procedure. Scalpel handles are available in a variety of lengths and sizes.

31. Blades are commercially prepackaged and are sterile. Blades may have a rounded, tapered, or hooked cutting edge. (Figure 9-1) They are dispensed to the sterile field by the circulating nurse and contained on a magnetic mat or other receptacle designed to prevent accidental injury. At the end of surgery all blades are placed on the needle mat, and the mat is disposed of in a designated sharps containers.

32. To prevent accidental injury to the scrub person, the blade should be firmly grasped with a needle holder during attachment to the knife handle. Blades must not be handheld during

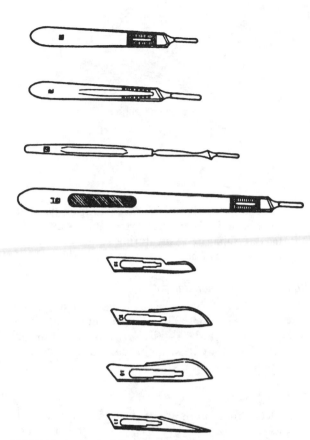

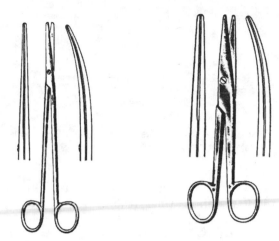

FIGURE 9-2 Scissors: Metzenbaum and Mayo (side views showing straight and curved jaws).
Source: Courtesy of Jarit Instrument Company, Hawthorne, New York.

FIGURE 9-1 Scalpel Handles and Blades.
Source: Courtesy of Bard-Parker Blades, Becton Dickinson, Franklin Lakes, New Jersey.

attachment to or removal from the handle. Scalpels are handed to the surgeon with the cutting edge facing away from the surgeon's palm. The safest technique is to pass scalpels to and from the surgeon in an emesis basin. Another technique to prevent injury from the scalpel is to verbalize each time a scalpel is passed. For example, the surgeon may say, "Blade back," indicating to the scrub person that a scalpel is being returned. As a result of the 2000 Needlestick Safety and Prevention Act, the Occupational Health and Safety Administration (OSHA) amended the Bloodborne Pathogen Standard to require the use of safer devices to protect healthcare workers from sharps injury (OSHA, Nov. 27, 2001). As a result, many facilities have converted to recently developed products that offer shielded scalpel blades and they no longer permit use of the traditional scalpel handle that requires loading of the blade. Policies for safe handling of scalpels and other sharps may vary according to the institution; however, all facilities should have a related policy that is strictly enforced.

33. Scissors are manufactured in many different sizes and styles. Mayo and Metzenbaum scissors are used often and are contained in most general surgery instrument sets. (Figure 9-2) Mayo scissors have either a straight or curved tip. Curved Mayo scissors are used to cut heavy, tough tissue. Straight-tipped Mayo scissors are used for cutting sutures and may be used to cut gauze or a disposable drape as needed. Metzenbaum scissors have a rounded tip, are more delicate than Mayo scissors, and are used to cut or dissect delicate tissue. All of these scissors open and close in the same manner as household scissors. For more delicate surgeries, such as plastic, micro, or eye surgery, a spring-action scissor in which the jaws are held open may be used. In a spring-action scissor a single movement pressing the spring together with thumb and forefinger causes the jaws to close. Releasing the pressure causes the jaws to open. (Figure 9-3)

34. Examples of other sharp dissectors are osteotomes, chisels, and rongeurs, used for cutting bone; curettes, used for bone and soft tissue; and periosteal elevators, used to separate tissue from bone or from other tissue. (Figure 9-4)

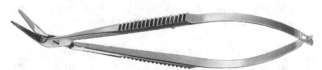

FIGURE 9-3 Castroviejo Scissors.
Source: Courtesy of Aesculap, Inc., Center Valley, PA. Used with permission.

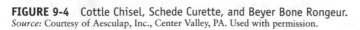
Cottle Chisel

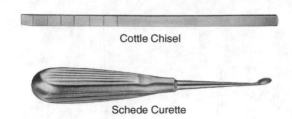
Schede Curette

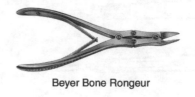
Beyer Bone Rongeur

FIGURE 9-4 Cottle Chisel, Schede Curette, and Beyer Bone Rongeur.
Source: Courtesy of Aesculap, Inc., Center Valley, PA. Used with permission.

35. Examples of blunt dissectors are the back end of a knife handle, a small peanut-shaped sponge, or a folded 4 × 4-inch gauze attached to an instrument. Curettes and elevators may also be blunt.

Clamps

36. Clamps are instruments that are designed to hold tissue or other materials. They are provided in a wide variety of shapes and sizes. The tips may be straight, curved, or angled. Some clamps are fine and delicate. Others are sturdy and appear more substantial.

37. Overall design is similar for all clamps. The design includes finger rings for holding the instrument, shafts of varying length, a joint (a screw or box lock) that joins the two halves of the instrument and permits opening and closing, a ratchet at the distal end for locking the instrument in a closed or partially closed position, and a distal tip or jaw. The design of the jaw determines the instrument's use. (Figure 9-5)

Hemostatic Clamps

38. Hemostatic clamps, commonly referred to as hemostats, are used to control bleeding. The clamping jaws of the instrument are horizontally serrated. This allows the clamp to compress the vessel with enough force to stop bleeding. The serrations also prevent the clamp from slipping off the tissue.

39. Common hemostat names are mosquito, Crile, Kelly (Rochester Peans), tonsil (Schnidt), and mixter. (Figure 9-6) Mosquitos are small clamps that may be curved or straight. They are most often used to clamp small bleeders in the superficial layers of tissue. Criles are curved and slightly longer and heavier than mosquitos. Tonsil clamps are curved and longer than Criles. They are used where additional length is needed. Kellys are straight or curved and are heavier than Crile or tonsil clamps. The tip of a mixter is in the shape of a right angle. Longer mixters

are useful for clamping and separating tissue in the abdominal cavity. Shorter mixters are often used to separate tissue during surgery on vasculature that is not deep within the body.

Noncrushing Vascular Clamps

40. The jaws of these clamps have opposing rows of fine serrations. They are used in vascular surgery to occlude a vessel without crushing it. The jaws may be straight, curved, rounded, or angled.

Occluding Clamps

41. Occluding clamps are used to clamp tissue, such as bowel or blood vessels, where prevention of leakage and minimization of tissue trauma is desired. The serrations on occluding clamps are vertical, close together, and arranged in multiple rows.

Grasping/Holding Clamps

42. Grasping or holding clamps are used on tissue for retraction and as aids during dissection and

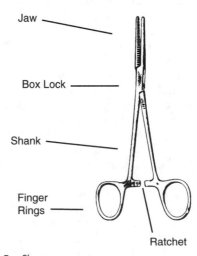
Jaw

Box Lock

Shank

Finger
Rings

Ratchet

FIGURE 9-5 Clamp.
Source: Courtesy of Jarit Instrument Company, Hawthorne, New York.

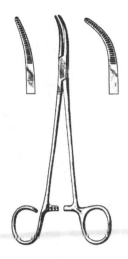

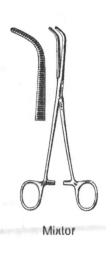

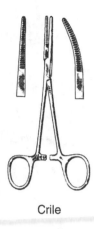

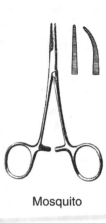

Tonsil (Schnidt)

Mixtor

Crile

Mosquito

FIGURE 9-6 Hemostats.
Source: Courtesy of Jarit Instrument Company, Hawthorne, New York.

suturing. They allow the surgeon to hold tissue with one hand and suture or dissect with the other. Some grasping clamps are used to hold sponges, suture needles, or ties.

43. Common grasping clamps are Allises, Babcocks, Kochers (Ochsners), sponge forceps, towel clips, tenaculum, and needle holders. (Figure 9-7)

44. The tips of an Allis have multiple teeth that do not crush and damage tissue. Babcocks have a curved and fenestrated tip and have no teeth. Babcocks and Allises are used on delicate tissue. A Babcock can be used to grip or enclose delicate structures such as a fallopian tube or ureter. A Kocher has transverse serrations and a single heavy tooth at its tip and is useful for grasping tough tissue. Sponge forceps can be used to hold tissue, but most often are used to hold a folded 4 × 4-inch gauze sponge that can be used to blot or sponge fluids or blood or to retract tissue. Towel clips are used to secure towels around the operative site and to hold drapes in place. Towel clips may have sharp tips that penetrate drapes or blunt tips that do not. Needle holders are designed to hold a needle securely in place so that the needle does not rotate or slip. Needle holders may or may not have a locking ratchet. The surface of the jaws may be smooth, diamond-cut made from tungsten carbide, or crosshatched. (Figure 9-8) Tungsten carbide diamond-cut jaws are designed to prevent the needle from twisting and turning. Needle holders with tungsten carbide jaws have gold-plated ring handles. Needle holders used for very fine sutures include a

spring action rather than a ratchet action. The needle is held in place by a single movement that presses the spring together between the surgeon's fingers. When the pressure is released, the jaws open and the needle is released.

Grasping Forceps

45. Grasping and holding instruments that are not shaped as clamps are referred to as forceps or pickups. (Figure 9-9) They are used to lift and hold tissue. The surgeon frequently holds forceps in one hand to grasp the tissue while using the other hand to cut, coagulate, or separate the tissue. Forceps are similar to tweezers. They have two arms and a spring action. A single movement that presses the arms together results in the tips of the forceps approximating. Forceps may have vertical or horizontal serrations, vary in length, and are available with or without one or more teeth on the tip. Toothed forceps are used to hold thick tissue, such as skin that may require extra grip. Nontoothed forceps hold more delicate tissue and cause minimal trauma.

Retractors

46. Retractors are designed to facilitate visualization of the operative field while preventing trauma to the surrounding tissue.

47. Retractors are available in various sizes and shapes. Some retractors require that the surgeon or assistant hold them while exerting pressure; others are self-retaining.

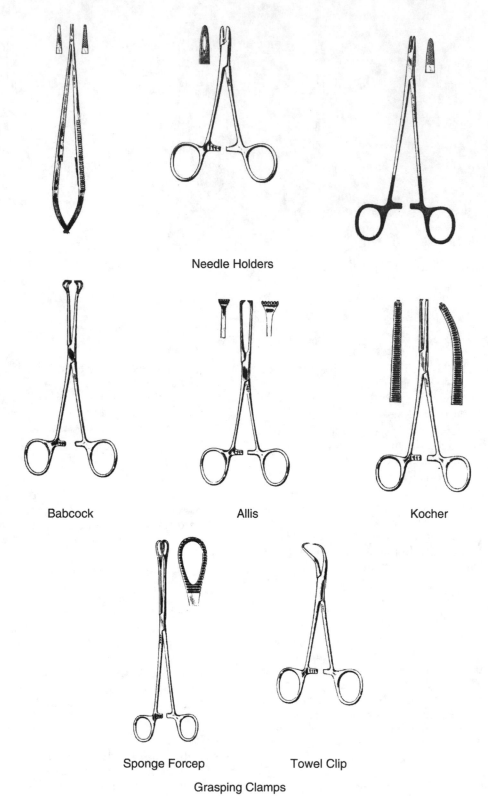

Needle Holders

Babcock

Allis

Kocher

Sponge Forcep

Towel Clip

Grasping Clamps

FIGURE 9-7 Common Needleholders and Grasping Clamps.
Source: Courtesy of Jarit Instrument Company, Hawthorne, New York.

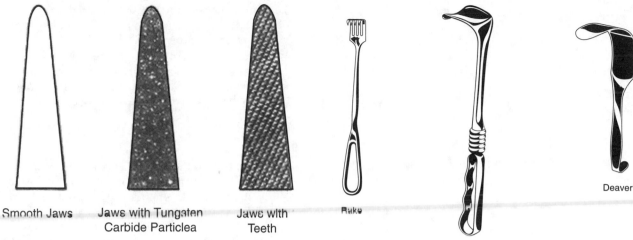

Smooth Jaws   Jaws with Tungsten   Jaws with
                 Carbide Particlea   Teeth

FIGURE 9-8   Needle Holder Jaws.
Source: Courtesy of ETHICON, Inc., Somerville, New Jersey.

48. Common non-self-retaining retractors are rakes, Richardsons, Deavers, Army-Navys, Parkers, malleables (ribbons), and loops. (Figure 9-10)

49. A Weitlaner, a Balfour with a blade, and a Bookwalter or a Thompson, both with multiple parts, are examples of commonly used self-retaining retractors. (Figure 9-11) Some self-retaining retractors, like the Thompson retractor, attach to the operating table and support blades of various length and configurations.

Suction

50. Suction instruments are used to remove blood and other fluids from the operative field.

51. Frazier, Yankauer, and Poole suctions may be included in a basic instrument set. (Figure 9-12)

52. A Frazier-tip suction is a right-angle tube that is supplied in a variety of diameters. A small-diameter Frazier suction is used where capillary bleeding and small amounts of fluid are encountered, in order to maintain a dry field with-

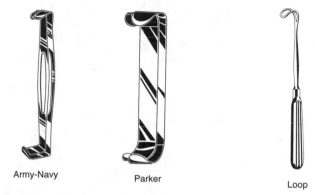

Deaver

Richardson

Army-Navy   Parker   Loop

FIGURE 9-10   Handheld Retractors.
Source: Courtesy of Jarit Instrument Company, Hawthorne, New York.

out the use of sponges. Some Frazier suctions incorporate an active electrode into the tip so they may be used to coagulate tissue as well as suction fluid.

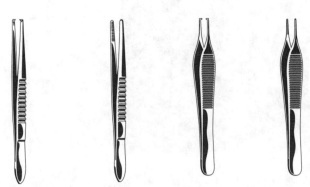

Figure 9-9   Tissue Forceps with and without Teeth.
Source: Courtesy of Jarit Instrument Company, Hawthorne, New York.

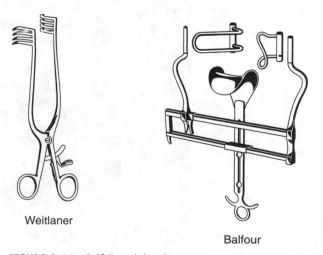

Weitlaner

Balfour

FIGURE 9-11   Self-Retraining Retractors.
Source: Courtesy of Jarit Instrument Company, Hawthorne, New York.

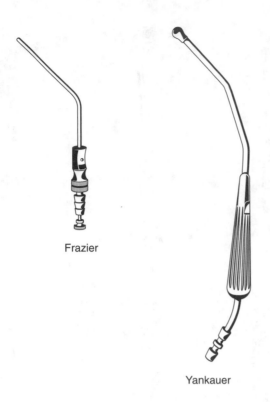

Frazier

Yankauer

FIGURE 9-12 Suction Instruments.
Source: Courtesy of Jarit Instrument Company, Hawthorne, New York.

53. A Yankauer suction is a slightly angled tube that is used in most general surgeries, including those involving the mouth and throat.

54. A Poole suction is a straight tube with an outer perforated shield that acts as a filter. It is useful where large amounts of blood or fluid collect and where the surgical area is deep, such as a body cavity.

Other

55. In addition to the instruments identified above, there are thousands of other surgical instruments, many of which are dedicated to a particular surgical specialty. For example, for a joint replacement, each implant manufacturer has developed a set of instruments specific to that implant. There are many powered instruments as well. Drills and saws of various types are available for orthopedic, neuro, and ear, nose, and throat (ENT) surgery.

56. The phenomenal growth in minimally invasive surgery has led to the development of a wide variety of rigid and flexible fiberoptic endoscopes and accessory instruments. Rigid scopes have become commonplace in the operating room and are used in every surgical specialty. Cystoscopes, hysteroscopes, arthroscopes, and laparoscopes

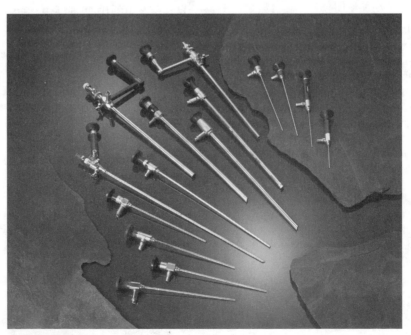

FIGURE 9-13 Laparoscopes.
Source: Courtesy of Aesculap, Inc., Center Valley, PA. Used with permission.

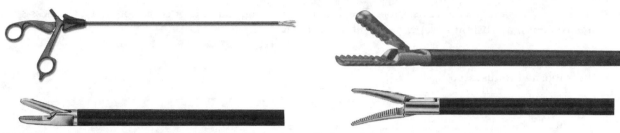

FIGURE 9-14   Laparoscopic Scissors, Laparoscopic Instrument Tip Examples.
Source: Courtesy of Aesculap, Inc., Center Valley, PA. Used with permission.

are the most widely used rigid endoscopes. An increasing number of small-diameter semirigid and flexible fiberoptic endoscopes are available as well.

57. Large-diameter flexible fiberoptic endoscopes are more commonly used in endoscopy units for gastrointestinal procedures.

58. In the early days of minimally invasive surgery, the surgeon inserted a rigid endoscope attached to a light source into the patient's body and observed the internal organ or site by looking though the endoscope eyepiece. (Figure 9-13) Today, the endoscope is coupled to a camera or incorporated into the endo-

scope and the image is displayed on a video monitor.

59. Accessory minimally invasive surgical instruments are designed to dissect, cut, grasp, cauterize, clip, suction, or suture tissue. Typical design includes a ring handle for holding the instrument, a long, small diameter, insulated shaft for insertion into the patient, and a tip or jaw engineered for a specific purpose. (Figure 9-14) Scissor, cautery, grasping, ligating clip holder, and suction tips are common.

60. The advent of robotic surgery has resulted in the development of another set of specialized instruments.

• •

SECTION QUESTIONS

Q1. List two injuries that the surgical patient is at risk for related to instrumentation that is not properly cared for. (Ref. 2)

_____

_____

Q2. When a patient incurs an infection following surgery, the cause is usually an improperly processed instrument. (Ref. 4)

True   False

Q3. Most surgical instruments are made of (Ref. 12):

a. titanium

b. stainless steel

c. vitallium

Q4. The term *stainless steel* is a misnomer. The degree of spotting, staining, or corrosion that a stainless-steel instrument may sustain is dependent on how instruments are (Ref. 17):

   a. used

   b. subjected to diseased tissue

   c. processed

   d. cared for

   e. manufactured

Q5. Instruments with an ebony finish are particularly useful in _____ surgery. (Ref. 22)

Q6. To attach a blade to a knife handle, the scrub person grasps the blade firmly with the thumb and fore-finger and slides the blade parallel to the handle into the grooves at the top of the handle. (Ref. 32)

   True   False

Q7. Metzenbaum scissors (Ref. 33):

   a. are intended to dissect delicate tissue

   b. are intended to cut suture

   c. have a straight tip

   d. have a rounded tip

   e. are used to cut heavy, tough tissue

Q8. Grasping or holding instruments are useful (Ref. 42):

   a. for retraction

   b. during dissection

   c. as an aid in suturing

Q9. Match the instrument name with the description. (Ref. 44)

   a. Kocher   _____   fenestrated tip, used to enclose delicate structures

   b. Allis   _____   transverse serrations, single heavy tooth

   c. Babcock   _____   multiple teeth at tip, does not crush tissue

   d. sponge forcep _____   designed to hold folded 4 × 4-inch gauze pad

Q10. A Weitlaner and a Balfour with blade are self-retaining retractors. (Ref. 49)

   True   False

Q11. _____, _____, and _____ are the names of suction instruments. (Ref. 51)

CARE AND HANDLING

Cleaning

61. Instruments contaminated with blood, body fluids, or tissue should be rinsed during and immediately following the procedure. When blood or other debris is permitted to dry on an instrument, it can harden in joints and become trapped in lumens or serrations or between scissor blades, which can cause malfunction, facilitate rusting and pitting, and make final cleaning more difficult.

62. During the procedure, instruments should be kept free of gross soil by wiping with a sponge moistened with sterile water (AORN, 2004, p. 309). Instruments with a lumen are kept open and free of debris by irrigating the lumen with sterile water. The scrub person should be provided with a syringe for this purpose. To prevent aerosolization of debris, lumens should be irrigated below the surface of the water.

63. Debris and organic material should not be permitted to dry on instruments. Material that has dried within lumens is particularly difficult to remove and may remain attached to the lumen during washing and sterilization, thus creating the potential for patient infection or foreign-body reaction. In one example, patient-to-patient transmission of pathogens was cited as a result of inadequate cleaning of flexible fiberoptic gastrointestinal endoscopes (Bronowicki et al., 1997, p. 237).

64. Instruments should be cleaned as soon as possible after surgery. When a delay is necessary, they should be treated with an enzymatic foam or gel spray that prevents adherence of debris. Instruments should be transported to the decontamination area in leak-proof containers, covered trays, or specially designed carts. It is preferable to wash instruments in an automated washer-disinfector or washer-decontaminator. In the absence of an automated system, instruments may be hand washed (Association for the Advancement of Medical Instrumentation [AAMI], 2002, p. 23).

65. In the presence of gross or dried-on debris, some precleaning may be necessary. Instruments that can tolerate immersion may be presoaked in a proteolytic enzymatic detergent according to the instrument and the detergent manufacturer's recommendations.

66. Personnel who are responsible for washing instruments should be attired in protective gloves, waterproof aprons, and face shields.

67. Ultrasonic cleaners may also be used to remove debris. Ultrasonic cleaning uses sound waves in a process called cavitation to remove debris from all parts of the instrument. Ultrasonic waves generate tiny bubbles that collapse creating tiny vacuums that pull soil from the instrument. Ultrasonic cleaning is not appropriate for all instruments. For example, the seal on lensed instruments will be destroyed by ultrasonic cleaning. Compatibility with the ultrasonic cleaning process must be determined before use. Ultrasonic cleaning is not microbicidal. Following ultrasonic cleaning, instruments are rinsed to remove loose debris, and instruments with movable parts are lubricated with an antimicrobial water-soluble lubricant. The lubricant should be used according to the manufacturer's instructions.

68. Some automated cleaning systems are designed to wash, rinse, sonicate (use ultrasound), disinfect, and lubricate.

69. Lensed instruments, flexible scopes, powered drills, and instruments that cannot tolerate high temperatures or immersion in water cannot be processed in an automated washing system. These devices are cleaned manually according to the manufacturer's instructions. For some specialized instruments, such as flexible endoscopes, specialized cleaning equipment is available.

General Guidelines for Care and Cleaning

70. All instruments should be handled and cleaned according to manufacturer's instructions. General guidelines for care and cleaning of instruments are as follows:

- Instruments are used only for the purpose for which they were designed. Misuse can readily result in improper alignment, dull blades, and cracking of joints or tips.

- During use, instruments are kept clean by wiping and frequent rinsing in sterile distilled water (immersion).

- Instruments are handled gently and individually or in small lots.

- Instruments are carefully put into the splash basin. They are not tossed. Entangled instruments can become misshapen or damaged.

- Lighter, more delicate instruments are placed on top of heavy, less delicate instruments. Delicate instruments can easily be damaged by the weight of heavy metal instruments.

- Following a surgical procedure, instruments are promptly cleaned. Prolonged exposure to blood and saline can cause corrosion and pitting of stainless steel. Instruments are washed and rinsed in water, not in saline. To reduce the potential for spotting that is caused by alkaline mineral deposits, demineralized or distilled rinse water is preferred.

- All instruments opened for a surgical procedure, whether or not they were actually used, are considered contaminated and must be decontaminated. Decontamination is the process whereby instruments are rendered safe to handle. In some circumstances cleaning alone may be sufficient to achieve decontamination; however, washing followed by a thermal or chemical disinfection cycle is programmed into most automated cleaning systems.

- In preparation for cleaning, all hinges and joints are opened to expose box locks and serrations where blood and debris may be concealed. Some automated cleaning systems provide special attachments for lumened instruments. Lumened instruments should be attached to irrigating ports within the washer when available.

- Some instrument sets, especially those intended for orthopedic surgery, are supplied in specialty trays imprinted with a template to indicate the name of the instrument and where in the set the instrument should be placed. The instrument fits snugly into the outlined slot. The template helps to identify the instrument and makes it easy for the scrub person to select the appropriate instrument upon surgeon request. While it is tempting to keep those instruments in their place throughout processing, best practice requires that the instruments are removed from their slots, washed, and then returned to their indicated slots.

- All instruments with removable parts are disassembled for cleaning.

- A noncorrosive, low-sudsing, free-rinsing detergent, with as neutral a pH as possible, is used for washing instruments. A high-sudsing detergent may not be completely removed during rinsing and can cause spotting and staining. Alkaline detergent is excellent for cleaning organic soil, and acid detergent is good for inorganic soil. However, a neutral pH is recommend because alkaline detergents can stain and corrode instruments and acid detergents can cause pitting. Enzyme detergents consist of a detergent and one or more enzymes that break down organic debris. Enzyme detergents may be designed to remove fats or protein and should be selected accordingly.

- During manual washing, only soft brushes are used to clean serrations and joints. Steel wool, scouring powder, and other abrasives are not used for cleaning. These can cause scratches and remove protective finishes. Instruments should be washed below the surface of the water in a manner that prevents splashing and aerosolization.

- Only water-soluble lubricants are used. Oil-based lubricants leave a residue that is not water-soluble and can compromise the sterilization process by preventing steam contact during the steam sterilization process (AAMI, 2002, p. 24).

Inspection

71. Instruments should be inspected prior to, during, and after surgery. The inspection process is an ongoing process, with the bulk of inspection taking place after decontamination and prior to assembly into sets in preparation for sterilization. Instruments should be inspected to ensure that they are clean and in proper working condition. Instruments that fail inspection should be removed and sent for repair.

72. Instruments should be inspected by the scrub person just prior to surgery. Although time may permit only a cursory inspection, this is sometimes sufficient to detect a defective instrument that could result in a delay in surgery or cause a patient injury.

73. During surgery, the surgeon may detect an instrument malfunction that is not immediately visible and only noticed when the instrument is used. When this occurs, the instrument should be set aside and indicated as needing repair.

74. Inspection should include the following:

- Clamps, scissors, and forceps are checked to ensure that tips are even and that they approximate. Tips should be in alignment and should not overlap.

- To be in perfect alignment, the serrations on the jaws of the clamps must mesh perfectly. To test how well the serrations mesh, clamps are fully closed and held up to a light. If the serrations mesh perfectly, no light will be visible between the jaws. Misalignment of hemostatic clamps is a common problem that is often caused by misuse of the instrument.

- Instruments that feature a tooth or teeth at the tips are checked to ensure that they approximate and open freely. Tips that are not aligned properly will stick together. Release will be sluggish and can result in torn tissue.

- Ratchets and hinges must close easily and hold firmly. If the jaws of clamps spring open during use, they may be misaligned, the ratchet teeth may be worn, or the shanks may be bent or have insufficient tension. To test the ratchet, the instrument is closed on the first ratchet tooth, held by the box lock, and the ratchet portion tapped against a solid surface. If the instrument springs open, the ratchets are faulty. A clamp that springs open when clamped on a blood vessel presents the potential for patient injury.

- Joints and hinges are checked to ensure that they move easily and are not stiff. Stiff joints may indicate inadequate cleaning, a need for lubrication, or a defective instrument.

- Box locks are inspected for cracks and looseness. Excessive play in the box lock indicates an alignment problem. Clamps with loose box locks will not hold tissue securely. Cracked box locks are an indication of impending breakage.

- Scissor cutting edges must be smooth and sharp. Blades are inspected for burrs and chips. Scissor blades with burrs and chips will not cut cleanly and can cause trauma to tissue. Tips of Mayo and Metzenbaum scissors should cut through four layers of gauze with little resistance.

- Edges of sharp instruments, such as osteotomes, chisels, and ronguers, should be inspected for chips, nicks, or dents.

- Needle holders should hold the needle securely without slipping or rotation. Testing is accomplished by securing a needle in the jaws and locking the instrument in the second ratchet tooth. If the needle can be easily moved by hand, the holder is worn and needs repair or replacement.

- If plated instruments are in use, they must be inspected for chips that can harbor microorganisms and for worn spots that can rust during autoclaving. (Although most instruments are made of stainless steel, a few plated instruments remain in use. Plated instruments are made by putting a chromium, cadmium, nickel, or silver coating directly on forged steel.)

- Rigid endoscopes should be held to the light while looking through the eyepiece, and the lens should be observed for clarity. A cloudy lens may indicate a leak in the lens seal with a subsequent accumulation of moisture inside. A partially blocked view may indicate a crack in one of the internal glass lenses or rods. There are several other more sophisticated tests that should be done to test the resolution, clarity, and projected image of rigid endoscopes. These are typically conducted by processing personnel just prior to packaging. Testing should also be done at the time of purchase and after repairs. Poor-quality repairs will result in expensive repeated repairs. The ability to compare scope quality after repair with baseline data will allow the person responsible for managing scopes to evaluate repair services. This is important because costs to repair rigid endoscopes can consume more of the annual OR instrument budget than purchase of new endoscopes.

- Flexible fiberoptic endoscopes should be inspected for obvious external defects to the outer sheath. Positioning controls should be rotated to ensure they move smoothly and easily. The lens should be held to the light while observing the distal end for tiny black spots. Black spots indicate a broken fiber, and broken fibers result in decreased light transmission.

- Fiberoptic cords should be inspected for nicks. They should be attached to a light source and the distal end observed for tiny black spots that indicate broken fibers that will result in diminished illumination.

- The camera should be connected to a video monitor, and the monitor observed for a picture. The coupler and the controls should move easily.

- Instruments are inspected to determine that all parts are present and that the instrument is intact. Pins and screws that are loose can cause an instrument to malfunction, and a part can be lost inside a patient.

- Instruments with insulation are inspected to verify that all insulation is intact. Insulation cracks or flaws can lead to inadvertent patient burn and serious injury such as peritonitis, which can lead to death (Perantinides, Tsarouhas, & Katzman, 1998, pp. 48, 51, 52). Insulation should always be checked by the scrub person before he or she permits use of the instrument in surgery.

• •

SECTION QUESTIONS

Q12. Cleaning of lumens is very important to patient safety. Inadequate cleaning can lead to what type of patient injury? (Ref. 63)

_____

Q13. List three pieces of personal protective attire that should be worn when cleaning contaminated instruments. (Ref. 66)

_____

Q14. Ultrasonic cleaning (Ref. 67):

    a. is the use of sound waves to remove debris

    b. should be followed with rinsing

    c. is an excellent method of destroying pathogenic microorganisms

Q15. Instruments should be cleaned in (Ref. 70):

    a. water

    b. saline

    c. low-sudsing detergent with neutral pH

    d. alkaline detergent

    e. acidic detergent

Q16. Why is it important that oil-based lubricants never be used to lubricate instruments? (Ref. 70)

_____

Q17. Instruments with multiple parts should remain assembled during processing to ensure that no part of the instrument is lost. (Ref. 70)

    True   False

Q18. What would someone be inspecting a clamp for while holding it up to the light in a closed position? (Ref. 74)

_____

_____

Q19. Tips of Mayo and Metzenbaum scissors should be sharp enough so that the tips cut through _____ layers of gauze with little resistance. (Ref. 74)

Q20. Describe how a rigid scope should be checked prior to use. (Ref. 74)

_____

• •

• • • References

Association for the Advancement of Medical Instrumentation (AAMI). (2002). Steam sterilization and sterility assurance in health care facilities. *ANSI/AAMI ST46:2002.* Arlington, VA: Author.

Association of periOperative Registered Nurses (AORN). (2004). Recommended practices for cleaning and caring for surgical instruments and powered equipment. In *Standards, recommended practices and guidelines* (pp. 309–317). Denver, CO: Author.

Bronowicki, J., Vernard, V., Botte, C., Monhoven, N., Gastin, I., Chone, L., et al. (1997). Patient to patient transmission of hepatitis C during colonoscopy. *New England Journal of Medicine, 337*(4), 237–240.

Centers for Disease Control. (1999). Bronschoscopy related infections and pseudoinfections. *MMWR Morbidity Mortality Weekly Report, 48*(26), 1–3.

Centers for Disease Control. (1998). Corneal decompensation after intraocular surgery—Missouri. *MMWR Morbidity Mortality Weekly Report, 47*(15), 306–309.

Occupational Safety and Health Administration (OSHA). (Nov. 27, 2001). Enforcement procedures for the occupational exposure to bloodborne pathogens, Directive CPL 02-02-069. Retrieved Oct. 22, 2004, from www.osha.gov/pls/oshaweb/owadisp.show_document?p_table=DIRECTIVES&p_id=2570.

Perantinides, P., Tsarouhas, A., & Katzman, V. (1998). The medicolegal risks of thermal injury during laparoscopic monopolar electrosurgery. *Journal of Healthcare Risk Management, 18*(1), 48, 51–52.

• • • Suggested Reading

Education Design. (2000). The care and handling of surgical instruments. Denver, CO: Author.

Spry, C. (2003). Care and handling of surgical instruments. In Tighe, S. (Eds.), *Instrumentation for the Operating Room* (pp. xv–xxix). St. Louis, MO: Mosby.

Appendix 9-A

• •

Chapter 9 Post Test

Instructions: Fill in the blank(s), mark the correct answer(s), or answer the question as appropriate.

1. List two potential patient problems that can arise if instruments are improperly handled and cared for. (Ref. 2)

   _____

   _____

2. All postoperative wound infections are the result of improperly cleaned instruments or poor aseptic technique. (Ref. 4)

   True   False

3. Stainless steel was developed at the same time that anesthesia was developed in the 1840s. (Ref. 10, 11)

   True   False

4. List two consequences to the operating room and the surgical team that can occur as a result of improper care and handling of surgical instruments. (Ref. 14)

   _____

   _____

5. To provide hardness and resistance to corrosion, most stainless steel instruments are made with alloys that are high in carbon and low in chromium. (Ref. 15)

   True   False

6. The 300 and 400 series of stainless steel are commonly used in the manufacture of surgical instruments. (Ref. 16)

   True   False

7. The finishing process in instrument manufacture is referred to as passivation and is the step prior to polishing. (Ref. 19)

   True   False

8. Instruments that have a bluish finish and are used primarily in microsurgical procedures are made from _____. (Ref. 23)

9. Describe two techniques for safely passing scalpels to and from the surgeon. (Ref. 32)

   _____

   _____

10. The two types of scissors used most often in general surgery are _____ and _____. (Ref. 33)

11. A periosteal elevator is used to _____. (Ref. 34)

12. Clamps used to control bleeding are often referred to as _____(Ref. 38)

13. A _____ is a grasping clamp with a single tooth at its tip and is used to grasp tough tissue. (Ref. 44)

14. Forceps _____ are most appropriate to hold skin while suturing. (Ref. 45)

    a. with teeth

    b. without teeth

15. What is the purpose of a Deaver, a Richardson, and an Army-Navy? (Ref. 46, 48)

    _____

16. Match the instrument to the description. (Ref. 35, 38, 44, 45, 48, 49)

    a. hemostat   _____ blunt dissector

    b. small peanut-shaped sponge   _____ controls bleeding

    c. Kocher   _____ non-self-retaining retractor

    d. Richardson   _____ grasps tough tissue

    e. Weitlaner   _____ two arms with spring action

    f. forceps   _____ self-retaining retractor

17. Instruments should be kept clean during surgery by wiping or rinsing with saline. (Ref. 62)

    True   False

18. For the majority of instruments, automated cleaning is preferable to manual cleaning. (Ref. 64)

    True   False

19. Lensed instruments should be cleaned in either a washer-decontaminator or an ultrasonic cleaner. (Ref. 67, 69)

    True   False

20. All instruments opened for a surgical procedure are considered contaminated even if they were not actually used. (Ref. 70)

    True   False

21. A high-sudsing, free-rinsing detergent with a neutral pH is best for washing surgical instruments. (Ref. 70)

    True   False

22. Describe a method to check a needle holder to determine if it is working properly. (Ref. 74)

    _____

    _____

Appendix 9-B

• •

Competency Checklist: Instrumentation—Care and Handling

Under "Observer's Initials," enter initials upon successful achievement of competency.
Enter N/A if competency is not appropriate for institution.

NAME _____

	OBSERVER'S INITIALS	DATE
1. Instrument inspection, prior to procedure:		
a. tips approximate	_____	_____
b. serrations mesh	_____	_____
c. ratchets hold securely	_____	_____
d. jaws open and close easily	_____	_____
e. cutting instruments are sharp	_____	_____
f. needle holders hold needle securely	_____	_____
g. scopes are clear	_____	_____
h. electrode insulation intact	_____	_____
i. camera relays image to monitor	_____	_____
2. Scalpel loaded safely.	_____	_____
3. Instruments handled carefully (placed, not tossed into basin).	_____	_____
4. Instruments cleaned periodically during procedure (rinsed, wiped, irrigated with water).	_____	_____
5. Instruments used only as intended (for example, does not open medication vial with a Kocher clamp).	_____	_____
6. Instruments contained/covered in preparation for transport to decontamination area.	_____	_____
7. Instruments awaiting washing are moistened with enzymatic instrument spray.	_____	_____
8. Wears personal protective equipment when washing instrument.	_____	_____
9. Washes instrument(s) below surface of the water.	_____	_____
10. Operates ultrasonic cleaner correctly.	_____	_____

OBSERVER'S SIGNATURE   INITIALS   DATE

_____

ORIENTEE'S SIGNATURE

_____

Chapter 9—Section Question Answers

Q1. Infection, retention of a foreign body
Q2. False
Q3. b
Q4. a, c, d, e
Q5. Laser
Q6. False
Q7. a, d
Q8. a, b, c
Q9. c, a, b, d
Q10. True
Q11. Frazier, Yankauer, Poole
Q12. Infection
Q13. Gloves, waterproof apron, face shield
Q14. a, b
Q15. a, c
Q16. Oil-based lubricants leave a residue that is not water-soluble, which can compromise the sterilization process
Q17. False
Q18. Alignment of the jaws
Q19. 4
Q20. Hold to the light, look through the eyepiece, check lens for clarity

Chapter 9—Post Test Answers

1. Infection, retention of foreign body
2. False
3. False
4. Delay in surgery, expensive repairs
5. True
6. True
7. True
8. Titanium
9. In an emesis basis, announce scalpel passing
10. Mayo, Metzenbaum
11. Separate tissue from bone or from other tissue
12. Hemostats
13. Kocher
14. a

(continues)

Chapter 9—Post Test Answers *(continued)*
15. Retraction
16. b, a, d, c, f, e
17. False
18. True
19. False
20. True
21. False
22. Secure needle in jaw, lock holder in second ratchet, attempt to move needle

10

Prevention of Injury—Wound Management

. . . .

Lesson Outline

I. NURSING DIAGNOSES—DESIRED PATIENT OUTCOMES
    A. Potential Injury
    B. Desired Patient Outcomes/Criteria
II. SURGICAL WOUNDS
    A. Surgical Wound Classification
    B. Wound Healing
        1. Primary, Secondary, and Tertiary Intention or Delayed Primary Closure
        2. Process of Wound Healing

III. SUTURE MATERIAL
   A. Classification of Suture Material
      1. Monofilament and Multifilament
      2. Absorbable Suture
      3. Nonabsorbable Suture
      4. Suture Diameter
   B. Suture Selection—Considerations
   C. Suture Package Information
IV. SURGICAL NEEDLES
   A. Needle Characteristics
   B. Needle Attachment
V. OTHER WOUND CLOSURE DEVICES
   A. Stapling Devices
   B. Skin Tapes, Skin Adhesives
   C. Drains
VI. DRESSINGS
VII. NURSING RESPONSIBILITIES RELATED TO WOUND MANAGEMENT

NURSING DIAGNOSES—DESIRED PATIENT OUTCOMES

Potential Injury

1. Patients undergoing surgery are at high risk for injury (compromised or interrupted wound healing) related to wound closure.

2. Patients are also at high risk for infection related to wound closure.

3. Wound dehiscence and wound evisceration are complications of wound healing. Wound dehiscence is the partial or complete separation of the wound edges after wound closure. Wound evisceration is the actual protrusion of the abdominal viscera through the incision. Although the incidence of either is relatively uncommon, it is a risk for patients who undergo abdominal surgery.

4. In patients under 30 years of age, wound dehiscence is rare. Occurrence in patients over 60 who undergo laparotomy is 5%. Overall occurrence is 1% to 3%, according to W. L. Way (cited in Long, 1993, p. 462).

5. There are many factors that determine the patient's risk for injury related to wound closure. Dehiscence or evisceration that occurs on days 1 to 3 postoperatively is usually the result of inadequate wound closure. Occurrences after the third postoperative day are often the result of excessive vomiting or coughing, infection, distention, or dehydration. A patient with a preexisting condition, such as obesity, diabetes, malignancy, immunocompromise, dehydration, or malnourishment with hypoproteinemia, may experience delayed or complicated wound healing. Wound separation that occurs 2 or more weeks postoperatively is generally a result of one or more of the above conditions.

6. Aseptic technique, suture materials, and surgical technique also influence wound healing. The majority of surgical wound infections are initiated along or adjacent to suture lines (Mangram, A., Horan, T., Pearson, M., Silver, L., & Jarvis, W., 1999, p. 251). A break in aseptic technique as well as poor surgical technique can contribute to wound infection. Suture materials vary in their ability to prevent infection.

Desired Patient Outcomes/Criteria

7. The desired outcomes for the patient who undergoes surgery are freedom from injury related to wound closure and freedom from infection related to wound closure. Evaluation criteria include absence of:

   • dehiscence or evisceration

   • excessive scar formation

   • wound site infection, including abscess, serous drainage, cellulitis, fever 72 hours postoperatively, redness, and pain or swelling 72 hours postoperatively

SURGICAL WOUNDS

Surgical Wound Classification

8. Surgical wounds are classified as clean (class I), clean contaminated (class II), contaminated

(class III), and dirty or infected (class IV). Wound classification is provided by the Centers for Disease Control.

9. A clean wound is one in which the gastrointestinal (GI), genitourinary, or respiratory tract is not entered. No inflammation is encountered, and there is no break in aseptic technique. Examples of clean surgical procedures include hernia repair, carpal tunnel repair, total joint replacement, and cataract extraction. Class 1 wounds usually do not have a drain and are closed by primary union. The wound edges are brought together, and healing occurs with minimal edema or discharge and no localized infection.

10. Approximately 75% of all surgical wounds fall into this category. Most are elective surgeries and are not predisposed to infection (Ethicon, 2002, p. 6).

11. A clean contaminated wound (class II) is one in which the GI, genitourinary, or respiratory tract is entered under planned, controlled means. The biliary tract, appendix, vagina, and oropharynx are included in this category provided there is no major break in aseptic technique, no spillage occurs, and no infection is present.

12. Examples of clean contaminated procedures include cholecystectomy, cystoscopy, hysterectomy, bronchoscopy, and intestinal resection when done under controlled circumstances.

13. A contaminated wound (class III) is one in which gross contamination is present but obvious infection is not present. Included in this category are incisions in which acute, nonpurulent inflammation or gross spillage from the GI tract is present, or when there is a major break in aseptic technique. Open fresh accidental wounds are included in this category.

14. Examples of contaminated procedures include gunshot wound, colon resection with GI spillage, and rectal procedures.

15. A dirty or infected wound (class IV) is one in which an old traumatic wound with dead tissue exists or an infectious process is present.

16. Examples of dirty or infected procedures include colon resection for ruptured diverticulitis, appendectomy for ruptured appendix, and amputation of a gangrenous appendage.

17. The overall rate of surgical site infection is estimated to be 2.6% (Fry, 2003, p. 15), with the lowest risk for class 1 procedures, followed by class II and class III. However, two efforts by the Centers for Disease Control have shown that depending upon the presence of risk factors other than the wound class, the rate of in-

fection for clean wounds can be as high as 15% (Mangram et al., 1999, p. 264). Because the majority of surgeries are performed on an outpatient basis, it is sometimes difficult to obtain accurate postoperative information regarding wound infection, and many wound infections may go unreported.

Wound Healing

Primary, Secondary, and Tertiary Intention or Delayed Primary Closure

18. Surgical wounds may heal by primary, secondary, or tertiary intention.

19. Wounds heal by primary intention when minimal tissue damage occurs, aseptic technique is maintained, tissue is handled gently, and all layers of the wound are approximated. The wound generally heals quickly with minimal scarring. This is the preferred method of healing.

20. Wounds heal by secondary intention when the wound cannot be sutured and is left open. An example is an ulcer where the edges cannot be sutured together. The wound heals from the bottom upward and is characterized by a red beefy appearance. Granulation tissue forms in the wound and gradually fills in the defect. The wound heals slowly, and there is considerable scarring. Because the wound is open, there is a greater risk for infection than if the wound were closed.

21. Wounds heal by tertiary intention or delayed primary closure when the wound is not sutured until several days after initial surgery. Extensive tissue loss from injury, or debridement of dirty or infected tissue, may result in a wound that cannot be closed at the time of the procedure. The open wound is packed with gauze that is typically changed twice a day. If within 3 to 5 days there is no sign of wound infection and if granulation tissue is present, the wound is closed.

Process of Wound Healing

22. Wound healing is generally divided into three overlapping stages: inflammatory, proliferation, and maturation.

23. The first phase of wound healing is the inflammatory stage, which begins when the incision is made and extends through the fourth or fifth postoperative day. This stage is marked by hemostasis and phagocytosis. The inflammatory response, not to be confused with infection, includes redness, swelling, and pain. Platelets form a clot, fibrin is deposited in the clot, and new blood vessels develop across the

sutured wound. A thin layer of epithelial cells bridge and seal the wound.

24. The inflammatory stage is followed by the proliferation stage, in which the epithelial cells are regenerated, collagen is synthesized, and new blood vessels form. The new highly vascular tissue is referred to as *granulation tissue*. The proliferation stage generally lasts 3 to 20 days. Toward the end of this stage, the wound begins to take on a raised pinkish scar and will have gained enough strength to permit suture removal.

25. The final stage of wound healing is the maturation or remodeling stage, which can last more than a year. Collagen continues to be deposited and is remolded, the wound shrinks and contracts, and a thin white scar line is formed. (Figure 10-1)

26. After 6 weeks, most wounds will have regained approximately 50% of their original tensile strength (the amount of strength provided by the suture material at the time of wound closure) (Wysocki, 1989, p. 508).

SUTURE MATERIAL

27. The word *suture* refers to a strand of material used to tie (ligate) a blood vessel so as to occlude the lumen or sew tissue together. Sutures are used to close wounds in a process referred to as *suturing*. Tissues are sutured together for the purpose of holding them until healing takes place.

28. Desired characteristics of all sutures are sterility, ease of handling, consistent tensile strength appropriate to the suture size, and minimal reactivity in tissue.

29. *Tensile strength* is the amount of tension or pull that a suture will withstand before it breaks. The tension or pull is expressed in pounds. Tensile strength determines the amount of wound support that the suture provides during the healing process. Suture tensile strength should be as strong as the tensile strength (ability to withstand stress) of the tissue in which it is placed. As suture diameter decreases, suture tensile strength decreases.

30. Suture materials must be sterile when they are placed inside the patient's body. This requires packaging that permits sterile presentation to the field and adherence to aseptic technique, thus maintaining sterility.

31. Suture material should be pliable, elicit minimal drag, slide easily through tissue, tie easily, and hold the knot securely.

32. Because suture material is a foreign body, some tissue reaction is inevitable. The foreign-body reaction will persist until the suture is either absorbed by the body or encapsulated. Suture is selected that offers the least potential for tissue reaction.

33. The surgeon's choice of suture is influenced by many factors. These are: the surgeon's familiarity with the suture; physical and biological characteristics of the suture material; healing characteristics of the tissue in which it will be placed; presence of infection or contamination;

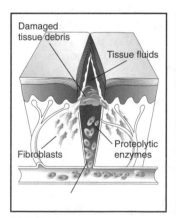
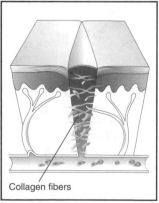
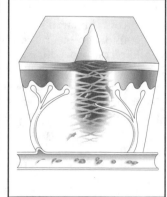

PHASE 1—
Inflammatory response and debridement process

PHASE 2 —
Collagen formation (scar tissue)

PHASE 3 —
Sufficient collagen laid down

FIGURE 10-1 Tissue Response to Injury.
Source: ETHICON, INC., 1996, Somerville, NJ.

patient characteristics such as age, weight, and state of health; and expected postoperative course of the patient.

34. Although suture selection is the surgeon's responsibility, the perioperative nurse must be familiar with suture material and its appropriate uses in order to plan for surgical procedures and to respond to unanticipated events, such as surgical complications, emergencies, and suture substitutions.

• •

SECTION QUESTIONS

Q1. Inadequate wound closure can result in what injury to the surgical patient? (Ref. 3, 5)

_____

_____

Q2. Suture material has no impact on surgical wound infection. (Ref. 6)

True   False

Q3. Surgery to repair an Achilles tendon, where no preexisting inflammation and no break in aseptic technique occurs, would be classified as (Ref. 9):

a. clean

b. clean contaminated

c. contaminated

Q4. Risk of infection for a class II procedure is _____ than the risk for a class I procedure. (Ref. 17)

a. lower

b. greater

Q5. The most desirable method of wound healing is by _____ intention. (Ref. 19)

a. primary

b. secondary

c. tertiary

Q6. Inflammation is a natural occurrence in the process of wound healing and extends through the fourth or fifth postoperative day. (Ref. 23)

True   False

Q7. Suture removal at the end of the proliferation stage of wound healing is appropriate. (Ref. 24)

True   False

Q8. A surgical wound will generally have regained approximately 50% of the strength provided by the suture material at the time of wound closure by (Ref. 26):

a. 1 week

b. 6 weeks

c. 1 year

Q9. Suture selection is influenced by (Ref. 33):

a. healing characteristics of the tissue in which it is placed

b. surgeon's familiarity with the suture

c. biological characteristics of the suture material

d. expected postoperative course

e. patient preference

• •

Classification of Suture Material

35. Standards and classification of suture are set by the United States Pharmacopeia (USP). Sutures are classified as monofilament or multifilament; absorbable or nonabsorbable; coated or uncoated.

Monofilament and Multifilament

36. Monofilament sutures are comprised of a single strand of material. Because they are a single strand, they incur little resistance as they are drawn through tissue and as they are tied. Knots made with monofilament suture have a tendency to loosen, and additional throws in the knot are needed to secure it. Monofilament sutures do not harbor bacteria and therefore reduce the potential for a suture-line infection.

37. Multifilament sutures are several strands twisted or braided together. They handle and tie securely and provide greater tensile strength than monofilament sutures. Multifilament sutures have a certain amount of capillarity. Capillarity is a process that allows tissue fluid to be soaked or absorbed into the suture and carried along the strand. A disadvantage of multifilament sutures is that microorganisms that may be contained in tissue fluid can be carried along the strand into the wound and result in infection. Multifilament sutures may be coated to improve their handling characteristics and to reduce capillarity.

Absorbable Suture

38. Absorbable suture is assimilated by the body during the healing process and is considered temporary. Assimilation time varies according to the type of suture material and to patient factors that may accelerate absorption. As the suture is absorbed, its tensile strength decreases.

39. Absorbable suture is made of material that is digested by body enzymes or is hydrolyzed (broken down by water in tissue fluids). Absorbable suture may be natural or synthetic. Natural absorbable sutures are highly purified collagen and are made from the submucosa layer of sheep intestine or the serosa layer of beef.

40. The most common natural absorbable suture is plain or chromatic surgical gut.

41. Plain surgical gut is natural suture. It has limited use and loses all of its tensile strength within approximately 7 days. Absorption takes place in approximately 70 days. This means it will take about 70 days for the suture to be absorbed; however, it will only provide support (progressively decreasing) for the wound for approximately 7 to 10 days. Therefore, plain gut suture is used primarily to ligate superficial blood vessels and to suture the subcutaneous tissue layer.

42. Surgical gut that has been treated in a chromium salt solution is referred to as *chromic gut*. Chromatization renders the gut more resistant to absorption.

43. Chromic gut retains tensile strength longer than plain gut. Tensile strength is retained for 10 to 14 days, enabling a wound to heal more slowly while providing support. It is absorbed in approximately 90 days.

44. Plain gut, chromic gut, and collagen sutures are digested by body enzymes through phago-

cytosis, which results in varying degrees of inflammatory reaction.

45. The rate of decline in tensile strength and absorption of surgical gut is influenced by the type of tissue in which it is used, the condition of the tissue, and the state of health of the patient. If the patient is anemic, malnourished, protein deficient, debilitated, or has an infection, the rate of absorption and the loss of tensile strength may be accelerated.

46. Surgical gut sutures are packaged in a conditioning fluid of alcohol and water. This conditioning fluid keeps the suture pliable. Surgical gut should be handled only when moist; therefore, it should be used immediately upon removal from the package. Gut suture that is removed from the package and allowed to dry will lose its pliability. Moistening it with sterile saline just prior to use will restore pliability. Gut suture should not be immersed or permitted to remain in saline or water because excessive moisture will reduce tensile strength.

47. Synthetic absorbable sutures are made from synthetic polymers of lactic and glycolic acid and polyester. They are absorbed through hydrolysis, which causes the polymer chain to break down. Hydrolysis results in less tissue reaction than enzymatic suture absorption. Synthetic suture is minimally affected by the presence of infection, the type of tissue, or the patient's state of health. Absorption time and loss of tensile strength are predictable.

48. The tensile strength of synthetic absorbable sutures is greater than for natural materials and varies from several weeks to several months. For some sutures, a 25% tensile strength remains after 6 weeks and for others, all tensile strength is lost in 2 weeks.

49. The selection of suture must be based on knowledge of the rate of tensile strength, degradation of the suture material, and time required for wound healing.

50. Synthetic absorbable sutures that provide the longest wound support times are appropriate for patients who heal slowly, such as the elderly, or patients with acquired immune deficiency syndrome (AIDS), or those receiving radiation therapy.

51. Synthetic absorbable sutures are packed dry and should not be immersed in solutions because this can reduce tensile strength.

52. Examples of synthetic absorbable sutures are DEXON® (polyglycolic acid), VICRYL® (polyglactin 910), PDS® (polydioxanone), MAXON® (polyglyconate), MONOCRYL® (poliglecaprone), and BIOSYN® (synthetic polyester).

53. An absorbable suture coated with the antibacterial agent triclosan (VICRYL Plus®), has recently been introduced to the market. This suture is useful in preventing bacterial colonization.

Nonabsorbable Suture

54. Nonabsorbable suture is made of either natural or synthetic material, is not assimilated, and is considered permanent once it is placed within the body.

55. Silk and cotton are natural nonabsorbable sutures. Cotton suture is made from cotton fibers that have been combed, aligned, and twisted into a multifilament strand. Because it is somewhat reactive in tissue, it is used very infrequently. Tensile strength is enhanced when the suture is moistened.

56. Surgical silk is a natural material made from thread spun by silkworms in their making of cocoons. The silk strands are twisted or braided and are usually dyed black. Silk loses its tensile strength within 1 year after implantation and cannot be used where very long-term support is needed, such as in a heart valve. Silk is not totally nonabsorbable and may dissolve after several years. On occasion, a silk suture will migrate to the wound surface. This action is referred to as *spitting*.

57. Silk is one of the most widely used nonabsorbable sutures and is often used in the gastrointestinal tract. It is pliable and holds the knot securely. Because of its capillarity, silk is treated to resist absorption of body fluids.

58. Nylon, polyester, polyethylene, polybutester, and polypropylene are some of the synthetic polymers used to manufacture synthetic nonabsorbable sutures. Synthetic fibers cause less tissue irritation, retain their strength longer, and have a higher tensile strength than do natural fibers.

59. Nylon suture (e.g., ETHILON®, DERMALON®, NUROLON®, and SURGILON®) has high tensile strength and is inert in the body. It is smooth and slides easily through tissue. Additional throws in the knot and square ties are necessary to provide knot security. Nylon is often used for skin closure and, because it can be manufactured into very fine strands, is suitable for ophthalmic surgery and microsurgery and is used in neurosurgery. Nylon suture used on the skin and neck areas is removed between 2 to 5 days. On other skin areas, suture removal is typically within 8 days

60. Polyester suture (e.g., Dacron, MERSILINE®, ETHIBOND®, TEVDEK®, and TI-CRON®) is closely braided, is available in a variety of

sizes, and is usually coated with a specially designed lubricant that reduces drag as the suture is passed through tissue. Polyester suture is often used in cardiac surgery and neurosurgery.

61. Polybutester suture (NOVAFIL®) is a monofilament suture with more flexibility and elasticity than other synthetic polymers.

62. Polypropylene suture (e.g., PROLENE®, SURGILENE®) is an inert monofilament, has good tensile strength, and slides smoothly through tissue. It is available in a variety of sizes including very fine strands. Its use is standard in cardiovascular surgery and other surgeries where prolonged healing is anticipated. Additional throws and square ties are necessary for knot security. Polypropylene suture should be gently stretched before use to eliminate memory and prevent kinking.

63. Polyester and polypropylene suture retain tensile strength and cause minimal inflammatory reaction, whereas silk will gradually lose tensile strength over time and does cause an inflammatory reaction.

64. Stainless-steel suture has the highest tensile strength and is the most inert of all sutures. It is particularly useful where strong permanent wound security is needed, such as the sternum following cardiovascular surgery. Metallic suture is difficult to handle and requires an exacting suture technique. It has very limited application.

Suture Diameter

65. Suture diameter ranges from a heavy size 7 to a very fine size 11-0. In decreasing thickness, suture begins with 7 and progresses as follows: 7, 6, 5, 4, 3, 2, 1, 0, 2-0, 3-0, 4-0, . . . 11-0. (Figure 10-2) Tensile strength decreases as suture diameter decreases. Sutures size 5-0 through 11-0 are finer than a human hair and are often used in microsurgery. They are fragile and must be handled with the utmost care.

66. The majority of sutures used in general surgery have diameters in the 1 to 4-0 range.

Suture Selection—Considerations

67. There are many factors that determine suture selection, such as expected length of time for healing, presence of contamination in the wound, desired cosmetic results, and surgeon preference.

68. Absorbable sutures are used in tissue that heals rapidly. Typical application includes the subcutaneous fat, stomach, submucosal layer of the colon, bladder, and biliary tract. Ordinarily nonabsorbable suture is used where extended

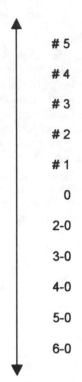

FIGURE 10-2 Size Progression of Sutures.

wound support is needed; however, absorbable suture with long-lasting tensile strength, such as polydioxanone (PDS II), is used where further tissue growth is expected, as in pediatric patients.

69. Nonabsorbable suture is used where extended wound support is needed, such as with fascia and tendons. It is routinely used in vascular, cardiac, and neurosurgery. Nonabsorbable suture that will be removed is used in ophthalmic surgery, for skin closure, and when temporary additional wound support is needed.

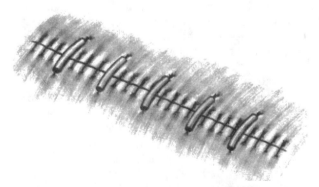

FIGURE 10-3   Retention Suture Bolster.
Source: Printed with permission from ETHICON, INC., Somerville, NJ.

70. When temporary additional abdominal wound support is needed, such as to support the primary suture line of an abdominal wound closure in an obese patient, to support healing by second intention, to eliminate dead space within the wound, or to prevent accumulation of fluid in an abdominal wound, retention sutures may be used. These nonabsorbable sutures are placed approximately 2 inches beyond the edge of the primary suture line and are passed through all layers of the abdominal wall. Once it is ascertained that the primary wound has healed sufficiently, the retention sutures are removed. (Figure 10-3)

• •

SECTION QUESTIONS

Q10. Monofilament suture resists harboring microorganisms. (Ref. 36)

True   False

Q11. Explain why capillarity with regard to suture material is a disadvantage. (Ref. 37)

_____

_____

_____

Q12. Suture that is assimilated by the body during the healing process is classified as (Ref. 38):

_____

Q13. Plain gut is used in tissue where very long-term support is necessary. (Ref. 41)

True   False

Q14. Chromic gut (Ref. 39, 40, 42, 43, 44):

a. is absorbed through phagocytosis

b. will support the wound for approximately 90 days

c. is not absorbable

Q15. List three patient conditions that may influence the rate of suture absorption and decline in tensile strength. (Ref. 45)

_____

_____

_____

Q16. Surgical gut (Ref. 46):

a. should be allowed to dry before being used for suturing

b. should be moist when used

c. may be moistened with sterile saline prior to use

Q17. List three advantages of synthetic absorbable suture over natural absorbable suture. (Ref. 47, 48)

_____

_____

_____

Q18. Suture that is considered permanent once it is placed within the body is classified as (Ref. 54):

_____

Q19. Surgical silk suture (Ref. 56):

   a. is made from thread spun by silkworms

   b. is a good choice for heart-valve replacement surgery

   c. is classified as nonabsorbable but may in fact dissolve over time

   d. may spit

Q20. Synthetic nonabsorbable sutures have a greater tensile strength and retain their strength longer than do natural nonabsorbable sutures. (Ref. 58)

   True   False

Q21. What may be done during the manufacturing process to reduce the drag on polyester-braided suture material? (Ref. 60)

_____

_____

Q22. A 4-0 suture has less tensile strength and is finer, that is, has a smaller diameter than a 5-0 suture. (Ref. 65)

   True   False

• •

Suture Package Information

71. Sutures are supplied sterile from the manufacturer in a double envelope package. The inner package contains the sterile suture(s). The outer package is a peel package designed to permit aseptic delivery of the suture to the sterile field.

72. Information required by the USP is printed on each suture package. This includes: material; trade name; generic name; product number; size, length, color; number of needles in the package if more than one; description of the needle; whether the suture is braided or monofilament, absorbable or nonabsorbable; coating material if used; manufacturer; date manufactured and expiration date; and compliance with USP standards. (Figures 10-4, 10-5)

73. Sutures are supplied in boxes containing multiple packages. They are commercially sterilized with ethylene oxide or ionizing radiation. Unused sutures should not be resterilized because product integrity cannot be guaranteed using hospital sterilization processes and cycles. Sutures are not intended to be resterilized; the original manufacturer does not supply reprocessing guidelines; and use of reprocessed suture could jeopardize patient safety.

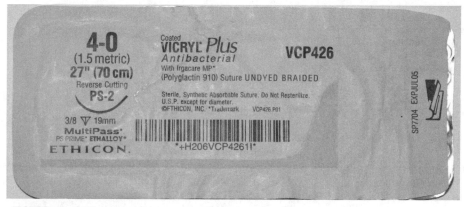

FIGURE 10-4   Suture package.
Source: Reprinted with permission from ETHICON, Inc., Sommerville, NJ.

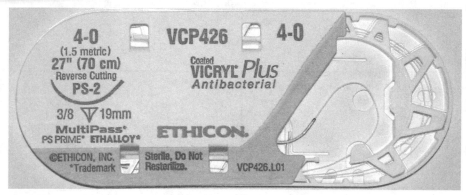

FIGURE 10-5   Suture package.
Source: Reprinted with permission from ETHICON, Inc., Sommerville, NJ.

SURGICAL NEEDLES

Needle Characteristics

74. Surgical needles are designed to carry suture material through tissue with minimum trauma. They are precision made to prevent excessive bending and still provide some flexibility without breaking. Surgical needles may be characterized by their shape, type of point, size, and how the suture material is attached.

75. The three basic parts of the needle are the point, shaft or body, and eye.

76. Needle points are tapered, cutting, or blunt. (Figure 10-6) Tapered needles are used in tissue, such as peritoneum or intestine, that offers little resistance to the needle as it is passed through. A taper-point needle is designed with the shaft gradually tapering to a sharp point so as to make the smallest possible hole in the tissue.

77. A cutting-point needle is designed with a razor-sharp tip and is used for tissue that is difficult to penetrate, such as skin or tendon. Cutting needles have cutting edges that extend along the shaft. There are variations of the cutting

needle that are used according to surgical preference in selected tissue.

78. Blunt-tip needles have a rounded end and are used in friable tissue, such as the liver or kidney, when neither piercing nor cutting is appropriate. Blunt needles are also used for safety purposes to reduce risk of exposure to bloodborne pathogens. They are especially useful for suturing in a deep cavity where visualization is difficult, as in gynecological surgery.

79. The shaft of the needle may be straight or curved. Curvatures are 1/4, 3/8, 1/2, and 5/8 circle. (Figure 10-7) Selection of needle shape and size is determined by the size and properties of the suture material, nature of the surgery, and the surgeon's preference.

80. The eye of the needle is where suture is either attached or threaded.

Needle Attachment

81. The needle may be attached to the suture needle during manufacture or may be threaded at the time of surgery. Needles that are attached are referred to as *swaged*, and the suture is re-

POINT/BODY SHAPE	APPLICATIONS
Conventional Cutting	ligament nasal cavity oral cavity pharynx skin tendon
Reverse Cutting	fascia ligament nasal cavity oral mucosa pharynx skin tendon sheath
MICRO-POINT Reverse Cutting Needle	eye
Precision Point Cutting	skin (plastic or cosmetic)
Side-cutting Spatula	eye (primary application) microsurgery ophthalmic (reconstructive)

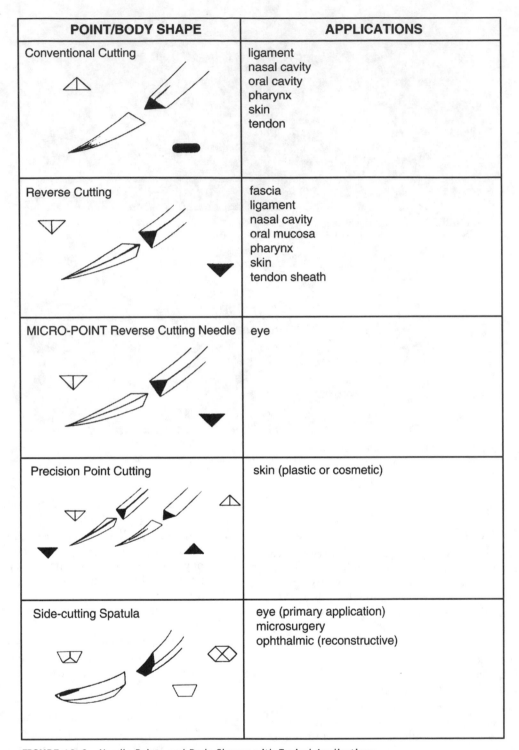

FIGURE 10-6 Needle Points and Body Shapes with Typical Applications.
Source: Reprinted with permission from ETHICON, INC., 1996, Somerville, NJ.

POINT/BODY SHAPE	APPLICATIONS	
TAPERCUT Surgical Needle	bronchus calcified tissue fascia ligament nasal cavity oral cavity ovary perichondrium periosteum	pharynx tendon trachea uterus vessels (sclerotic)
Taper	aponeurosis biliary tract dura fascia gastrointestinal tract muscle myocardium nerve peritoneum	pleura subcutaneous fat urogenital tract vessels
Blunt	blunt dissection (friable tissue) fascia intestine kidney liver spleen cervix (ligating incompetent cervix)	
CS ULTIMA Ophthalmic Needle	eye (primary application)	
PC PRIME Needle	skin (plastic or cosmetic)	

FIGURE 10-6 *continued*.

Straight

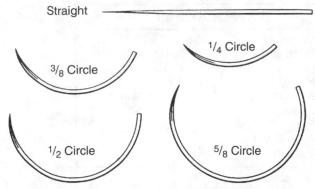

3/8 Circle

1/4 Circle

1/2 Circle

5/8 Circle

FIGURE 10-7 Needle Shapes. Surgical needles vary in shape, size, type of point, body and how suture is attached (swaged or threaded).
Source: Reprinted with permission from *Perspectives on Sutures,* p. 52, © 1978, Davis and Geck.

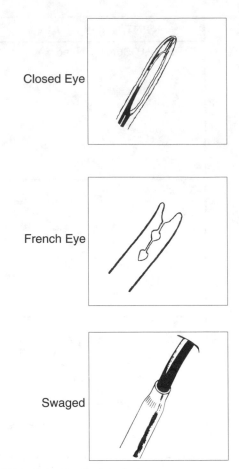

Closed Eye

French Eye

Swaged

FIGURE 10-8 Needle Attachments.
Source: Reprinted with permission from ETHICON, INC., 1996, Somerville, NJ.

ferred to as *swaged* or *atraumatic*. Needle and suture strand are a continuous unit in which needle diameter and suture diameter are matched as closely as possible, thus minimizing tissue trauma. Atraumatic suture eliminates the need for threading. Almost all sutures used in surgery are atraumatic.

82. A modification of the permanently swaged suture is the controlled-release suture, sometimes referred to as a *pop off*. Needle and suture are one continuous unit; however, they may be separated by means of a light tug. Controlled-release sutures facilitate rapid interrupted suturing techniques.

83. Suture may be attached to a needle with a round, oval, or square eye. It is threaded in much the same manner as a household needle. (Figure 10-8)

84. A French-eyed needle has a slit from the inside of the eye to the proximal end of the needle. Suture is forced, rather than threaded, through this slit.

85. Use of an eyed needle necessitates two strands of suture being pulled through tissue. This bulk causes tissue trauma and for this reason is rarely used.

OTHER WOUND CLOSURE DEVICES

Stapling Devices

86. Stapling devices are available for approximation of internal tissues and for fascia and skin closure. Staples are made of stainless steel or titanium. Stapling devices are designed for stapling specific tissue and are not interchange-

able. Staples may be applied individually, as in skin or fascia staplers, where clips or staples are delivered one at a time. Stapling devices that deliver multiple staples simultaneously are used in intestinal and thoracic surgery.

Skin Tapes, Skin Adhesives

87. Adhesive skin tapes (Steri Strips®, Proxistrips®) are used to approximate surgical incision wound edges. (Figure 10-9) They are used in conjunction with subcuticular sutures to approximate incision edges. Used in this manner they are an alternative to suture or staple skin closure. Skin tapes may also be used as a complement to suture or staple closures. They are used to replace skin staples or sutures that have been removed several days postoperatively.

88. Skin tapes are available in widths of 1/8, 1/4, and 1/2 inch and in lengths from 1 1/2 to 4 inches.

89. Skin adhesives (DERMABOND®, INDERMIL®) are used to glue skin edges together. Skin adhesives are useful where cosmetic con-

that are anticipated to produce fluid sufficient to place undue stress on closure may be drained.

91. Three types of drains are passive, active, and sump. Passive drains function through gravity and capillary action. Active drains employ negative pressure. Sump drains are double lumen devices that may be attached to either continuous or intermittent low suction.

92. The most commonly used passive drain is a Penrose. A Penrose drain is a simple lumen drain made from rubber or silicone. The external end of the drain empties because of gravity or capillary action through the drain to a surgical dressing where drainage is captured. Disadvantages of the Penrose drain are that it provides a pathway for microorganisms to migrate from the surrounding environment into the wound, and wound drainage cannot be accurately measured.

93. Commonly used active drains are the Hemovac and the Jackson Pratt. (Figure 10-10) Drainage flows from the end inside the wound through tubing that exits adjacent to the incision site and is attached to a closed reservoir. The reservoir is collapsed before being attached to the drain. The resultant negative pressure directs drainage out of the wound to fill the reservoir. The reservoir may be emptied and negative pressure reinstated to collect additional drainage. Unlike the Penrose drain, Hemovac or Jackson Pratt drains permit accurate measurement of drainage, and because they are closed systems they provide less of a pathway for microorganisms to migrate into the wound.

94. Sump drains are double lumened. One lumen provides for the passage of filtered air into the wound, and the other permits passage of drainage material from the wound. In the presence of copious drainage, the sump pump may be connected to an external suction.

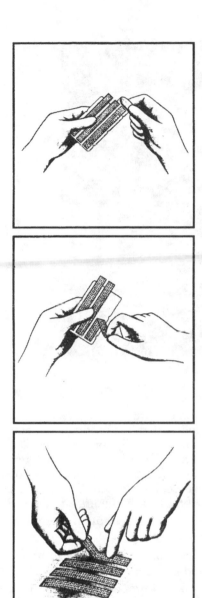

FIGURE 10-9 Skin Tapes.
Source: Reprinted with permission from ETHICON, INC., 1996, Somerville, NJ.

siderations are important. Unlike sutures, they leave no suture tracks along a healed incision line. Skin adhesives are used to seal the incision to prevent entry of microorganisms and are particularly useful in traumatic surgery where risk of infection is greatest.

Drains

90. Some surgical wound closures will incorporate a drain. Drains are used primarily to obliterate dead space where tissue may not have been adequately approximated or to remove foreign or harmful materials, i.e., infected or necrotic tissue, or when hemostasis is uncertain. Wounds

DRESSINGS

95. Most surgical incisions are closed primarily and are covered with a sterile surgical dressing. Typically, a nonadherent dressing that will not stick to the wound and cause trauma is applied first (Telfa®), followed by a gauze dressing. In the case of a large wound or one in which some additional absorbency is needed, the gauze layer will be covered with an absorbent pad. The final layer is then taped.

96. Alternately, the surgeon may choose to dress a clean wound using a nonadherent dressing (Telfa®), followed by application of a thin

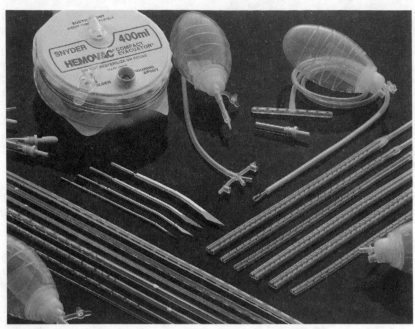

FIGURE 10-10 Self-Contained Wound Drainage Systems.
Source: Courtesy of Zimmer, Inc., Dover, Ohio.

transparent semipermeable dressing that is oxygen permeable but is a barrier to bacteria and water (Tegaderm™, OpSite®).

97. Other types of dressings may be used for a variety of incisions or wounds, and surgeon preference will dictate the choice. Among the variety of dressings available are mesh nonadherent dressings, dressings impregnated with petrolatum, and dressings impregnated with an antimicrobial.

NURSING RESPONSIBILITIES RELATED TO WOUND MANAGEMENT

98. Although the selection and use of wound-closure material and devices is primarily the surgeon's responsibility. However, the nurse delivers suture to the sterile field and the nurse in the scrub role passes suture to the surgeon. The perioperative nurse with a knowledge and understanding of suture and needle characteristics can help prevent patient injury. For example, a cutting needle used in a vascular procedure, where a tapered point is desired and anticipated, can cause trauma to the patient and result in additional bleeding; and an absorbable suture used where permanent wound support is desired can result in wound separation.

99. The more knowledgeable the nurse is regarding wound closure materials and devices, the less likely it is that inappropriate materials and devices that can compromise patient safety will be utilized. The nurse who understands sutures, drains, and dressings will be able to anticipate the surgeon's needs and assist in keeping surgery time to a minimum.

100. The following are nursing responsibilities related to use of suture:

- Select sutures according to preference card and anticipated need.
- Count sutures according to suture package information and verify upon opening.
- Arrange suture in order of anticipated use.
- Prepare one or two sutures for immediate use, i.e., load them on needle holders, keep remainder in package until needed.
- Place loaded needle holders so as to prevent accidental exposure.
- To prevent recoil, gently tug suture strands prior to passing to surgeon. Do not tug at point of needle attachment.
- Pass suture so as to prevent accidental exposure.
- Place used needles on appropriate collection pad.
- Close needle collection pad and deposit into sharps container.

SECTION QUESTIONS

Q23. List three types of surgical needle points. (Ref. 76)

_____

Q24. Name the needle point most appropriate for suturing liver tissue. (Ref. 78)

_____

Q25. Suture to which the needle is permanently attached is referred to as _____ or _____.
(Ref. 81)

Q26. Describe a disadvantage to using an eyed needle that must be threaded. (Ref. 85)

_____

_____

Q27. Explain the three primary purposes of a wound drain. (Ref. 90)

_____

_____

_____

Q28. Describe the benefit of a Hemovac or Jackson Pratt drain over a Penrose drain. (Ref. 93)

_____

_____

Q29. The perioperative nurse's knowledge and understanding of wound closure material can help prevent patient injury. Explain an instance of how this is possible. (Ref. 98, 99)

_____

_____

• • • References

Ethicon. (2002). *Wound closure manual.* Selangor Darul Ehsan, Malaysia: Author.

Fry, D. (2003). Surgical site infection: Determinants, diagnosis and prevention. *Point of View,* 42(1), 15–22.

Long, B. (1993). Postoperative intervention. In B. Long, W. Phipps, & V. Cassmeyer (Eds.), *Medical surgical nursing.* St. Louis, MO: Mosby Year Book.

Mangram, A., Horan, T., Pearson, M., Silver, L., & Jarvis, W. (1999). Guideline for prevention of surgical site infection, 1999. *Infection Control and Hospital Epidemiology,* 20(4), 247–278.

Wysocki, A. (1989). Surgical wound healing: A review for perioperative nurses. *AORN Journal,* 49(2), 508.

• • • Suggested Reading

Phillips, N. (2000). Hemostasis and wound closure. *Berry & Kohn's Operating Room Technique* (10th ed., pp. 528–551). St. Louis, MO: Mosby.

Tomaselli, N. (2003). Prevention and treatment of surgical site infections. *Infection Control Resource,* 2(1), 1–5.

Appendix 10-A

· ·

Chapter 10 Post Test

Instructions: Fill in the blank(s), mark the correct answer(s), or answer the question as appropriate.

1. List two potential patient injuries related to wound closure. (Ref. 1, 2, 3)

   _____

   _____

2. The majority of surgical wound infections are initiated along or close to the suture line. (Ref. 6)

   True   False

3. Match the wound classification with the surgery type. (Ref. 9, 11–16)

   a. class I   _____ amputation of a gangrenous foot

   b. class II   _____ cataract extraction

   c. class III   _____ bilateral inguinal hernia repair

   d. class IV   _____ removal of an inflamed (but not ruptured) appendix

                           _____ bronchoscopy

4. When a wound cannot be sutured together following surgery, it is left open to heal from the bottom upward and fills in with granulation tissue. This is referred to as wound healing by (Ref. 20):

   a. primary intention

   b. secondary intention

   c. tertiary intention

5. The amount of pull that a suture will withstand before it breaks is defined as _____ strength. (Ref. 29)

6. Suture that is assimilated by the body during the healing process is classified as _____. (Ref. 38)

7. What may be done to multifilament suture during manufacture to reduce capillarity? (Ref. 37)

   _____

8. Monofilament suture (Ref. 36, 37):

   a. resists capillarity

   b. tends to loosen and requires extra throws in the knot to secure it

   c. incurs more resistance than multifilament suture when drawn through tissue

9. The rate of absorption of gut suture is affected by (Ref. 45):

   a. the patient's state of health

   b. the presence of infection

   c. the type of tissue in which it is placed

   d. the condition of the tissue in which it is placed

10. Synthetic absorbable suture is absorbed by (Ref. 47):

    a. the action of enzymes

    b. hydrolysis

11. Nylon suture (Ref. 59):

    a. is often used in surgery of the GI tract

    b. is often used for skin closure

    c. can be provided in fine sutures suitable for ophthalmic surgery

    d. is absorbed by enzymes

12. Where prolonged healing is anticipated, such as in cardiovascular surgery, and minimal reactivity is desired, appropriate suture material is (Ref. 62):

    a. chromic gut

    b. Vicryl

    c. Prolene

    d. silk

13. The suture strand with the smallest diameter is (Ref. 65):

    a. 4–0

    b. 6–0

    c. 2–0

    d. 2

14. Retention sutures are primarily used in orthopedic surgical procedures. (Ref. 70)

    True   False

15. List eight items of information that may be obtained from the suture package. (Ref. 72)

    _____   _____

    _____   _____

    _____   _____

    _____   _____

16. A taper needle is most appropriate for suturing (Ref. 76):

    a. skin

    b. liver

    c. intestine

    d. peritoneum

17. What is an atraumatic suture? (Ref. 81)

    _____

18. A stapling device may be used to close fascia. (Ref. 86)

    True   False

19. A Penrose drain permits leakage of drainage onto dressings and provides a pathway for migration of microorganisms. (Ref. 92)

    True   False

20. The perioperative nurse may utilize knowledge about wound closure materials to (Ref. 99, 100):

    a. anticipate needed suture

    b. help to minimize surgery time

    c. help prevent injury to patient tissue

Appendix 10-B

• •

Competency Checklist: Prevention of Injury: Wound Management

Under "Observer's Initials," enter initials upon successful achievement of competency.
Enter N/A if competency is not appropriate for institution.

NAME _____

	OBSERVER'S INITIALS	DATE

1. Suture selected according to preference card and anticipated need.   _____   _____

2. Suture counted correctly.   _____   _____

3. Package contents verified when opened.   _____   _____

4. Suture arranged on back table in order of anticipated use.   _____   _____

5. Suture loaded in anticipation of need—remaining suture maintained in package.   _____   _____

6. Loaded suture placed on Mayo/back table in manner to avoid accidental exposure.   _____   _____

7. Suture with memory (e.g., prolene) pulled gently before passed to surgeon to prevent rebound (no pull exerted on needle attachment).   _____   _____

8. Suture passed in safe manner (sharp announced, etc.).   _____   _____

9. Needles removed from suture in safe manner.   _____   _____

10. Needles placed carefully on magnetic needle mat or other appropriate receptacle.   _____   _____

11. Needles deposited in sharps box following procedure.   _____   _____

OBSERVER'S SIGNATURE   INITIALS   DATE

_____

ORIENTEE'S SIGNATURE

_____

Chapter 10—Section Question Answers

Q1. Dehiscence, evisceration
Q2. False
Q3. a
Q4. b
Q5. a
Q6. True
Q7. True
Q8. b
Q9. a, b, c, d
Q10. True
Q11. Capillarity can cause pathogenic microorganisms to be soaked or absorbed into the suture and carried along the strand
Q12. Absorbable
Q13. False
Q14. a
Q15. Type of tissue in which it is used, condition of the tissue, patient's state of health, presence of infection
Q16. b, c
Q17. Less tissue reaction, minimally affected by presence of infection, type of tissue, or patient's health, absorption rate is predictable
Q18. Nonabsorbable
Q19. a, c, d
Q20. True
Q21. Coat with specially designed lubricant
Q22. False
Q23. Taper, cutting, blunt
Q24. Blunt
Q25. Swaged, atraumatic
Q26. Two strands (double thickness) must be pulled through the tissue, which causes tissue trauma
Q27. Obliterate dead space, remove harmful materials, determine adequacy of hemostasis
Q28. Permits accurate measurement of drainage, is a closed system—lessens opportunity for migration of organisms into the wound
Q29. Knowing which suture/needle is appropriate for the tissue can prevent use of inappropriate suture materials or needles that could cause injury

Chapter 10—Post Test Answers

1. Infection, compromised wound healing, wound dehiscence, wound evisceration
2. True
3. d, a, a, c, b
4. b
5. Tensile
6. Absorbable
7. Coating to prevent capillarity
8. a, b
9. a, b, c, d
10. b
11. b, c
12. c
13. b
14. False
15. Material, trade name, generic name, product number, size, length, color, number of needles, type of needles, whether braided or monofilament, whether absorbable or nonabsorbable, whether coated, date of manufacture, expiration date
16. c, d
17. Needle and suture strand are one continuous unit, needle is swaged
18. True
19. True
20. a, b, c

Prevention of Injury—Anesthesia

• • • • • • • • • • • • •

Lesson Outline

I. POTENTIAL INJURY—DESIRED PATIENT OUTCOMES
    A. Nursing Diagnoses
    B. Desired Patient Outcomes
    C. Outcome Criteria
    D. Overview of Nursing Responsibilities
II. PREANESTHESIA
    A. Assessment Data
    B. American Society of Anesthesiologists Classification
    C. Patient Teaching
    D. Patient Instructions
    E. Selection of Anesthetic Agents and Technique

III. ANESTHESIA TECHNIQUES—OVERVIEW
IV. PREMEDICATION
   A. Goals
   B. Medications/Protocols
V. MONITORING
   A. Practice Recommendations and Standards
   B. Monitoring Devices
     1. Precordial or Esophageal Stethoscope
     2. Electrocardiagram (ECG)
     3. Pulse Oximetry
     4. Blood Pressure
     5. Temperature
     6. Capnography
VI. GENERAL ANESTHESIA
   A. Inhalation Agents
   B. Anesthesia Machine
   C. Intravenous Agents
     1. Barbiturate Induction Agents
     2. Nonbarbiturate Induction Agents
     3. Dissociative Induction Agent
     4. Narcotics
     5. Tranquilizers—Benzodiazepines
     6. Neuromuscular Blockers (Muscle Relaxants)
   D. Stages of Anesthesia
   E. Preparation for Anesthesia—Nursing Responsibilities
   F. Sequence for General Anesthesia—Nursing Responsibilities
VII. MALIGNANT HYPERTHERMIA
   A. Overview
   B. Treatment
   C. Nursing Responsibilities
VIII. MODERATE SEDATION/ANALGESIA
   A. Overview
   B. Nursing Responsibilities
IX. REGIONAL ANESTHESIA
   A. Overview
   B. Spinal
   C. Epidural and Caudal
   D. Intravenous Block (Bier Block)
   E. Nerve Block
   F. Local Infiltration
   G. Topical
   H. Regional Anesthesia—Nursing Responsibilities

POTENTIAL INJURY—DESIRED PATIENT OUTCOMES

1. A little over a hundred years ago, anesthesia technique was a crude open-drop ether administration. Depth of anesthesia and physiologic response were inconsistent and poorly controlled. The risk of complication was high. The recent development of sophisticated anesthesia and airway management techniques, new anesthetic agents, refined preanesthesia assessment, and technologically advanced monitoring devices have all made delivery of anesthesia a highly refined process and have dramatically reduced the associated risk.

2. The number of anesthetics administered yearly in the United States is estimated to be 25 million, and most patients suffer no significant consequences as a result of anesthesia. In the 1900s, the death rate from anesthesia was 1 in 500. Today, estimates range between 1 in 126,000 to 1 in 300,000 for healthy patients (Lema, 2003, p. 1)

Nursing Diagnoses

3. Although the death rate associated with anesthesia is extremely low, the risk of complication remains. Anesthetic agents can compromise ventilation, perfusion, and cardiac output, and can alter hypothalamic thermoregulation. Appropriate nursing diagnoses for the patient undergoing anesthesia are high risk for injury (untoward drug reaction or interaction, ineffective airway, decreased cardiac output, electrolyte or fluid imbalance, ineffective breathing pattern, alteration in thought process, and ineffective thermoregulation or hypothermia) related to anesthesia. Other diagnoses may be appropriate based on the patient's condition as identified during assessment.

4. The type of anesthesia, the anesthetic agents employed, the surgical procedure, and the patient's preanesthesia physiological condition all impact the degree of risk for the above conditions. For example, the ambulatory patient who undergoes a minor surgical procedure with local anesthetic or moderate sedation/analgesia is at minimal risk for hypothermia compared to the patient who undergoes open abdominal surgery with general anesthesia, where anesthetic agents cause dilation of blood vessels and the nature of the procedure exposes the patient's gut to room temperature.

Desired Patient Outcomes

5. The desired outcome for the patient who undergoes anesthesia is successful recovery and a return to the preanesthesia physiological state, including normothermia, unimpeded air exchange, adequate ventilation, maintenance of cardiac output and fluid volume, electrolyte and fluid balance, absence of allergic reaction, and unimpaired thought processes.

6. The time frame in which these desired outcomes is expected to be achieved will vary according to the procedure, anesthetic agents, and anesthesia technique (i.e., local, regional, or general). For example, in the immediate postoperative period, the patient may or may not be expected to breathe unassisted. Goals for when independent breathing should be expected to occur are determined by the patient's preexisting respiratory condition, the intent of the anesthesia care provider, the anesthetic agents employed, and the nature of the surgery.

Outcome Criteria

7. There are several postanesthesia scoring systems used to evaluate the patient's recovery. The most common is the Aldrete postanesthesia scoring system, which is used to evaluate the recovery of patients who have received general anesthesia. It evaluates patient activity, respiration, circulation, and oxygen saturation. Points are assigned to patient responses, and discharge from the postanesthesia care unit is dependent on the patient's achieving an acceptable score. (Exhibit 11-1)

8. The acceptable score varies with institutional policy, anticipated recovery, and unit to which the patient is discharged. A patient being transferred from the postanesthesia-care unit to a step-down unit may not require as high a score as a patient who is returning to a regular unit. For obvious reasons, a patient who is discharged on the same day of surgery must achieve a high score.

Overview of Nursing Responsibilities

9. Anesthesia may be administered by a certified registered nurse anesthetist (CRNA) or an anesthesiologist. A CRNA is a registered nurse with at least 2 years of anesthesia training after basic nursing school and acute care training. An anesthesiologist is a medical doctor with at least 4 years of anesthesia training after medical school.

10. Preoperatively the CRNA or anesthesiologist will perform a patient assessment, determine the anesthetic agents to be employed, and in collaboration with the surgeon and patient, select the anesthetic technique. Intraoperative responsibility includes delivery of anesthesia, with all the necessary physiological support throughout the procedure and through transport to the postanesthesia-care unit. Postoperatively the CRNA or anesthesiologist evaluates the patient's readiness for discharge and writes a discharge order.

11. Primary responsibility for assisting the anesthesiologist or nurse anesthetist rests with the perioperative nurse in the circulating role. In situations where moderate sedation/analgesia is administered by the surgeon and an anesthesiologist or nurse anesthetist is not present, the responsibility for patient monitoring increasingly belongs to the perioperative nurse.

12. Overall responsibilities of the perioperative nurse related to anesthesia delivery include but are not limited to:

   • Preanesthesia assessment—In addition to the assessment performed by the CRNA or anesthesiologist, the perioperative nurse performs a patient assessment. Information that is obtained serves as a safety check to ensure that significant patient data are known to the surgical team. The information also provides

Exhibit 11-1   Aldrete Score

Activity	Able to move four extemities voluntarily on command	1
	Able to move two extremities voluntarily on command	1
	Able to move no extremities voluntarily on command	0
Respiration	Able to breathe deeply and cough freely	2
	Dyspnea or limited breathing	1
	Apneic	0
Circulation	BP + 20 of preanesthetic level	2
	BP + 20–49 of preanesthetic level	1
	BP + 50 of preanesthetic level	0
Consciousness	Fully awake	2
	Arousable on calling	1
	Not responding	0
O_2 Saturation	Able to maintain O_2 saturation > 92% on room air	2
	Needs O_2 inhalation to maintain O_2 saturation > 90%	1
	O_2 saturation < 90% even with O_2 supplement	0

Source: From Aldrete, A.J., and Wright, A. *Anesthiology News,* 18(11): 17, 1992. In Litwack, K. (Ed.), *Post Anesthesia Care Nursing.* St. Louis: Mosby Year Book, Inc., 1995.

guidelines for anticipating problems, for the course of treatment, and for recovery.

- Patient support—Emotional support is provided in the preoperative period. Emotional support may consist of answering questions, providing a reassuring touch, and/or remaining close to the patient. Physiological support that is provided throughout the perioperative period is accomplished by applying patient monitoring devices, interpreting monitoring data, being alert to patient physiological status and changes, and implementing interventions, such as providing oxygen or preparing and administering intravenous fluids as appropriate. Assistance is given to the anesthesia care provider by anticipating and providing needed equipment and pharmacological agents in a timely manner. The perioperative nurse accompanies the patient to the postanesthesia-care unit and provides physiological and emotional support as needed. In the postoperative period, the perioperative nurse may assist both the anesthesia care provider and the postanesthesia-care unit nurse to stabilize the patient in the unit.

- Communication—Data obtained during the patient assessment are communicated to and verified with the anesthesia care provider prior to delivery of anesthesia. In addition to the documentation requirements of the institution, the perioperative nurse gives a report to the postanesthesia-care unit nurse that provides information necessary to prepare for the reception of the patient and the patient's recovery from anesthesia. Report to the postanesthesia-care nurse should include at least the following:

  1. patient name and age
  2. surgical procedure
  3. surgeon and anesthesiologist/CRNA
  4. anesthetic agents/technique
  5. intraoperative medications
  6. estimated blood loss
  7. fluid and blood administration
  8. urine output
  9. response to surgery/anesthesia
  10. lab results
  11. chronic and acute health history
  12. drug allergies

13. concerns, possible problems, desired patient outcomes not met

14. discharge plan

The perioperative nurse may share responsibility for report with anesthesia personnel and must be knowledgeable of patient status in the above entities and be able to communicate the information to the postanesthesia-care unit nurse.

- Patient teaching—In preparation for anesthesia, the perioperative nurse will provide and reinforce information regarding routines, preanesthesia preparations, instructions for the day of surgery, and procedure-specific postoperative instructions.

13. In many institutions, particularly in small rural facilities, the perioperative nurse provides care throughout the recovery period as well as preoperatively and intraoperatively. Staffing variances and limited resources have resulted in the need for many perioperative nurses to demonstrate competence in postanesthesia care as well as in perioperative nursing. The field of postanesthesia nursing is a specialty in itself and requires significant specialty training. Perioperative nurses who have responsibility for the recovery phase must be skilled in this specialty. Even where responsibility does not include postanesthesia care, the perioperative nurse must be skilled in the use of monitoring equipment and in the interpretation of the data. The perioperative nurse must also be familiar with anesthetic agents and techniques in order to anticipate patient events, quickly implement nursing interventions, and assist the anesthesia care provider.

• •

SECTION QUESTIONS

Q1. The risks associated with anesthesia delivery have been dramatically reduced with the advent of (Ref. 1):

a. technologically advanced monitoring systems

b. sophisticated airway management devices

c. new anesthetic agents

d. improved monitoring of waste anesthetic gases

e. refined patient assessment

Q2. Death as a direct result of anesthesia occurs in approximately 1 out of every 100,000 patients. (Ref. 2)

True   False

Q3. An appropriate nursing diagnosis for the patient who undergoes anesthesia is high risk for injury such as (Ref. 3):

a. ineffective airway

b. altered self-image

c. decreased cardiac output

d. altered thought process

e. ineffective thermoregulation

Q4. List five desired patient outcomes for the patient who undergoes anesthesia (Ref. 5):

_____

_____

_____

_____

_____

Q5. The name of the common postanesthesia scoring system that is used to evaluate the recovery of the patient who has received general anesthesia is (Ref. 7):

_____

Q6. When moderate sedation/analgesia is administered in the absence of an anesthesiologist or CRNA, the responsibility for monitoring may appropriately belong to the perioperative nurse. (Ref. 11)

True   False

Q7. Relative to anesthesia, the perioperative nursing responsibilities may include (Ref. 12):

a. patient assessment

b. patient support

c. patient data communicated to the anesthesiologist

d. patient data communicated to the postanesthesia care provider

e. administration of fluids

f. patient teaching

Q8. In addition to patient name and age, list seven pieces of information that the perioperative nurse should include in the report to the postanesthesia care nurse. (Ref. 12)

_____

_____

_____

_____

_____

• •

PREANESTHESIA

Assessment Data

14. In preparation for surgery and anesthesia, the patient may be required to undergo assessment and preoperative testing several days prior to surgery. Diagnostic testing may include a chest X-ray; an electrocardiogram (ECG); blood chemistry, including a clotting profile; urine analysis; and other tests as deemed necessary by any of the physicians who are attending to the patient's care. The choice of diagnostic studies is determined by the patient's medical and surgical history, the results of the physical examination, and the intended surgical procedure.

15. At the time of preoperative testing, the patient may be interviewed and examined by the anesthesia care provider, who may request additional laboratory and diagnostic testing. During preoperative testing, a perioperative nurse may also interview, assess, and prepare the patient for surgery.

16. The trend today is toward minimal preoperative testing, and the healthy patient may require no laboratory or diagnostic procedures. There is a lack of evidence that routine laboratory testing impacts patient outcomes, and for this reason most diagnostic testing today is patient and procedure specific.

17. With the continuing movement to ambulatory surgery, the patient may not be seen by the anesthesia care provider or perioperative nurse until the day of surgery. Preoperative instructions may be provided by the nurse who is present at the time that the decision for surgery is made. Instructions may also be reinforced by telephone by a perioperative nurse a day or so prior to surgery.

18. Guidelines from the American Society of Anesthesiologists, coupled with institutional requirements, may require an ECG and chest X-ray for patients over a certain age who will undergo general anesthesia or moderate sedation/analgesia. Preoperative diagnostic requirements will vary according to institutional policy and anesthesia care provider preference.

19. During preoperative assessment, the perioperative nurse will review the patient's chart and previously obtained assessment data and assess the patient's readiness for surgery. In addition to the nursing assessment data that are relevant to planning intraoperative care, particular attention is given to data that are significant to anesthesia.

20. Information should be solicited about coexisting disease, history of asthma, previous surgeries, anesthetics, and complications. Family history with anesthetics should be investigated. Such data may provide information suggestive of possible adverse reactions, such as malignant hyperthermia, that can be prevented.

21. Current medications, including herbal medications, and drug allergies must be noted. This information is critical to prevent drugs that may react unfavorably with current medications or that will cause an allergic reaction from being administered to the patient. Allergies to contrast dyes, iodine solutions, adhesive tape, and latex should also be noted, as should any history of drug or substance abuse.

22. The patient should be checked for cracked lips, lacerations in or around the mouth, loose or chipped teeth, and dentures. This is important for patients who will undergo general anesthesia and intubation.

23. Female patients of childbearing age should be assessed to determine whether or not they are pregnant. Often this will necessitate a urine pregnancy test.

24. Smoking history is important because smoking may contribute to postoperative pulmonary complication in patients who receive general anesthesia. However, the benefits of smoking cessation of as little as 12 hours have been demonstrated, and patient teaching should encourage cessation for as long as possible prior to surgery (Brooks-Braun, 1995, p. 343).

25. Diagnostic testing that was previously ordered should be checked to ensure that the tests were actually performed and that the results are on the chart. In the event that abnormalities are noted, the perioperative nurse should confirm that all team members are aware of the test results.

American Society of Anesthesiologists Classification

26. The anesthesia care provider will assign the patient a physical status in accordance with the American Society of Anesthesiologists (ASA) classification. Patients may be assigned a physical status (PS) from 1 to 5 as follows (ASA, 2004):

- P1 patients—healthy, no organic disease
- P2 patients—mild systemic disease (e.g., obesity, controlled hypertension)
- P3 patients—severe systemic disease (e.g., poorly controlled hypertension or history of myocardial infarction)
- P4 patients— severe systemic disease that is a constant threat to life (e.g., renal or cardiac failure

- P5 patients—moribund and not expected to survive—surgery performed as a last recourse (e.g., ruptured aneurysm)
- P6 patients—brain dead—organs harvested
- E—if the procedure is an emergency, the physical status is followed by "E" (for example, "P2E")

This classification system is useful in determining the anesthesia technique to be employed. For example, some institutional policies do not permit class III patients to undergo surgery under general anesthesia as an ambulatory surgery patient, and class III and above patients must have an anesthesiologist or CRNA present during surgery even where anesthesia technique is moderate sedation/analgesia only.

Patient Teaching

27. Patient teaching is ideally initiated at the time that the decision is made to have surgery. Instruction in preoperative routines, expected outcomes, and day-of-surgery instructions may be given in the physician's office or the clinic where the decision for surgery was made. Teaching and/or reinforcement should occur when and if the patient is instructed to report for a presurgical examination or diagnostic workup. Teaching during the presurgical workup may be initiated by a nurse other than the perioperative nurse. In some facilities, a preanesthesia clinic nurse or a postanesthesia-care unit nurse initiates preoperative teaching in preparation for anesthesia and reinforces the instructions with a phone call the night before surgery. The patient who is already hospitalized may be instructed by the nurse on the patient's unit.

28. Regardless of where the teaching was accomplished or who was responsible for preanesthesia instructions, the perioperative nurse should reinforce teaching just prior to surgery and should verify that the patient is in compliance with instructions for the day of surgery.

Patient Instructions

29. Preanesthesia instructions will vary according to the intended surgical procedure and patient condition, and must be individualized. Instructions should include but not be limited to the following:

- postoperative routines—length of surgery, expected recovery time, postoperative anesthesia care and routines

- preoperative preparation (if indicated)—preoperative shower or enema
- preoperative medications—medications to be taken on the day of surgery, both routine and single-dose medications. (On occasion, specific medications will be ordered for a period prior to surgery and other medications that the patient routinely takes will be held.)
- food and liquid intake—traditionally, patients receiving general anesthesia have been instructed to take nothing by mouth (NPO) for 6 to 8 hours prior to surgery. For the patient who is admitted on the day of surgery, typical instructions are "NPO after midnight." With the loss of a protective airway reflex under general anesthesia, a patient who vomits or regurgitates incurs a high risk of aspiration pneumonitis. Aspiration of even a small amount of acid from the stomach can cause severe pneumonitis. A pH of 2.5 and a volume of 0.4 mL is considered an amount that exposes the patient to risk. Ongoing studies, however, indicate that extended periods of fasting do not guarantee an empty stomach (Roth, 1995, p. 214). Protocols generally restrict solid food intake to 6 to 8 hours before surgery, with clear liquids permitted up to 2 to 3 hours before. NPO restrictions will vary with patient age (infant and young child restrictions are generally shorter), institutional protocol, and anesthesia care provider preference.

Selection of Anesthetic Agents and Technique

30. Many factors influence the selection of anesthetic agents and technique. Each patient is unique, and an assessment must be made to determine those drugs that best meet the surgical requirements and that provide for the patient's well-being. Factors that are considered include but are not limited to the following:

- age
- medical history
- current physical status
- intended surgical procedure and expected length of recovery from anesthesia
- patient preference
- surgeon preference/requirements
- anesthesia care provider preference and expertise

- patient's previous anesthesia/recovery experience
- whether surgery is elective or emergent
- considerations for postoperative pain management

ANESTHESIA TECHNIQUES—OVERVIEW

31. Anesthesia may be general, regional, local, or moderate sedation/analgesia.

32. General anesthesia depresses the central nervous system. The patient is unconscious and reflexes are obtunded. Physiologic status is controlled by the anesthesia care provider. This state is characterized by amnesia, analgesia, and muscle relaxation.

33. Moderate sedation/analgesia is also referred to as conscious sedation, monitored anesthesia care (MAC), anesthesia standby, or local standby. In moderate sedation/analgesia the patient is given a local anesthetic at the site of surgery. Medications are administered intravenously to provide sedation and analgesia. The decision as to whether an anesthesia care provider is needed is based on the patient's condition, ASA classification, the procedure, and institutional policy.

34. Moderate sedation/analgesia may be administered to ill patients who cannot tolerate general anesthesia and is referred to as *monitored anesthesia care*. Moderate sedation/analgesia is also appropriate for healthy patients who undergo a minor procedure and who do not require the presence of an anesthesia care provider.

35. In the absence of an anesthesia care provider, the perioperative nurse has the responsibility for monitoring the patient. Institutional policy, in conjunction with the state's Nurse Practice Act, determines whether the responsibility for intravenous drug administration belongs to the nurse, the surgeon, or both.

36. Regional anesthesia blocks the conduction of pain impulses from a specific region of the body. The patient is awake but does not feel pain during surgery. In regional anesthesia, a major nerve block, such as spinal, epidural, or orbital, is anesthetized. Regional anesthetics, such as lidocaine (Xylocaine), bupivacaine (Marcaine), chloroprocaine (Nesacaine), and tetracaine (Pontocaine) are used. Because the patient is awake, additional agents may be administered to reduce anxiety and provide sedation.

37. Local anesthesia is actually a form of regional anesthesia; however, only a small, localized area is infiltrated using an anesthetic such as lidocaine (Xylocaine) or bupivacaine (Marcaine).

PREMEDICATION

Goals

38. The practice of preoperative medication is controversial, and protocols vary between institutions and between anesthesia care providers. Current practices support the evaluation of each patient's needs prior to ordering and administering medications, rather than relying on standard medication protocols.

39. At one time it was standard practice to medicate the patient in preparation for anesthesia and surgery. Today it is not unusual for the patient to receive no preoperative medication. This is particularly true for ambulatory surgery patients, in whom premedication may prolong recovery and delay discharge. In addition, residual effects of medication cannot be monitored after discharge.

40. Goals of premedication may include one or more or all of the following:

- reduction of anxiety
- sedation
- analgesia
- amnesia
- prevention of nausea and vomiting
- reduction in gastric volume and acidity
- facilitation of induction
- reduction of risk of allergic reaction
- decrease of secretions

Medications/Protocols

41. Oral premedications are usually given 60 to 90 minutes prior to surgery, with IV agents requiring 30 to 60 minutes. Some agents, such as metoclopramide (Reglan), which is used to promote gastric emptying and lower stomach pH, fall outside these guidelines. These are given 15 to 30 minutes before induction.

42. Depending on the desired outcome, the following agents are appropriate for use in the preoperative period:

43. Benzodiazepines, such as midazolam (Versed), diazepam (Valium), and lorazepam (Ativan), reduce anxiety, provide sedation and some amnesia.

44. Barbiturates, such as secobarbital (Seconal) and pentobarbital (Nembutal), provide sedation

with minimal cardiac or respiratory depression.

45. H$_2$ receptor blocking agents, such as ranitidine (Zantac, Glaxo), cimetidine (Tagamet), and famotidine (Pepcid), raise gastric pH and reduce the risk of and complications from aspiration.

46. Nonparticulate antacid, such as sodium citrate (Bicitra), raises gastric pH.

47. Dopamine antagonist, such as metoclopramide (Reglan), increases gastric emptying. Agents that raise pH or increase gastric emptying are particularly useful for patients at high risk for aspiration. Conditions that suggest high risk for aspiration include:

- morbid obesity
- old age
- pregnancy
- history of hiatal hernia with reflux
- uncertain NPO status with the need for emergency surgery
- history of diabetes with gastroparesis
- history of partial bowel obstruction
- history of peptic ulcer disease

48. Anticholinergics, such as atropine, scopolamine, and glycopyrrolate (Robinul), decrease oral and tracheobronchial secretions and prevent bradycardia, which can occur during parasympathetic stimulation or with certain anesthetic agents during induction.

- These drugs are particularly useful with patients who exhibit excessive salivation problems that put them at risk for aspiration. They are also appropriate for toddlers and young children, who have a tendency to increase salivation up to tenfold when oral mucous membranes are stimulated (Litwack, 1995, p. 118).
- Anticholinergics, once given routinely as a preoperative medication, are now ordered only for selected patients. Patients who are given anticholinergics may complain of a very dry mouth. A moistened 4 × 4-inch gauze pad can be provided to moisten lips and tongue and provide patient comfort.

49. Antiemetics, such as droperidol (Inapsine), are given to prevent nausea and vomiting. These are particularly useful for patients who report a history of nausea and vomiting after anesthesia and surgery.

50. Antibiotics, such as Cefazolin (Ancef, Kefzol), Cefoxitin (Mefoxin), or Cefotetan (Cefotan), are being utilized more frequently as a prophylaxis to prevent infection in clean operative procedures. Many institutions have a policy that calls for antibiotic administration in selected procedures from between 1 to 2 hours prior to incision. For some orthopedic procedures, doses many be repeated every 2 to 3 hours after the initial dose. Although preoperative antibiotics, if timed properly, have been shown to reduce infection (Barie, 2002, p. S-13) and are recommended in selected circumstances in the CDC Guideline for Prevention of Surgical Site Infection (Mangram, Horon, Pearson, Silver, Jarvis, 1999, p. 267), implementation remains controversial and protocols do vary between institutions. Institutional policies and protocols regarding antibiotic utilization should be consulted.

51. Narcotics, such as meperidine (Demerol), fentanyl (Sublimaze), hydromorphine (Dilaudid), and morphine, provide relief from pain. Morphine, hydromorphine (Dilaudid), and meperidine (Demerol) are respiratory depressants and occasionally cause nausea and vomiting. Narcotics are primarily indicated in patients who are experiencing pain. Patients who have received narcotics must be closely observed for adequate ventilation.

52. It is not uncommon for patients who anticipate general anesthesia to mistakenly believe that the premedication they received should have put them to sleep for the surgery. Patients may be anxious because they are still awake. It is important to provide reassurance by informing patients that they will be given additional anesthetic agents for surgery, will be asleep, and will not feel pain.

53. Fear of the unknown, fear of having to relinquish control, and fear of never awakening are some of the concerns expressed by patients in the preoperative period. Perioperative nurses need to be aware of patients' fears, take the time to listen, stay close to the patient, and provide emotional support and reassurance. The period just prior to surgery may be the most stressful for the patient and is a time when the presence of a nurse is crucial to alleviate anxiety.

MONITORING

54. Patient monitoring is essential during anesthesia to detect physiologic changes in response to

both the anesthesia and the surgical procedure. Ongoing monitoring is critical to providing appropriate and timely interventions in order to maintain satisfactory physiologic status.

55. The degree of monitoring that is required is determined by the intended procedure and the patient's history and state of health. As a minimum, monitoring for all surgical patients should include ECG, blood pressure, heart rate, and pulse oximetry. When general anesthesia is administered, end tidal volume carbon dioxide, oxygen analysis of anesthesia gases, and core body temperature monitoring are added.

Practice Recommendations and Standards

56. The Association of periOperative Registered Nurses (AORN) has adopted practice recommendations for the nurse who monitors the patient receiving local anesthesia and the patient receiving moderate sedation/analgesia. The AORN recommendations state that monitoring should include (AORN, 2004a,b, p. 214):

    - blood pressure
    - cardiac rate and rhythm
    - respiratory rate
    - oxygen saturation
    - skin condition
    - level of consciousness
    - comfort level/tolerance to procedure

57. The American Society of Anesthesiologists has standards for basic intraoperative monitoring. Qualified anesthesia personnel shall be present in the room throughout the conduct of all general anesthetics, regional anesthetics, and monitored anesthesia care. During all anesthetics, the patient's oxygenation, ventilation, circulation, and temperature shall be continually monitored (Delamar, 2003, p. 225):

    - oxygenation—to ensure adequate oxygen concentration in the inspired gas and the blood during all anesthetics
    - ventilation—to ensure adequate ventilation of the patient during all anesthetics
    - circulation—to ensure the adequacy of the patient's circulatory function during all anesthetics
    - body temperature—to aid in the maintenance of appropriate body temperature during all anesthetics

Monitoring Devices

58. Monitoring devices may be invasive or noninvasive. Noninvasive monitoring devices do not penetrate a body orifice.

59. Examples of noninvasive monitors are ECG electrodes, blood pressure cuffs, and pulse oximeters. Invasive monitors are introduced beneath the skin or mucosa or do enter a body cavity. Examples of invasive monitors are an arterial line and central venous catheter.

60. The choice of monitoring device is determined by the intended procedure, the patient's history and state of health, the anesthesia care provider, the surgeon's judgment, and anticipated postoperative management.

61. Patients undergoing complex, critical, and extensive surgical procedures and patients with complex health problems will require extensive monitoring. A combination of invasive and noninvasive monitors will be employed. Examples where invasive monitoring is appropriate are in cardiac surgery, in surgeries or in patients where repeated blood samples will be required, and in patients in whom wide variations in blood pressure are anticipated. The healthy patient who undergoes a simple procedure will require noninvasive monitoring only.

62. The perioperative nurse must have a knowledge of monitoring equipment and the ability to interpret data. In situations where the entire responsibility for monitoring rests with the perioperative nurse, such as with local anesthesia or moderate sedation/analgesia, monitoring is especially critical. In these situations, many institutions have supplementary monitoring competency requirements that must be met before the perioperative nurse is permitted to monitor independently. However, even where an anesthesiologist or CRNA is present, the perioperative nurse must be able to recognize normal and abnormal physiologic responses, to administer oxygen and pharmacologic therapy, and to anticipate and assist in pharmacologic and emergency interventions.

63. There are several monitors that are considered standard for patients who receive general anesthesia.

Precordial or Esophageal Stethoscope

64. A stethoscope taped to the patient's chest or an esophageal stethoscope placed within the patient's esophagus provides the capability for continuous auscultation of the chest in order to monitor cardiac rate and rhythm and breath sounds.

Electrocardiogram (ECG)

65. ECG monitoring is essential to detect changes in cardiac rate and rhythm and to detect dysrhythmia and myocardial ischemia. Myocardial ischemia in the perioperative period may lead to myocardial infarction postoperatively. Early detection and identification of cardiac irregularities permit timely and specific interventions that can prevent further complications.

66. ECG leads should be placed on clean, dry skin surfaces, and adherence should be checked.

Pulse Oximetry

67. Pulse oximetry measures the oxygen saturation of arterial hemoglobin, which is an indication of the oxygen transfer at the alveolar-capillary level. A photodetector with one end attached to the pulse oximeter is placed on a vascular bed, such as a finger, toe, or an ear lobe. The photo detector consists of a light source side and a receptor side. Two different wavelengths (a red and an infrared) are transmitted through the tissue from the light source side of the photodetector. The receptor side of the photodetector measures the optical density of light that is passed through tissue. Optical density is influenced by the amount of oxygen in the hemoglobin. The absorption of light for each color indicates the ratio of saturated blood to unsaturated blood.

68. Oxygen saturation readings should be near 100%, and readings below 90% are generally indicative of significant hypoxemia. Hypoxemia may lead to cardiac arrest. Pulse oximetry permits the prompt recognition of pending hypoxemia and possible prevention. In the event of decreased oxygen saturation, the perioperative nurse must be prepared to provide ventilatory support and to administer oxygen.

69. Satisfactory oxygen saturation readings from pulse oximetry are not a guarantee that tissues are being adequately perfused with oxygen. Other factors such as hemoglobin level must also be considered. Hemoglobin carries oxygen; however, the hemoglobin may be saturated with oxygen and there may still be insufficient hemoglobin for transport to tissues.

70. Bright lights can interfere with photodetector performance. Exposure to surgical and fluorescent light should be avoided by placing the finger or toe with the attached probe under a blanket or drape.

71. Intravascular dyes, such as methylene blue, will impair the photodetector's ability to measure O_2 saturation. Conditions causing vasoconstriction, such as Raynaud's disease or severe peripheral vascular disease, can also prevent an accurate reading (Delamar, 2003, p. 227).

72. Photodetectors should not be placed or secured so tightly that localized tissue ischemia results.

Blood Pressure

73. Blood pressure measures pressure in the heart during contraction and relaxation. Blood pressure monitoring may be accomplished manually or with an automatic monitor that takes readings at preset intervals. Automatic monitors that measure blood pressure and cardiac rate and that display rhythm are considered standard equipment in the operating room and postanesthesia-care unit. These monitors are also incorporated into all general anesthesia delivery machines.

74. Care must be taken to prevent IV lines from being compressed with a blood-pressure cuff. The site of cuff application should be periodically inspected to ensure that adequate deflation has taken place between readings. Extended inflation periods may lead to neurological injury.

Temperature

75. Anesthetic agents affect the patient's temperature by dilating blood vessels and by inhibiting the temperature-regulating mechanism in the hypothalamus. Patient exposure, open surgery, and cool irrigating fluids also affect body temperature. Hypothermia, defined as body temperature less than 36°C, can reduce the effectiveness of certain anesthetic agents, lead to shivering, and adversely affect pulse oximetry readings.

76. Temperature may be monitored with an external patch thermometer or a more accurate internal esophageal or rectal probe.

77. Warm prep solutions prior to surgery and/or use of a forced-air warming blanket throughout the procedure may decrease the risk of hypothermia. Other interventions to maintain normal body temperature include limiting patient exposure and use of warm irrigation fluids.

78. Keeping patients warm can also prevent surgical site infection. Recent studies have shown that mild hypothermia can triple the infection rate and prolong hospital stays. Regardless of the length of the operation, it is recommended that all patients be warmed with the use of a forced-air warming blanket (OR Manager, 2004, p. 11). Other measures utilized to maintain normothermia are warm blankets, warmed fluids, and head coverings such as

towels. For infants, a head covering made from a stockinette and use of Webril to wrap the arms and legs can help to maintain normal body temperature.

Capnography

79. Capnography measures the percentage of carbon dioxide exhaled during mechanical ventilation. Capnography is useful as a check to ascertain endotracheal rather than esophageal intubation and to detect acute changes in metabolic function that indicate the possibility of hypothermia or malignant hyperthermia.

80. Most capnography units provide a digital display of end tidal CO_2 and a waveform readout of expired CO_2 partial pressure versus time.

· ·

SECTION QUESTIONS

Q9. To avoid possible missed diagnoses, there is a trend today to perform an increasing number of diagnostic tests in preparation for surgery. (Ref. 16)

True   False

Q10. All patients who are scheduled for general anesthesia, regardless of their age, should have a preoperative ECG. (Ref. 18)

True   False

Q11. During assessment, the following should be noted (Ref. 20, 21, 22):

a. allergies to drugs

b. allergies to tape

c. family history with anesthesia

d. current medications

e. history of substance abuse

f. loose teeth

Q12. Preoperative teaching (Ref. 27, 28, 29):

a. may be performed by the postanesthesia care nurse

b. may be performed by the perioperative nurse

c. should be reinforced just prior to surgery

d. should include medications to take on the day of surgery

e. should include expected recovery time

f. may be performed in the surgeon's office

Q13. Aspiration pneumonitis is a possible consequence of the aspiration of less than 5 mL of stomach contents. (Ref. 29)

True   False

Q14. General anesthesia is characterized by amnesia, analgesia, and muscle relaxation. (Ref. 32)

True   False

Q15. Medications administered during moderate sedation/analgesia are intended to provide (Ref. 33):

    a. muscle relaxation

    b. sedation

    c. analgesia

Q16. Moderate sedation/analgesia should be reserved for healthy patients only. (Ref. 34)

    True   False

Q17. Spinal anesthesia is an example of regional anesthesia. (Ref. 36)

    True   False

Q18. An example of a local anesthetic is (Ref. 37, 43, 47):

    a. lidocaine (Xylocaine)

    b. diazepam (Valium)

    c. metoclopramide (Reglan)

Q19. List four goals of preoperative medication. (Ref. 40)

_____

_____

_____

_____

Q20. Patients who are pregnant are at a higher risk of aspiration than patients who are not pregnant. (Ref. 47)

    True   False

Q21. Anticholinergic drugs, such as atropine, are particularly useful for toddlers as a preoperative medication to reduce oral secretions. (Ref. 48)

    True   False

Q22. Monitoring for all patients should include oxygen saturation and ECG. (Ref. 55, 56)

    True   False

Q23. Explain the purpose of an esophageal stethoscope. (Ref. 64)

_____

_____

Q24. Pulse oximetry (Ref. 56, 67, 68, 69, 70):

    a. measures arterial hemoglobin oxygen saturation

    b. should read 80% or higher to be within the normal range

c. should be monitored on every patient who undergoes anesthesia

d. permits prompt recognition of pending hypoxemia

e. readings that are above 90% are a guarantee that the patient's tissues are being adequately perfused with oxygen

f. may be faulty in the presence of bright lights

Q25. List three factors during surgery under anesthesia that put the patient at risk for below-normal temperature. (Ref. 75)

_____

_____

_____

Q26. Describe a means to prevent heat loss in an infant in preparation for surgery. (Ref. 78)

_____

Q27. Measuring the percentage of carbon dioxide exhaled during mechanical ventilation is a useful means to check that the endotracheal tube is properly placed. (Ref. 79)

True   False

• •

GENERAL ANESTHESIA

81. Effective general anesthesia includes amnesia (sleep and/or hypnosis), analgesia, and skeletal-muscle relaxation. Because different anesthetic agents produce different amounts of these responses, it is usual for more than one agent to be administered.

82. Inhalation and intravenous injection are methods used to deliver general anesthetic agents.

Inhalation Agents

83. Nitrous oxide (N_2O), halothane (Fluothane), enflurane (Ethrane), isoflurane (Forane), desflurane (Suprane), and sevoflurane are the most commonly used inhalation anesthetic agents. (Table 11-1) They enter the system by inhalation and are removed by lung ventilation.

84. Nitrous oxide is a sweet-smelling gas that acts rapidly but lacks potency. It is nonirritating, produces few aftereffects, and recovery is rapid. Because it is a relatively weak anesthetic agent, it is often used as a supplement to other inhalation agents and narcotics. In combination with oxygen alone, it is sufficient only for minor procedures that do not produce intense pain.

85. For major procedures, nitrous oxide is used with other agents to potentiate the anesthetic state.

86. A major precaution with the administration of nitrous oxide is to prevent too high a concentration, which can lead to hypoxia.

87. Halothane, enflurane, isoflurane, and sevoflurane are liquid anesthetics that are vaporized as they pass through a vaporizer on the anesthesia machine. They are inhaled.

88. Halothane is sweet smelling, is nonirritating to the respiratory tract, and is a bronchodilator. Induction and recovery are rapid. It is often used with children.

89. Halothane is also a cardiopulmonary depressant, and side effects include bradycardia, peripheral vasodilation, hypotension, and decreased tidal volume.

90. Halothane has a significant depressant effect on the hypothalamus, which controls body temperature, thus making the patient unable to regulate body temperature to compensate for environment temperature. As a result, if the

TABLE 11-1	Inhalation Agents		
Agent	**Use**	**Advantages**	**Disadvantages**
Oxygen	Sustain life		
Nitrous oxide	Induction of anesthesia; maintenance of anesthesia	Rapid induction and recovery; few aftereffects; nonirritating to respiratory tract	Poor relaxation, insufficient potency for general surgery, hypoxia a potential hazard
Halothane (Fluothane)	Maintenance of anesthesia; may be used for induction	Rapid smooth induction; nonirritating to respiratory tract; useful for patients with bronchia; asthma; pleasant odor	Potential toxicity to liver; cardiovascular depressant—hypotension, bradycardia, sensitizes myocardium to catecholamines; may cause ventricular arrhythmias if epinephrine used; affects body temperature control—hypothermia
Enflurane (Ethrane)	Maintenance of anesthesia; may be used for induction	Rapid induction and recovery; minimal aftereffects; potentiates nondepolarizing muscle relaxants; provides some relaxation; pharyngeal and laryngeal reflexes obtunded	Slightly irritating odor; decreased blood pressure and respirations with deepening anesthesia; abnormal electroencophalographic pattern at high concentrations
Isoflurane (Forane)	Maintenance of anesthesia; may be used for induction	Rapid induction and recovery; minimal aftereffects, obtunds laryngeal and pharyngeal reflexes; good relaxation, potentiates all muscle relaxants; protects heart against catecholamine-induced arrhythmias; cardiovascular system remains stable	Expensive, profound respiratory depressant
Sevoflurane	Maintenance of anesthesia; may be used for induction	Most rapid induction and emergence; no ether smell; easy to breathe; protects heart against myocardial irritability	Metabolizes to inorganic fluoride; raises fluoride level in patients with renal disease—unknown consequences; mild and transient chills, fever, nausea; contraindicated in patients susceptible to malignant hyperhermia
Desflurane (Suprane)	Maintenance for short period	Rapid emergence, good relaxation	Irritating to respiratory tract; can cause transient increase in heart rate and blood pressure

room is cold the patient may shiver during emergence from halothane inhalation. Hypothermia is a possible complication.

91. Halothane can sensitize the myocardium to catecholamines and cause ventricular arrhythmia to occur if epinephrine is used as a local injection for vasoconstriction. Therefore, when halothane is used, even small doses of epinephrine are administered with extreme caution.

92. There is a question as to whether the metabolites of halothane affect liver function; therefore, it is generally not given to patients with known liver disease or to patients who will require several surgical procedures within a short period of time.

93. Enflurane provides rapid induction and rapid emergence. Heart rate is not generally affected. Enflurane provides good muscle relaxation and potentiates other muscle relaxants.

94. Enflurane decreases blood pressure, and hypotension is a common occurrence.

95. Isoflurane provides excellent relaxation and potentiates muscle relaxants. Induction and

emergence are rapid. The cardiovascular system remains stable, and electrocardiographic abnormalities are not associated with isoflurane inhalation.

96. Isoflurane does not sensitize the myocardium to catecholamines and therefore epinephrine may be used for local vasoconstriction.

97. Isoflurane causes peripheral vasodilation. Hypotension is common at induction; however, blood pressure rapidly returns to normal.

98. Desflurane provides good relaxation and offers rapid onset and emergence. A transient increase in cardiac rate and blood pressure may occur. It cannot be used for induction because of its pungent odor, which can cause gagging and laryngospasm.

99. Sevoflurane allows a more rapid induction and emergence than other inhaled anesthetic agents. Because sevoflurane is not irritating to the respiratory tract and does not irritate the myocardium, it may replace halothane as the inhalation of choice for children. Its rapid induction and emergence may also promote use for ambulatory surgery procedures.

Anesthesia Machine

100. Inhalation agents are directed to the patient from an anesthesia machine.

101. Oxygen, nitrous oxide, and air are supplied through hoses from a central source within the healthcare facility or from cylinders attached to the machine. For safety purposes, the hoses and cylinders are color-coded and their fittings are not interchangeable. Oxygen cylinders and hoses are color-coded green, nitrous oxide is blue, and air is yellow.

102. Flowmeters attached to the machine measure the amount and flow of nitrous oxide and oxygen being delivered to the patient. The anesthesia care provider selects the ratio of oxygen and nitrous oxide. Flowmeters are also color-coded.

103. Another safety feature is a shutoff device that prevents nitrous oxide from being delivered if oxygen is not also delivered.

104. The anesthesia machine is equipped with an oxygen flush button that allows 100% oxygen to be delivered to the patient. The machine includes a mechanical ventilator and monitoring devices for blood pressure, ECG, inspired oxygen, and end tidal carbon dioxide. An alarm system to signal apnea or a disconnection from the breathing circuit attached to the machine is also included.

105. The anesthesia machine includes a vaporizer for vaporizing and delivering liquid anesthetics (halothane, enflurane, isoflurane, sevoflurane, and desflurane).

106. Oxygen and other anesthetic inhalation agents may be mixed and directed to and from the patient through corrugated rubber or plastic tubes. These tubes are joined with a built-in Y connector that may be attached to a face mask or an endotracheal tube. Anesthetic gases are directed to the patient through a one-way valve in one tube, and expired gases are returned through the other tube. A reservoir bag, similar to a balloon, is part of this delivery system. When this reservoir bag is manually compressed, oxygen and inhalation agents may be forced into the lungs and the patient's ventilation may be controlled.

107. As the expired gases are returned from the patient, the carbon dioxide passes through a carbon-dioxide system and is absorbed. Oxygen is added to the remaining exhaled gases, and these are returned to the patient for rebreathing.

108. Anesthesia machines are equipped with a scavenger system that controls the collection of excess expired gases, which are then eliminated through a suction line.

109. Studies indicate that the presence of nitrous oxide, as well as other anesthetic gases in the atmosphere, presents a serious health hazard to operating room staff. Decreased mental performance, reduced fertility, spontaneous abortion, and neurological, renal and liver disease have been associated with exposure. The National Institute for Occupational Safety and Health has set limits of exposure for anesthetic gases. Every effort must be made to prevent the escape of these gases into the atmosphere.

110. Limits are as follows (NIOSH, 1994):

- nitrous oxide—25 parts per million (ppm) over an 8-hour time-weighted average
- halothane—0.5 ppm when used in combination with nitrous oxide, 2 ppm when used alone, per hour

111. The level of anesthetic waste gases is periodically tested to determine an institution's compliance with NIOSH recommendations. The perioperative nurse should be aware of these limits and of testing results.

112. In addition to required periodic testing to monitor the amount of waste gas in the operating room, anesthetic gases should be shut off except during delivery to the patient. Routine testing of anesthesia equipment for leaks and

reviews of anesthesia technique can help prevent overexposure.

Intravenous Agents

113. Intravenous agents are introduced directly into the circulatory system, usually through a peripheral vein in the arm or hand.

114. Intravenous agents are most often used as a supplement to inhalation agents.

115. Unlike inhalation agents, which can be easily removed from the system by ventilating the lungs, intravenous agents must be metabolized by the liver or kidneys and excreted.

Barbiturate Induction Agents

116. Barbiturates are commonly used for induction of anesthesia.

117. The most commonly used barbiturates are thiopental sodium (Sodium Pentothal), sodium thiamylal (Surital), and methohexital sodium (Brevital). They are short acting and result in a rapid progression from sedation to loss of consciousness. They do not provide analgesia.

118. Barbiturates are potent respiratory depressants, and initial transient apnea is expected. For this reason, before barbiturates are administered, preparations are made to provide oxygen and to assist or control the patient's ventilation.

119. Barbiturates also depress the cardiovascular system, and a degree of hypotension can be expected.

Nonbarbiturate Induction Agents

120. The nonbarbiturate drug propofol (Diprivan) has achieved popularity as an induction and maintenance agent. It is a hypnotic-sedative agent that produces rapid induction.

121. Propofol is delivered in a milky white intralipid emulsion. This medium supports microbial growth, and outbreaks of infection have been associated with its use (Wang, 1997). Propofol must be used within 6 hours of preparation, and handling requires strict aseptic technique. The patient may experience pain upon injection. Recovery from propofol is more rapid than with barbiturates, and it is therefore often utilized for ambulatory surgery. There are minimal aftereffects and less incidence of postoperative nausea and vomiting.

122. Etomidate (Amidate) is a nonbarbiturate induction agent that has minimal effects on myocardial metabolism, cardiac output, and peripheral or pulmonary circulation. It is short acting and is generally utilized for patients with a positive cardiac history and/or patients who cannot tolerate dramatic changes to blood pressure. Etomidate does not provide analgesia.

Dissociative Induction Agent

123. Ketamine hydrochloride (Ketalar) is a dissociative agent that produces a catatonic state and provides amnesia and analgesia. The patient will breathe unassisted, may move, and may appear to be awake. However, an anesthetized state has been achieved and surgery may be performed without patient response. Ketamine is rapidly metabolized, and patients emerge quickly from its effects.

124. Ketamine may be given intravenously or intramuscularly. It is useful for diagnostic procedures and procedures where it is desirable to have the patient breathe unassisted. It is sometimes used for children who undergo short procedures that do not require muscle relaxation.

125. Because ketamine is a dissociative agent, patients may experience hallucination postoperatively. This is more common in adults and may be minimized when diazepam or midazolam is given. A quiet, darkened area for recovery is advised.

Narcotics

126. Narcotics may be used preoperatively as a premedication or intraoperatively during induction and maintenance.

127. The narcotics meperidine hydrochloride (Demerol), and morphine sulfate are frequently used premedications.

128. Narcotics that are used intraoperatively are fentanyl (Sublimaze), sufentanil (Sufenta), alfentanil (Alfenta), morphine, hydromorphone (Dilaudid), and meperidine (Demerol). Fentanyl is 80 to 100 times more potent than morphine, and sufentanil is more potent than fentanyl.

129. Small doses of narcotics are used intraoperatively as adjuncts to other drugs and to provide relief from pain in the early postoperative period.

130. Narcotics provide profound analgesia with little influence on blood pressure, cardiac rate, and cardiac output. They are of particular value in cardiac surgery.

131. Narcotics are respiratory depressants, and patients who have received high doses of narcotics intraoperatively must be closely monitored to ensure that they are breathing adequately. A patient who has received a high dose of narcotic intraoperatively may appear to be awake and alert postoperatively but may suddenly begin to hypoventilate and lose consciousness.

Tranquilizers—Benzodiazepines

132. Tranquilizers commonly used intraoperatively are diazepam (Valium) and midazolam (Versed).

133. Tranquilizers are used for induction and as adjuncts to other anesthetic agents. Their use permits lower doses of other agents.

134. Diazepam produces amnesia, and midazolam provides excellent amnesia.

135. Flumazenil (Romazicon) is an important drug that is used to reverse the effects of benzodiazepines. It reverses sedation and respiratory depression without cardiovascular effects. Patients who are reversed must be closely monitored because flumazenil may lose its effect sooner than the underlying benzodiazepine, and hypoventilation can then occur.

Neuromuscular Blockers (Muscle Relaxants)

136. Muscle relaxants (Table 11-2) commonly used intraoperatively are succinylcholine (Anectine), tubocurarine chloride (curare), pancuronium bromide (Pavulon), atracurium besylate (Tracrium), cisatracurium besylate (Nimbex), mivacurium (Mivacron), rocuronium bromide (Zemuron), and vecuronium bromide (Norcuron).

137. Two primary indications for neuromuscular blockers are: (1) to relax the jaw and larynx in order to facilitate controlled breathing and tracheal intubation, and (2) to increase muscle relaxation to permit ease of tissue handling during surgery.

138. Muscle relaxants vary in terms of onset and duration. Intubation is accomplished with neuromuscular blockers that have rapid onset and are short acting.

139. Neuromuscular blockers paralyze the neuromuscular junction and block impulses from motor nerves to skeletal muscle. The patient becomes paralyzed. Neuromuscular blockers are depolarizing or nondepolarizing.

140. Succinylcholine is a depolarizing muscle relaxant. When it reaches the neuromuscular junction it acts like acetylcholine, producing a depolarization of the membrane at the motor end plate. The depolarization causes a muscle contraction that is followed by a neuromuscular block. The drug prevents repolarization, and the muscle remains relaxed and paralyzed. The muscle contractions are sometimes obvious and appear similar to twitching. This twitching, referred to as *fasciculation*, progresses in cephalocaudal sequence as the drug circulates through the patient's body.

141. Succinylcholine produces paralysis within seconds and is used for intubation. Because of its rapid onset, it is valuable in emergency situations where rapid intubation is required.

142. Nondepolarizing muscle relaxants block the action of acetylcholine at the neuromuscular junction but do not cause depolarization at the motor end plate, so fasciculation does not occur.

143. Nondepolarizing agents have a slower onset than depolarizing agents and their effect lasts longer.

144. The anesthesia care provider continually monitors the patient to determine the amount of paralysis present. Applying a nerve stimulator to a peripheral nerve, such as the ulnar nerve or a branch of the facial nerve, and observing for absence of contractions is helpful in determining the amount of paralysis present.

145. The anticholinergic agents pyridostigmine (Regonol) or neostigmine (Prostigmin) are used when necessary to reverse the action of nondepolarizing agents. These two drugs are usually used in combination with atrophine sulfate or glycopyrrolate (Robinul), to counteract the muscarinic effects (bradycardia and salivation) of the anticholinesterases.

TABLE 11-2	Muscle Relaxants		
Agent	**Use**	**Advantages**	**Disadvantages**
Depolarizing Muscle Relaxant—Rapid Onset, Short Duration			
Succinylcholine (Anectine, Quelicin)	Intubation Short procedures	Rapid onset; brief duration	Can cause muscle fasciculation, postoperative myalgia; requires refrigeration, contraindicated in patients with recent bum, muscle trauma, or recurrent neuromuscular disorder; can trigger malignant hyperthermia; prolonged effect in patients with serum cholinesterase deficiency.
Nondepolarizing Muscle Relaxants—Intermediate Onset, Intermediate Duration			
Atracurium (Tracrium)	Intubation Maintenance of muscle relaxation	No significant cardiovascular effects	Required refrigeration; slight release of histamine
Vecuronium (Norcuron)	Intubation Maintenance of muscle relaxation	No significant cardiovascular effects; no release of histamine	Must be mixed
Mivacurium (Mivacron)	Intubation Maintenance of muscle relaxation		Expensive; prolonged effect in patients with serum cholinesterase deficiency
Rocuronium (Zemuron)	Intubation Maintenance of muscle relaxation	Provides excellent intubating conditions; rapid onset	May increase heart rate; eliminated via liver, contraindicated in patients with hepatic disease, contraindicated for rapid intubation for cesarean sections
Nondepolarizing Muscle Relaxants—Delayed Onset, Loger Duration			
Tubocurarine (curare)	Maintenance of muscle relaxation		Strong histamine release; automatic blockade can cause hypotension
Pancuronium (Pavulon)	Maintenance of muscle relaxation	Long duration	Can cause hypertension and increased heart rate

• •

SECTION QUESTIONS

Q28. Nitrous oxide is a useful supplement to other inhalation agents and is seldom used in combination with oxygen alone. (Ref. 84)

True   False

Q29. Inhalation agent(s) commonly used for children are (Ref. 88, 99):

   a. halothane

   b. enflurane

   c. isoflurane

   d. desflurane

   e. sevoflurane

Q30. Oxygen cylinders, hoses, and flowmeters are color-coded _____.
Nitrous oxide cylinders, hoses, and flowmeters are color-coded _____. (Ref. 101, 102)

Q31. Explain why is it important for anesthesia delivery machines to be equipped with a scavenger system. (Ref. 109)

_____

_____

Q32. Inhalation and intravenous agents may be used in combination to achieve general anesthesia. (Ref. 114)

True   False

Q33. Thiopental sodium (Sodium Pentothal), sodium thiamylal (Surital), and methohexital sodium (Brevital) are barbiturates that are used for induction because they cause rapid loss of consciousness. (Ref. 117)

True   False

Q34. Propofol (Ref. 120, 121):

   a. is a narcotic

   b. is a rapid induction agent

   c. provides muscle relaxation

   d. may cause pain to the patient upon injection

   e. handling requires strict aseptic technique because it is supplied in a medium that supports bacterial growth

   f. results in minimal aftereffects

Q35. What adverse reaction might a patient have following ketamine? (Ref. 125)

_____

Q36. Narcotics such as fentanyl (Sublimaze) may be administered intraoperatively to provide relief of pain postoperatively. (Ref. 129)

True   False

Q37. Explain why patients who have received high doses of narcotics should be closely monitored postoperatively to ensure that they are breathing adequately. (Ref. 131)

_____

_____

_____

Q38. Flumazenil (Romazicon) is a reversal agent for (Ref. 135):

a. narcotics

b. tranquilizers

c. muscle relaxants

Q39. Neuromuscular blockers (Ref. 137, 139):

a. cause paralysis

b. produce sleep

c. are useful for jaw relaxation to facilitate intubation

d. permit ease of tissue manipulation

Q40. Succinylcholine (Ref. 140, 141):

a. is a depolarizing muscle relaxant that causes a muscle contraction followed by a neuromuscular block that results in paralysis

b. can cause fasciculation

c. has a slow onset

d. is useful where emergency rapid intubation is needed

• •

Stages of Anesthesia

146. In 1720, Arthur Guedel integrated the four stages of anesthesia with their signs and symptoms into a system that until recent times was used to estimate the depth of anesthesia. By observing the patient's physiological changes and reflex responses, the depth of anesthesia was determined. The system applied to patients who were not premedicated, breathed spontaneously, and were administered ether.

147. The stages are as follows:

• Stage I, Relaxation—from administration of anesthesia to loss of consciousness. Patient response—dizziness, drowsiness, exaggerated hearing, and a decreased sense of pain.

• Stage II, Excitement—from loss of consciousness to onset of regular breathing. Patient response—irregular breathing, increased muscle tone and involuntary motor activity, thrashing and struggling activity (susceptible to auditory and tactile stimulation).

• Stage III, Surgical Anesthesia—from onset of regular breathing to cessation of respiration. Patient response—regular thoracoabdominal breathing, a relaxed jaw, a loss of pain and auditory sensation, and loss of eyelid reflex.

- Stage IV, Danger—from cessation of respiration to circulatory failure and death. Patient response—pupils that are fixed and dilated, a rapid and thready pulse, and paralyzed respiratory muscles.

148. Because anesthetic agents that are used today quickly bring the patient to stage III, the untoward responses of stage II are seldom seen and Guedel's system is not suitable for evaluating the depth of anesthesia. Perioperative nurses, however, should have an appreciation of the depth of anesthesia. It should be noted that the excitement phase in Stage II may still be seen with the induction and emergence of children, especially during a mask induction of anesthesia. An awareness of the patient's level of anesthesia allows the nurse to plan for and provide safety measures. Recovery from anesthesia occurs in reverse order.

Preparation for Anesthesia—Nursing Responsibilities

149. As much as possible, the room should be made ready and preparations for surgery completed before the patient is brought into the operating room suite. Once the patient is in the room, it is important that the circulating nurse be immediately available to provide emotional support, ensure patient dignity, institute safety measures, and assist the anesthesia care provider.

150. In preparation for induction, nursing responsibilities may include transfer of the patient from the stretcher to the operating room table, placement of electrocardiographic leads, application of blood-pressure cuff, placement of the intravenous line, application of the safety strap, and adjustment of the patient's gown and sheets. Because these preparatory activities have the potential for exposing the patient, nursing interventions at this time should focus on maintaining patient dignity. The perioperative nurse can limit exposure of the patient by immediately closing the operating room doors and keeping unnecessary personnel from the room.

151. As preparations are made for anesthesia induction, patients can experience feelings from mild anxiety to acute fear. The perioperative nurse can help allay these feelings by being at the patient's side, speaking calmly, answering questions, and explaining activities. Nonverbal support, such as holding the patient's hand, can be the most supportive intervention.

152. Efforts should be made not to stimulate the patient or interrupt the calming effect of the preoperative medication. All unnecessary noise should be avoided. It is the responsibility of the perioperative nurse to provide and maintain a quiet atmosphere in the operating room; however, all team members must participate in the effort. All unnecessary conversation should be curtailed. The operating room door should remain closed. Instrument counting should not be performed within range of the patient's hearing. Overhearing "blades," "needles," "mosquitoes," and so forth can be frightening to the patient. Hearing is the most difficult sense to anesthetize, is the last sensation lost before unconsciousness, and noise should be kept to a minimum.

In rare instances anesthesia awareness may occur when an anesthetized patient experiences unintended intraoperative awareness and has direct recall of those events. Incidence is estimated to be between 0.1 percent and 0.2 percent of all patients undergoing general anesthesia or between 20,000 to 40,000 cases each year. Forty-eight percent of these patients report hearing during their sugery (JCAHO, 2004, p. 1). Conversation during the intraoperative period should always be respectful of the patient's dignity.

153. Prior to anesthesia induction, the perioperative nurse should check the suction to ensure that it is turned on and working properly. The suction catheter should be placed within easy reach of the anesthesia care provider.

154. Induction is the period from when an anesthetic is first administered until the patient loses consciousness and is then stabilized at the desired level of anesthesia (Delamar, 2003, p. 231).

155. Induction is a critical time during the administration of anesthesia, and it is essential for patient safety that the perioperative nurse be present and available to assist the anesthesia care provider with suctioning and intubation and, if necessary, to restrain the patient (particularly children).

156. In young children who may not tolerate the placement of an intravenous line, and in patients with a tracheostomy tube, induction is usually begun with an inhalation agent.

Sequence for General Anesthesia—Nursing Responsibilities

157. In patients who have an intravenous line, a typical sequence for general anesthesia might progress as follows:

- If the patient can tolerate it, a mask is placed over the nose and mouth while the patient breathes 100% oxygen for a few minutes. The oxygenation serves as a safety margin in the event of an airway obstruction or brief period of apnea during insertion of the endotracheal tube.

- A narcotic and/or a benzodiazepine is injected and ventilation is monitored.

- A barbiturate (thiopental sodium or thiamylal sodium) or a nonbarbiturate (propofol or etomidate) is injected to produce sleep. Sleep may be judged by the lack of eyelid movement when the eyelid is stroked. Sleep will usually occur within 1 or 2 minutes.

- With the mask over the patient's nose and mouth, the anesthesia care provider will ventilate the patient and observe the chest rise. If the chest does not rise, the head and mandible are repositioned until a patent airway is maintained.

- When it is established that the airway is clear, a paralyzing dose of muscle relaxant is administered to facilitate intubation. (Muscle relaxants with a longer onset may be injected before the patient is asleep, as the effect will not occur until after sleep is achieved.)

- A laryngoscope is used to visualize the vocal cords, and the patient is intubated. (An endotracheal tube is inserted into the trachea.) The perioperative nurse can assist the anesthesia care provider by pulling outwardly on the corner of the patient's mouth to permit better visualization of the vocal cords and placement of the endotracheal tube. The perioperative nurse can also assist by passing the endotracheal tube to the anesthesia care provider so he or she does not have to interrupt visualization to pick up the tube, and by providing a 10-mL syringe to inflate the endotracheal tube cuff.

- Correct endotracheal tube placement is confirmed by:

  1. observing fog in the clear endotracheal tube

  2. observing the patient for bilateral chest excursion without epigastric enlargement

  3. listening for bilateral breath sounds

  4. identifying carbon dioxide expiration through end-tidal monitoring

158. If the patient is not intubated, a combination of inhalation agents will be administered via a mask or laryngeal mask airway (LMA). For short procedures and procedures where paralysis is not necessary, the patient is usually not intubated. The mask is strapped or held over the patient's nose and mouth and connected via anesthesia tubing to the anesthesia machine. The patient may breathe spontaneously, or breathing and delivery of anesthetic agents may be accomplished manually by compressing a reservoir bag on the anesthesia machine. This is also referred to as *bagging the patient.*

159. The LMA is a device that provides good airway protection without intubation. It is inserted into the patient's mouth, positioned securely over the larynx, and inflated to keep it securely in place. The patient is connected to the anesthesia machine via an anesthesia circuit. The patient may breathe spontaneously or be mechanically ventilated. (Figure 11-1)

160. If the patient is intubated, the endotracheal tube is inserted directly into the larynx and secured in place by inflating a cuff that is attached to the tube. The endotracheal tube is connected to the anesthesia machine via tub-

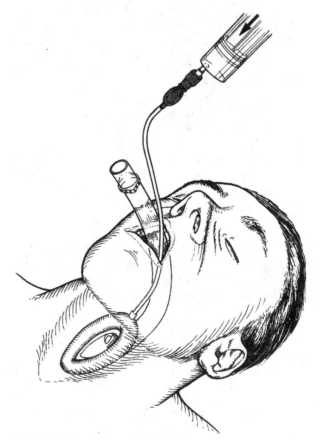

FIGURE 11-1   Laryngeal Mask Airway.
Source: Reprinted with permission from ETHICON, INC., 1986, Somerville, NJ.

ing, and inhalation agents are delivered automatically according to preset parameters.

161. When a barbiturate or hypnotic is given at the start of induction, it will quickly reach the patient's brain and apnea will usually result. The patient's pharyngeal muscles and tongue relax, and airway obstruction can occur. If a clear airway is not maintained, the patient will attempt to breathe as the drug washes out of the brain. The abdominal muscles may strain and pull the diaphragm down, compressing the stomach and causing the patient to regurgitate. If the patient regurgitates and attempts to breathe, he or she can aspirate gastric contents into the lungs, with resultant aspiration pneumonia. The perioperative nurse must be prepared to immediately provide suction, turn the patient's head to the side, adjust the table into the Trendelenburg position, and assist the anesthesia provider as needed.

162. Patients who have not been NPO for the required period of time are not given general anesthesia unless it is an emergency situation wherein regional anesthesia is not appropriate. The patient who ate and then became ill, the trauma victim with blood in the stomach, or the patient with a hiatal hernia is at risk for aspiration. Aspiration of stomach contents can prove fatal. The perioperative nurse's first priority is to remain at the patient's side at the head of the table, prepared to assist the anesthesia care provider until intubation is complete and assistance is no longer needed. A suction catheter or tip, a nasogastric tube, an emesis basin, and a towel should be immediately available.

163. During intubation the perioperative nurse may be asked to assist by firmly pressing the cricoid cartilage posteriorly with the index finger or thumb and forefinger. This maneuver is referred to as the *Sellick maneuver*. It compresses the esophagus between the cricoid cartilage and the vertebral column. It aids in visualization of the tracheal lumen for intubation and occludes the esophagus to prevent regurgitation. Pressure must begin when the patient is awake and must be maintained until the endotracheal tube is in place, inflated, and placement verified by an anesthesia provider. (Figure 11-2)

164. Once the cuff is inflated, the endotracheal tube is connected to the anesthesia machine from which the inhalation agents are delivered and by which ventilation is controlled.

165. General anesthesia depresses the hypothalamus, thus preventing the patient from compensating for the temperature in the room. If the operating room is cold, the anesthetized patient can become hypothermic. Nursing interventions should be directed toward maintaining the patient's body temperature within normal limits. Maintaining normal body temperature has been identified as a means to reduce risk of infection (OR Manager, 2004, p. 11). Appropriate interventions include providing a warming blanket, covering the patient with a warm blanket, limiting skin exposure, and supplying warm fluids for irrigation during surgery.

Automated forced air warming devices should be used strictly in accordance with the manufacturer's instructions. The air hose should never be used without being connected to the warming blanket provided with the device. Severe patient burns have been reported when the air hose alone has been used (Kressin, 2004).

166. Injury related to improper positioning is a risk for the anesthetized patient. Patients who are improperly positioned can sustain injury of the integumentary, respiratory, circulatory, or musculoskeletal system. Peripheral nerves, eyes, skin, and digits are especially susceptible to injury. Injury resulting from improper positioning may be temporary or can be permanent.

167. Following the induction of anesthesia, the perioperative nurse should scan the patient from head to foot and, if necessary, take corrective action to ensure that the patient is properly positioned. This is a critical review because once the patient is draped, positioning cannot be visualized.

168. If the patient is moved or repositioned during the procedure, a check should again be made to ensure a safe and proper position.

169. Before repositioning the patient, the perioperative nurse should confer with the anesthesia care provider to determine that the patient can be moved without compromise to the airway and to ventilation, and that he or she is ready to assist in repositioning by guiding and securing the patient's head to prevent accidental extubation or disconnection from the ventilator.

170. During the surgical procedure, the perioperative nurse monitors fluid output and replacement, blood loss, blood and blood product replacement, and the amount of irrigating solution used.

171. Emergence from anesthesia, particularly from extubation, is a critical period when the perioperative nurse must be at the patient's side and immediately available to assist the anesthesia care provider.

172. Extubation can initiate bronchospasm or laryngospasm reflex. The airway may become

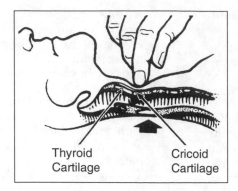

Using the index finger to displace the cricoid cartilage posteriorly thus obstructing the esophagus

Thyroid Cartilage   Cricoid Cartilage

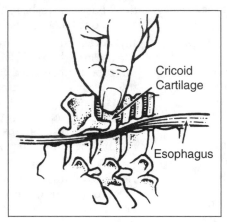

Cricoid Cartilage

Esophagus

Two-finger technique that obstructs the esophagus between the sixth cervical vertebra and the cricoid cartilage

FIGURE 11-2   The Sellick Maneuver.
Source: Courtesy of Gensia Pharmaceuticals, Inc., San Diego, California.

obstructed, and vomiting can occur. Airway management and adequate ventilation are priorities. Prior to extubation, the perioperative nurse should check to make sure that a suction catheter is within reach of the anesthesia care provider and that suction is turned on and working.

MALIGNANT HYPERTHERMIA

Overview

173. Malignant hyperthermia is an emergency complication of general anesthesia. It is characterized by a rapid rise in temperature, with temperatures rising as high as 109.4°F (43°C).

174. Exact incidence of malignant hyperthermia is unknown; however, some experts believe 1 in 10,000 may be affected (Malignant Hyperthermia Association, n.d.). It is considered to be,

according to H. Hein, the leading cause of anesthetic deaths in healthy young adults (cited in Beck, 1994, p. 367). Approximately 10% of patients who experience a malignant hyperthermia episode may die (Genetic Information and Patient Services, n.d.).

175. In patients who experience malignant hyperthermia, the sarcoplasmic reticulum (calcium-storing membrane of the muscle cell) is unable to regulate calcium within the muscle cell in the presence of certain anesthetic agents.

176. When malignant hyperthermia occurs, intracellular calcium increases, and the result is sustained contracture of skeletal muscle. The contractions cause muscles to consume higher than normal amounts of oxygen, which then produces lactic acid and heat. The patient's temperature rises rapidly and dramatically. Electrolytes, enzymes, and myoglobin leak from the cells. Hyperkalemia may result and lead to cardiac arrhythmias. The loss of myoglobin can result in renal failure.

177. Symptoms may be multifocal and include sudden inappropriate tachycardia with tachypnea, unstable blood pressure, generalized rigidity, masseter muscle spasm, metabolic and respiratory acidosis, increased end-tidal CO_2, fever, profuse sweating, cyanotic mottling of the skin, and dark unoxygenated blood in the field. Temperature can rise as much as 1.8°F (1°C) every 5 minutes.

178. Tachycardia and increased end-tidal CO_2 are often the first symptoms to appear and may be attributed to causes other than malignant hyperthermia. The classic symptom of fever may occur after the appearance of other symptoms.

179. Certain inhalation agents and depolarizing muscle relaxants are known to be malignant hyperthermia triggers. The inhalation agent fluothane (Halothane) and the muscle relaxant succinylcholine (Anectine) are primary triggering agents. Enflurane, isoflurane, desflurane, and sevoflurane are also contraindicated for patients susceptible to malignant hyperthermia.

180. When succinylcholine is the triggering agent, a sudden severe rigidity of the jaw may be seen following administration of the drug.

181. Depending on the patient and the triggering agent, malignant hyperthermia can occur immediately or as late as 24 hours following the administration of anesthesia.

182. There are multiple causes of malignant hyperthermia; however, inheritance is believed to be a significant factor. Certain muscle disorders, such as Duchenne's muscular dystrophy, have been associated with malignant hyperthermia.

183. Patients who are susceptible to malignant hyperthermia can sometimes be identified through preoperative assessment. Assessment risk factors are:

    - personal or family history of malignant hyperthermia or complications arising from anesthesia
    - a family history of suspicious anesthesia experience
    - history of unexplained muscle cramps with fever
    - inherited skeletal muscle disorders

184. If it is suspected that the patient is susceptible to malignant hyperthermia, the surgery may be postponed until a skeletal muscle biopsy test is performed to confirm the diagnosis.

Treatment

185. If a patient experiences a malignant hyperthermia episode during surgery, initial treatment is to immediately discontinue all triggering anesthetic agents, hyperventilate with 100% oxygen, administer dantrolene sodium (Dantrium), and rapidly terminate surgery. Dantrolene sodium is a skeletal muscle relaxant that blocks the release of calcium from the sarcoplasmic reticulum that in turn decreases muscle contractions.

186. If it is impossible to terminate surgery, anesthesia is continued with nontriggering agents.

187. Cooling of the patient is achieved by wound irrigation with cold saline, administration of cold intravenous solutions, surface cooling with ice or a cooling blanket, and a cold gastric and rectal lavage.

188. The anesthesia circuit and carbon-dioxide absorbent should be changed to reduce risk from residual triggering agents.

189. Dantrolene sodium is administered at 2.5 mg/kg until the patient responds or a maximum of 20 doses is given. The patient will generally respond within minutes. Acidosis is treated with sodium bicarbonate.

190. Additional treatment is governed by blood gas, electrolyte, creatine phosphokinase (CPK), lactic dehydrogenase (LDH), and blood-clotting analysis.

191. Following an episode of malignant hyperthermia, the patient must be closely monitored for a possible recurrent episode. Dantrolene sodium is continued for 48 hours or more.

192. Every operating room where general anesthesia is administered should have immediate access to dantrolene sodium and a written, readily accessible protocol for the management of malignant hyperthermia. A cart containing supplies needed to manage a malignant hyperthermia occurrence should be readily available, and staff should be familiar with the contents and the treatment protocol.

193. In addition to a posted policy and a cart with necessary supplies, many operating room departments have an anesthesia machine reserved for use in the event of a malignant hyperthermia episode. Should an episode occur, the reserved anesthesia machine is brought to the room to replace the one in use. This saves time by eliminating the necessity to change the anesthesia circuit and replace the carbon-dioxide absorbent on the existing machine.

194. Dantrolene sodium is supplied in a 20-mg vial and requires 60 mL of sterile water for reconstitution. The water should contain no preservative. Reconstitution of dantrolene sodium is difficult and requires vigorous shaking. The malignant hyperthermia supply cart should

contain 36 vials of dantrolene and sufficient sterile water for reconstitution. (Thirty-six vials are required to reach a maximum dose for a 175-pound patient.)

Nursing Responsibilities

195. During the preoperative interview, the perioperative nurse should assess the patient for risk factors associated with malignant hyperthermia.

196. The perioperative nurse should be familiar with the malignant hyperthermia protocol and be able to institute prompt and appropriate treatment. Competencies include the ability to:

    • assess the patient preoperatively for malignant hyperthermia risk factors

    • prepare the room with appropriate supplies for a patient known to be susceptible to malignant hyperthermia

    • recognize signs and symptoms of malignant hyperthermia

• rapidly supply and reconstitute dantrolene sodium

• provide necessary supplies without hesitation

• assist the anesthesia care provider with intravenous line setup and placement, drug preparation and administration, implementation of laboratory testing, and as otherwise directed

• cool patient—surface, intravenous, and lavage

197. If the patient is known or considered to be susceptible to malignant hyperthermia, regional anesthesia or only nontriggering anesthetics are administered, and fresh anesthesia circuitry and CO_2 absorbent are used. Other interventions are the preparation of the operating room table with a cooling blanket, transfer of the malignant-hyperthermia cart and supplies into the room, and, depending on institutional policy, prophylactic administration of dantrolene sodium.

• •

SECTION QUESTIONS

Q41. Describe two nursing interventions to assist the patient to maintain dignity while in the operating room just prior to anesthesia induction. (Ref. 150)

_____

_____

Q42. During induction, the perioperative nurse (Ref. 149, 151, 152):

   a. may provide significant support by holding the patient's hand

   b. must be immediately available to assist the anesthesia care provider

   c. should maintain quiet in the room

Q43. The laryngeal mask airway protects the patient's airway without intubation. (Ref. 159)

   True   False

Q44. In the event that the patient aspirates stomach contents, the perioperative nurse must be prepared to immediately place the table in reverse Trendelenburg position. (Ref. 161)

   True   False

Q45. The Sellick maneuver is performed (Ref. 163):

   a. to occlude the esophagus to prevent regurgitation

   b. to visualize the tracheal lumen

   c. only by the anesthesia care provider

   d. to assist patient ventilation

Q46. Extubation may initiate (Ref. 172):

   a. bronchospasm

   b. laryngospasm

   c. vomiting

Q47. Malignant hyperthermia is a disorder of the hypothalamus, which regulates temperature. (Ref. 175, 176, 182)

   True   False

Q48. The neuromuscular blocker _____ is a primary triggering agent of malignant hyperthermia. (Ref. 179)

Q49. The treatment drug for malignant hyperthermia is _____ and it is administered at _____ mg/kg until the patient responds or a maximum of 20 doses is given. (Ref. 185, 189)

Q50. Describe two interventions to cool the patient during a malignant hyperthermia crisis. (Ref. 187)

_____

_____

Q51. Describe two nursing interventions to prepare the room if the patient is considered to be susceptible to malignant hyperthermia. (Ref. 197)

_____

• •

MODERATE SEDATION/ANALGESIA

Overview

198. Moderate sedation/analgesia, also known as conscious sedation, is a drug-induced depression of consciousness. The patient is able to respond purposefully to verbal commands, either alone or accompanied by light tactile stimulation. No interventions are required to maintain a patent airway. Spontaneous ventilation is adequate (Phillips, 2000, p. 404).

199. Moderate sedation/analgesia is frequently employed for diagnostic procedures or minor surgery where the presence of an anesthesiologist is not routinely necessary. Examples of procedures are colonoscopy, incision and drainage of an abscess, excision of small mass, face-lift, vasectomy, and the reduction of a dislocation with a cast application.

200. The goals of moderate sedation/analgesia are to:

   • allay fear and anxiety
   • maintain consciousness and the ability to respond to verbal stimulation
   • maintain respirations unassisted
   • provide adequate analgesia
   • maintain stable vital signs
   • achieve partial amnesia
   • facilitate prompt return to activities of daily living

201. Each institution should develop criteria to identify which patients are suitable candidates for moderate sedation/analgesia. Physiological sta-

tus and psychological maturity should be evaluated. The assessment should include an airway assessment to determine if the patient would be difficult to intubate if necessary. Factors that could make intubation difficult include but are not limited to: significant obesity, significantly recessed or protruding jaw, limited range of neck motion, short thick neck (less than 3 finger breadths), small mouth opening (< 3 cm in adult), tracheal deviation, large tongue, and protruding teeth (Hall, 2004, p. 7).

202. Sedatives and analgesic agents are delivered intravenously. Commonly used agents include diazepam (Valium), midazolam (Versed), morphine sulfate (Duramorph), meperidine (Demerol), and fentanyl (Sublimaze).

203. Reversal agents include naloxone hydrochloride (Narcan) for narcotics and flumazenil (Romazicon) for benzodiazepines.

204. Desired effects of moderate sedation/analgesia are relaxation, cooperation, and intact protective reflexes. Verbal communication is diminished; the patient breathes unassisted and is easily aroused.

205. Undesirable effects are nystagmus (may be normal with large doses of diazepam), slurred speech, unarousable sleep, hypotension, agitation, combativeness, respiratory depression, airway obstruction, and apnea (AORN, 2004b, p. 214).

Nursing Responsibilities

206. The registered nurse who monitors the patient receiving moderate sedation/analgesia should have no other responsibilities during the procedure that would leave the patient unattended and compromise monitoring (AORN, 2004b, p. 211). An additional nurse should be present to function in the circulating role.

207. The patient who receives moderate sedation/analgesia must be continuously monitored for any reaction to drugs and for physiologic and psychologic changes that may cause a patient to progress to a state of deep sedation. Deep sedation may be characterized by extremely slurred speech, not easily being aroused, inability to independently maintain a patent airway, and nonresponsiveness to verbal commands. In the event that a patient progresses to a state of deep sedation and cannot be easily aroused and cannot maintain independent ventilatory function, the nurse must be competent to provide rescue measures.

208. In addition to the ability to perform a thorough preoperative assessment, the nurse who is monitoring the patient should have a working knowledge of resuscitation equipment and the function and use of monitoring equipment, and should be able to interpret any data that are obtained.

Monitoring equipment should include oxygen delivery device, pulse oximeter, blood pressure monitor, and electrocardiograph. Suction should be immediately available, turned on, and functioning. The patient should have an established intravenous line, and reversal agents should be in the room and immediately available. The crash cart should be immediately available.

209. Necessary knowledge and/or skills include the following:

- knowledge of anatomy and physiology
- knowledge of airway management, including the use of oxygen delivery devices and equipment
- use of monitoring equipment for determining oxygen saturation, blood pressure, cardiac rate and rhythm, respiratory rate, and level of consciousness
- interpretation of monitoring data, including interpretation of cardiac dysrhythmia
- knowledge of pharmacology and action of moderate sedation/analgesia agents
- knowledge of desirable and undesirable effects of moderate sedation/analgesia agents
- recognition of complications related to moderate sedation/analgesia
- use of resuscitative equipment (AORN, 2004b, p. 212).

210. Some institutions require advance life-support certification for nurses who monitor patients receiving moderate sedation/analgesia.

211. Patients who are discharged to another unit should be monitored for several hours to ensure the maintenance of a satisfactory level of consciousness, a patent airway, and stable vital signs.

212. Ambulatory surgery patients should not be discharged until the following criteria have been met:

- Vital signs are stable.
- Airway is patent.
- Alert level of consciousness is maintained.
- Mobility and sensory functions are intact.
- Protracted vomiting is absent.
- Surgical site and dressing are satisfactory.

- Pain is manageable.
- Hydration is adequate (AORN, 2004b, pp. 215–216).

213. Patients should be given written postoperative instructions because medications used in moderate sedation/analgesia can diminish the ability to recall information that has been given verbally.

REGIONAL ANESTHESIA

Overview

214. Regional anesthesia is preferable for patients who require emergency surgery and have a full stomach. It is also used where general anesthetic agents are contraindicated in patients who have metabolic, renal, or hepatic disease. The respiratory and cardiac systems remain relatively stable with regional anesthesia. Sometimes a regional anesthetic is utilized in conjunction with a general anesthetic.

215. Regional anesthesia techniques include spinal, epidural, and caudal block, intravenous block, nerve block, local infiltration, and topical administration.

Spinal

216. Spinal anesthesia is obtained when the anesthetic agent is injected into the cerebrospinal fluid in the subarachnoid space. Injection is made through a lumbar interspace usually between L2 and L3, or below, so that the needle is not inserted into the spinal cord, which normally ends at L1 to L2. As the anesthetic is absorbed by the nerve fibers, nerve transmission is blocked. Spread of the anesthetic agent and the subsequent level of anesthesia is determined by cerebrospinal pressure, injection site, amount, concentration, and specific gravity of the anesthetic solution, speed of injection, and the position of the patient during and immediately following the injection.

217. Spinal anesthetic solutions are generally a mixture of local anesthetic and dextrose. These solutions settle in accordance with gravity. The block can be directed up, down, or to one side of the spinal cord by adjusting the patient's position. After 10 or 15 minutes the block is set and does not extend further.

218. Agents frequently used for spinal anesthesia are lidocaine (Xylocaine), pontocaine (Tetracaine), and bupivacaine (Marcaine).

219. Spinal anesthesia is used for lower abdominal, pelvic, lower extremity, and urologic procedures, and for cesarean sections.

220. The administration of spinal anesthesia requires patient cooperation. Proper positioning is the key to successful placement of the anesthetic injection. Nursing intervention should be directed toward positioning the patient and providing support during administration of the spinal.

221. Injection of the anesthetic is accomplished with the patient in a sitting or lateral decubitus position. In the sitting position, the patient is assisted to sit on the operating table with the legs over the side and the feet on a stool. The stool should be high enough to cause the patient's knees to be raised above the level of the waist. The patient should be encouraged to arch the back outward and lower the chin to the chest. (Figure 11-3) In the lateral decubitus position, the hips, back, and shoulders are aligned parallel with the edge of the table. The patient is instructed to bring the knees up toward the chest and to flex the head and neck. These maneuvers assist in spreading the vertebrae and exposing the desired interspaces to facilitate correct needle insertion.

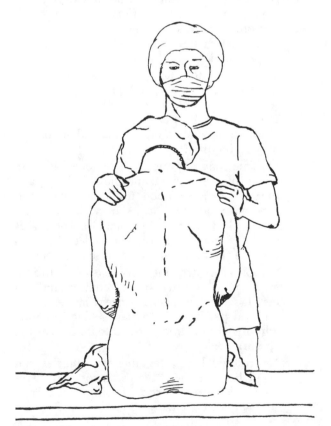

FIGURE 11-3 Position for Spinal Anesthesia.
Source: Courtesy of Andrew Maillard.

222. During preparation for spinal anesthesia, the perioperative nurse should help to position the patient, assist the anesthesia care provider as needed, and provide assurance to the patient. The patient in the lateral decubitus position is very close to the edge of the table, and safety measures to prevent falling are necessary. The perioperative nurse should remain with the patient, institute measures to prevent falling, and help the patient feel secure.

223. When administering spinal anesthesia, strict attention to asepsis is important in order to prevent entry of pathogens that can cause meningitis into the subarachnoid space.

224. Complications of spinal anesthesia include a rapid drop in blood pressure, nausea and vomiting, total spinal anesthesia, postdural headache, and neurological or integumentary positioning injury.

225. Sudden hypotension is caused by vasodilation when sympathetic nerves that control vasomotor tone are blocked. Peripheral pooling, decreased venous return, and decreased cardiac output can also result. Ephedrine may be administered to restore normotension.

226. Nausea and vomiting can occur as a result of hypotension or as a reaction to sedation medication. Suction should be immediately available, and an emesis basin and wet towel should be provided.

227. Total spinal anesthesia occurs when the level of anesthesia becomes so high that paralysis of respiratory muscles results and respiratory distress occurs. This is an emergency situation. Ventilation must be supported, and intubation may be required.

228. Patients may experience headache 24 to 48 hours following spinal anesthesia if the dura at the site of injection does not seal itself off and cerebrospinal fluid leaks into the epidural space. The loss of cerebrospinal fluid decreases cerebrospinal pressure, leaves less fluid to cushion the brain, and can cause headache.

229. In most cases, treatment consists of hydration, intravenous or oral caffeine, sedation, and bed rest. If symptoms persist longer than 24 hours, a blood patch of the patient's blood may be administered at the puncture site to seal the epidural leak.

230. Neurological or integumentary injuries can occur because the patient's sensory pathways are blocked and improper positioning or pressure cannot be felt.

Epidural and Caudal

231. Epidural anesthesia is achieved by injection of the anesthetic agent into the epidural space.

(Figure 11-4) The agent may be injected through the interspaces of the thoracic or cervical vertebrae; however, the lumbar region is the usual site of injection.

232. Epidural anesthesia is useful in anorectal, vaginal, and perineal procedures and is often used in obstetric surgery.

233. For caudal anesthesia, the anesthetic is injected into the epidural space through the caudal canal in the sacrum.

234. Commonly used epidural and caudal anesthetic agents are lidocaine hydrochloride (Xylocaine), bupivacaine (Marcaine), and chloroprocaine (Nesacaine).

235. Epidural anesthesia can be delivered as a single dose, or a small catheter can be left in place for continuous infusion. Continuous infusion is useful for pain management in the postoperative period.

236. Anesthetic agents that are injected into the epidural space are not as affected by positioning as in spinal anesthesia.

237. Complications of epidural anesthesia are:

- dural puncture—postdural headache
- inadvertent subarachnoid injection—total spinal anesthesia
- inadvertent intravascular injection—extreme hypotension and cardiac arrest

Intravenous Block (Bier Block)

238. Intravenous block involves intravenous injection of a local anesthetic agent into the vein of

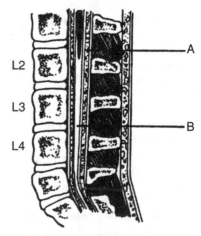

FIGURE 11-4 Regional Anesthesia Sites. A. An Epidural anesthesia is achieved by injection of the anesthetic into the epidural space. B. Spinal anesthesia is achieved when the anesthetic agent is injected into the cerebrospinal fluid in the subarachnoid space. Injection is made between L2 and L3 or below.

a tourniquet-occluded extremity. In this procedure, an intravenous catheter is inserted into the operative extremity. Two side-by-side tourniquets, or one double-cuffed tourniquet, are applied, but not inflated, on the extremity. The extremity is elevated and drained of blood with an Esmarch or elastic bandage. The proximal tourniquet or cuff is then inflated, and a fixed amount of anesthetic agent is injected. The anesthetic agent infiltrates and is confined to the tissues that are distal to the tourniquet. To alleviate tourniquet pain, the second distal cuff is inflated after the anesthetic agent has taken effect. The proximal cuff is then deflated.

239. After the procedure, the tourniquet is released and the remaining anesthetic is absorbed into the general circulation. If absorption is too rapid, cardiovascular collapse or central nervous system toxicity can occur.

240. This technique is used most often for surgeries of the upper extremity that last an hour or less.

241. Lidocaine (Xylocaine) is used for intravenous block.

Nerve Block

242. In nerve block, the anesthetic agent, usually lidocaine (Xylocaine), is injected into and around a nerve or nerve group that supplies sensation to a small area of the body.

243. Nerve blocks can be used for purposes of surgical intervention but are more commonly used for sustained relief in patients with chronic pain and to increase circulation in some vascular diseases.

244. Nerve blocks can be minor or major. Major blocks involve multiple nerves or a plexus. Minor blocks block a single nerve.

245. Major nerve blocks used in operative procedures are brachial-plexus block for procedures of the arm, orbital block for eye procedures, and cervical block for procedures involving the neck.

246. Common minor blocks are radial and ulnar nerve blocks for procedures of the elbow, wrist, or digits.

247. The perioperative nurse may assist during nerve block by aspirating the needle during placement to check for inadvertent vascular injection. The nurse may also be asked to inject the local anesthetic while the anesthesia care provider secures the placement of the needle. Whether or not it is appropriate for the nurse to inject the anesthetic will depend upon institutional policy, state board of nursing regulations, and demonstrated competency.

Local Infiltration

248. Local infiltration involves the injection of the anesthetic agent into subcutaneous tissue at, or close to, the anticipated incision site.

249. Local infiltration is useful for minor, superficial procedures.

250. The most frequently used local anesthetic is lidocaine (Xylocaine). Epinephrine may be added to the lidocaine to cause vasoconstriction, reduce bleeding, and slow absorption of the drug.

251. Toxic reactions from local anesthetics can occur if too rapid an absorption from a vascular site occurs or if there is an inadvertent intravascular injection. Toxic reactions include central nervous system and cardiovascular depression. The nurse needs to be alert to the possibility of a toxic reaction. Initial signs of central nervous system toxicity are restlessness, lightheadedness, visual and auditory disturbances, dizziness, tremors, and convulsions. This may be followed by unconsciousness, apnea, and cardiac arrest. Patients who say that they hear unusual sounds or express a feeling of uneasiness may be experiencing a toxic reaction. Initial treatment consists of establishing and maintaining an airway, assisting or controlling ventilation with oxygen, and administering sedation.

252. It is the responsibility of the perioperative nurse to ensure that resuscitation equipment is available when local anesthetics are administered.

253. During local anesthesia, the perioperative nurse should monitor the patient's blood pressure, cardiac rate and rhythm, respiratory rate, oxygen saturation, skin condition, and mental status (AORN, 2004a, p. 214).

Topical

254. In topical anesthesia, the anesthetic is applied directly to a mucous membrane or an open wound. Topical anesthesia is often used for nasal surgery, cystoscopy, and procedures of the respiratory tract in which it is advantageous to eliminate cough and laryngeal reflex.

255. Commonly used topical anesthetics are pontocaine (Tetracaine), cocaine, and lidocaine (Xylocaine).

256. Cocaine is used in nasal passages; pontocaine in the eye; and lidocaine in the throat, nose, esophagus, and genitourinary tract.

257. Lidocaine may be supplied as a liquid, liquid spray, or jelly.

258. Topical anesthetics are readily absorbed by mucous membranes and therefore act rapidly.

Sudden cardiovascular collapse is possible following the application of topical anesthetic in the respiratory tract. Resuscitation equipment should be immediately available.

Regional Anesthesia—Nursing Responsibilities

259. Responsibilities of the perioperative nurse will vary according to the type of regional anesthesia being administered.

260. Patients who are scheduled to receive regional anesthesia may be apprehensive about being awake during surgery. They may mistakenly believe that their being awake will result in inevitable pain or that they will be unable to avoid observing the surgery. Providing assurance, answering questions, and remaining close to the patient will, in most instances, significantly reduce anxiety. Even patients who are sedated should be aware that the nurse is close by and is available to provide support.

261. For some surgeries it is important that the patient be alert and cooperate with the surgeon to facilitate the procedure. The perioperative nurse can provide encouragement, support, and information that the patient needs during these times.

262. Patients who receive regional anesthesia are awake, and conversation in the operating suite should reflect this consideration. Regional anesthesia patients are usually given supplemental tranquilizers and may sleep. However, they are arousable and may be startled by noise or made anxious by inappropriate conversation. It is appropriate to place a sign on the door of the operating suite stating that the patient is awake. This will serve as a reminder to persons who enter.

263. During placement of the needle for spinal, epidural, caudal, and nerve block, the patient should be protected from unnecessary exposure to prevent embarrassment and cooling. Pillows and blankets should be provided to increase patient comfort.

264. Preparation of the incision site with an antiseptic scrub may necessitate exposing the patient and may cause the awake patient to become embarrassed or anxious. It is important to maintain the patient's dignity and minimize exposure.

265. Every patient receiving some type of regional anesthesia should be monitored. The extent of monitoring and the person responsible for monitoring is determined by the anesthesia technique, the results of preoperative assessment, the surgical procedure, the recognized anesthesia standards and practices, and the institution's policy. Administration of topical and local infiltration anesthetics is the surgeon's responsibility. During spinal, epidural, caudal, intravenous block, and nerve block, an anesthesia care provider is present. However, during local anesthesia it is unusual for an anesthesia care provider to be present, and monitoring is the responsibility of the perioperative nurse. The AORN recommended practice for the patient receiving local anesthesia states, "Patients receiving local anesthesia during a surgical procedure should be assessed throughout the perioperative experience by an RN. The RN managing the care of the patient receiving local anesthesia should monitor the patient's physiological and psychosocial status throughout the procedure" (AORN, 2004b, pp. 325, 326).

266. The nurse who monitors the patient receiving local anesthesia must be able to recognize a normal baseline and any changes that occur. Baseline data must include blood pressure, cardiac rate and rhythm, respirations, oxygen saturation, skin condition, and mental status. In addition, a knowledge of the drugs used as well as possible reactions to them is necessary in order for the perioperative nurse to be able to provide appropriate nursing interventions.

267. During local anesthesia, the perioperative nurse should track and monitor the amount of anesthetic agent given. The maximum recommended dose of 1% lidocaine, without epinephrine, for adults is 300 mg (4.5 mg/kg). The maximum recommended dose of lidocaine with epinephrine is 500 mg (7 mg/kg). The amount that is administered should be reported to the surgeon.

268. Nursing intervention for all patients who receive regional anesthesia should include preparation for toxic systemic reactions of the central nervous system and cardiovascular collapse. Resuscitation equipment must be immediately available, and the perioperative nurse monitoring the patient must be competent in the use of the equipment and preparation and action of related medications. Current cardiopulmonary resuscitation (CPR) certification is an essential requirement for the perioperative nurse.

• •

SECTION QUESTIONS

Q52. During moderate sedation/analgesia, the patient should be sedated enough not to respond to verbal stimuli. (Ref. 198)

True   False

Q53. Morphine is the most common drug used in moderate sedation/analgesia. (Ref. 202)

True   False

Q54. List four undesirable effects of moderate sedation/analgesia. (Ref. 205)

_____

_____

_____

_____

Q55. Patients who have had moderate sedation/analgesia should be given written postoperative instructions because the medications they received may diminish their recall ability. (Ref. 213)

True   False

Q56. Respiratory and cardiac systems remain relatively stable under regional anesthesia. (Ref. 214)

True   False

Q57. Regarding spinal anesthesia (Ref. 216, 220, 221, 222, 224):

a. the level of anesthesia is influenced by the patient's position immediately following administration

b. injection is at or above L2 to L3

c. the primary nursing responsibility is assistance in positioning and support

d. it is always administered with the patient in a sitting position

e. a sudden rise in blood pressure is a complication of spinal anesthesia

Q58. Total spinal anesthesia is an emergency. Explain why. (Ref. 227)

_____

_____

Q59. A headache 24 to 48 hours after spinal anesthesia is usually the result of an increase in cerebrospinal pressure. (Ref. 228)

True   False

Q60. Epidural anesthesia is useful for labor and delivery. (Ref. 232)

True   False

Q61. Intravenous block (Ref. 238, 240, 241):

a. is useful for procedures on the shoulder

b. includes the injection of lidocaine into a vein

c. includes the application of a tourniquet to an extremity

d. is useful for procedures of the hand

Q62. Nerve blocks (Ref. 242, 245):

a. are useful in patients with chronic pain

b. are useful for abdominal procedures

c. involve application of a tourniquet

Q63. The perioperative nurse who assists the anesthesia care provider during a nerve block may be asked to inject the local anesthetic. Depending upon institutional policy, state board of nursing regulations, and competency, this may or may not be an appropriate responsibility. (Ref. 247)

True   False

Q64. When lidocaine with epinephrine is administered as a local anesthetic, absorption of the drug is _____ and as a result, a _____ dose may be given than can be given when lidocaine without epinephrine is used. (Ref. 250, 267)

a. accelerated/lower

b. slowed/higher

Q65. During a procedure under local anesthetic, the perioperative nurse should monitor the patient's cardiac rate and rhythm and mental status. (Ref. 253)

True   False

Q66. Topical anesthetics are absorbed slowly by mucous membranes and are therefore safe. (Ref. 258)

True   False

Q67. An airway assessment (Ref. 201):

a. is useful in identifying patient who may not be suitable for moderate sedation/analgesia

b. should include assessment of obesity, neck length, and size of mouth opening

c. is not necessary if the patient has been classified according to the ASA Classification System

Q68. It is possible for patients receiving moderate sedation/analgesia to progress to a state of deep sedation. List three characteristics of deep sedation. (Ref. 207)

_____

_____

_____

••• References

American Society of Anesthesiologists. (2004). ASA physical status classification system. Retrieved June 25, 2004, from www.asahq.org/clinical/physicalstatus.htm

Association of periOperative Registered Nurses (AORN). (2004a). Recommended practices for managing the patient receiving local anesthesia. In *Standards, recommended practices and guidelines* (pp. 211–217). Denver, CO: Author.

(AORN). (2004b). Recommended practices for moderate sedation/analgesia. In *Standards, recommended practices and guidelines* (pp. 211–217). Denver, CO: Author.

Baric, P. (2002). Surgical site infections: Epidemiology and prevention. *Surgical Infections, 3,* S-9–S-19.

Beck, C. (1994). Malignant hyperthermia: Are you prepared? *AORN Journal, 59*(2), 367–390.

Brooks-Braun, J. A. (1995). Postoperative atelectasis and pneumonia. *American Journal of Critical Care, 4*(5), 340–347.

Delamar, L. (2003). Anesthesia. In M. Meeker & J. Rothrock (Eds.), *Alexander's care of the patient in surgery* (12th ed., pp. 219–251). St. Louis, MO: Mosby.

Genetic Information and Patient Services, Inc. (n.d.) Malignant hyperthermia. Retrieved July 4, 2004 from www.icomm.ca/geneinfo/mh.htm

Hall, K. (2004). Frequently asked questions. *SGNA News, 22*(2), 7.

JCAHO. (2004). Sentinel Event Alert, Issue 32, Oct. 6, pp. 1–3. Retrieved Oct. 27, 2004, from www.asahq.org/news/SEAfinal.pdf

Kissen, K. (2004). Burn injury in the operating room: A closed claims analysis. ASA Newsletter, 68(6) retrieved October 27, 2004 from www.asahq.org/Newsletters/2004/06_04/kressin06_04.html

Lema, M. (2003). Safe anesthetic practice—Fact, fantasy or folly. *Ventilations, ASA Newsletter, 67*(6). Retrieved June 25, 2004, from www.asahq.org/newsletter/2003/06_03/ventilations06_03.html

Litwack, K. (1995). *Post anesthesia nursing care.* St. Louis, MO: Mosby Year Book.

Malignant Hyperthermia Association. (n.d.) About malignant hyperthermia. Retrieved June 25, 2004, from www.mhacanada.org/about/htm

Mangram, A., Horan, T., Pearson, M., Silver, L., Jarvis W. (1999). Guideline for prevention of surgical site infection, 1999. *Infection Control and Hospital Epidemiology, 20*(1), 247–278.

National Institutes of Occupational Safety and Health (NIOSH). (1994). Controlling exposures to nitrous oxide during anesthesia administration (NIOSH Alert, Publication No. 94-100). Retrieved June 25, 2004. from www.cdc.gov/niosh/noxidalr.html

OR Manager. (2004). *Preventing surgical infections by keeping patients warmed, 20*(4), 1, 11–16.

Phillips, N. Berry and Kohn's operating room technique, 10th ed. (pp. 401–442). St. Louis, MO: Mosby.

Roth, R. A. (Ed.). (1995). *Perioperative nursing care curriculum.* Philadelphia: W. B. Saunders.

Wang, V. (1997). Propofol. *Clinical Toxicology Review 19*(8). Retrieved June 25, 2004, from www.maripoisoncenter.com/ctr/970Spropofol.html

••• Suggested Reading

Phillips, N. (2004). *Berry and Kohn's operating room technique,* 10th ed. (pp. 401–442). St. Louis, MO: Mosby.

Appendix 11-A

Chapter 11 Post Test

Instructions: Fill in the blank(s), mark the correct answer(s), or answer the question as appropriate.

1. Possible patient injury related to anesthesia includes an ineffective airway, an untoward drug reaction, decreased cardiac output, and an ineffective breathing pattern. List two additional possible injuries related to anesthesia. (Ref. 3)

   _____

   _____

2. An anesthesiologist, a certified nurse anesthetist, or a perioperative nurse may be responsible for monitoring the patient who is receiving moderate sedation/analgesia. (Ref. 11)

   True   False

3. Because patient assessment in preparation for anesthesia is performed by an anesthesiologist or a CRNA, it is not necessary for the perioperative nurse to also perform an assessment. (Ref. 12)

   True   False

4. During the assessment it is important that the patient be asked about family history with anesthetics. Explain why this information is important. (Ref. 20)

   _____

   _____

5. Preoperative teaching should include encouraging a patient who smokes to refrain from smoking prior to surgery because that may reduce the risk of postoperative pulmonary complications. (Ref. 24)

   True   False

6. List six factors that influence selection of anesthesia agents and technique. (Ref. 30)

   _____

   _____

   _____

   _____

   _____

   _____

7. The primary goal of preoperative medication is to put the patient to sleep. (Ref. 40, 52)

   True   False

8. Agents that promote gastric emptying and lower stomach pH, such as metoclopramide (Reglan), should be given 90 minutes or more before surgery. (Ref. 41)

   True   False

9. Match the medications with the effects. (Ref. 43, 45, 48, 51)

   a. midazolam (Versed)   ___ raises gastric pH

   b. ranitidine (Zantac)   ___ reduces anxiety, provides some amnesia

   c. glycopyrrolate (Robinul)   ___ decreases oral secretions

   d. fentanyl (Sublimaze)   ___ relief from pain

10. Monitoring for all patients who receive anesthesia should include (Ref. 55, 56):

    a. ECG

    b. blood pressure

    c. heart rate

    d. oxygen saturation

11. An internal esophageal probe may be used to monitor patient temperature. (Ref. 76)

    True   False

12. Some anesthetic agents, such as isoflurane and halothane, dilate blood vessels or interfere with the tempera-ture-regulating mechanism in the hypothalamus and can cause the patient' temperature to drop. (Ref. 90, 97)

    True   False

13. Nitrous oxide (Ref. 84, 85, 86, 109, 110):

    a. is sufficient for most surgeries

    b. is a potential hazard to operating room staff

    c. is used in combination with other inhalation agents

    d. is a neuromuscular blocker

    e. exposure limit is 35 ppm over 8 hours

14. Inhalation agents are removed from the patient's system through_____ (what mechanism?).
    IV agents are metabolized by the _____ and _____. (Ref. 115)

15. Match the medications with the description. (Ref. 117, 120, 121, 122)

    a. thiopental sodium (Sodium Pentothal)   ___ nonbarbiturate induction agent

    b. propofol (Diprivan)   ___ barbiturate

    c. etomidate (Amidate)   ___ minimal aftereffects such as vomiting

                                              ___ medium supports bacterial growth

                                              ___ short-acting induction agent

                                              ___ utilized for cardiac patients

                                              ___ rapid loss of consciousness

                                              ___ minimal effects on myocardial metabolism

16. Fentanyl is a powerful narcotic that provides relief from pain and is given during surgery as an adjunct to other drugs and to relieve pain in the postoperative period. (Ref. 128, 129)

    True   False

17. Succinylcholine (Anectine), atracurium besylate (Tracrium), tubocurarine chloride (curare), mivacurium (Mivacron), pancuronium bromide (Pavulon), and vecuronium bromide (Norcuron) are neuromuscular blockers. Name the one that is a depolarizing agent and causes fasciculation. (Ref. 140)

_____

18. Neuromuscular blockers (Ref. 137, 138, 139, 141, 143):

    a. are useful to relax the jaw and larynx at intubation

    b. are delivered from the anesthesia machine

    c. cause paralysis

    d. are all short acting

    e. are given to facilitate tissue manipulation intraoperatively

19. The aspiration of stomach contents can be fatal. List three immediate interventions that the perioperative nurse should be prepared to take in the event of regurgitation. (Ref. 161, 162)

_____

_____

_____

20. The Sellick maneuver is an appropriate intervention for the patient with a hiatal hernia. (Ref. 162, 163)

    True   False

21. It is a nursing responsibility to ensure that the anesthetized patient is properly positioned. (Ref. 166, 167, 168, 169)

    True   False

22. List four symptoms other than muscle rigidity that may be seen in malignant hyperthermia. (Ref. 177, 178)

_____

_____

_____

_____

23. _____ is usually one of the first signs of malignant hyperthermia crisis. (Ref. 178)

    a. rapid rise in temperature

    b. increased end-tidal CO_2 volume

    c. profuse sweating

24. The treatment drug for malignant hyperthermia is _____ and it is administered at _____ mg/kg until the patient responds or a maximum of 20 doses is given. (Ref. 185, 189)

25. Goals of moderate sedation/analgesia are to allay patient fear and anxiety, to maintain consciousness, to elevate the pain threshold, and to maintain stable vital signs. (Ref. 200)

    True   False

26. Naloxone hydrochloride (Narcan) enhances the effect of narcotics. (Ref. 203)

    True   False

27. It is appropriate to have resuscitative equipment available when local infiltration, nerve block, and intravenous block are being administered because cardiovascular collapse is a possible adverse reaction to these forms of anesthesia. (Ref. 239, 251, 252, 253)

    True   False

28. List two reasons why regional anesthesia might be more appropriate for a patient than general anesthesia. (Ref. 214)

    _____

    _____

    _____

29. Describe the benefit derived by encouraging the patient to arch the back and lower the chin in preparation for spinal anesthesia. (Ref. 221)

    _____

    _____

30. The perioperative nurse should remain in contact with the patient during spinal anesthesia administration in the lateral position because the patient may feel in danger of falling from the table. (Ref. 222)

    True   False

31. Explain why patients under spinal anesthesia are at risk for neurologic or integumentary injury. (Ref. 230)

    _____

    _____

32. Epidural anesthesia can be delivered as a single dose, or a small catheter may be left in place for continuous infusion and pain management. (Ref. 235)

    True   False

33. Appropriate anesthesia technique for a cataract surgery is (Ref. 245):

    a. nerve block

    b. intravenous block (Bier)

34. What reaction should the perioperative nurse suspect if a patient receiving local anesthesia states he or she feels lightheaded, hears voices, or is restless, and what interventions should the nurse be prepared to take? (Ref. 251)

    Reaction:

    _____

    Interventions:

    _____

    _____

35. The nurse who is monitoring the patient who is receiving local anesthesia must be able to recognize and interpret normal baseline data and changes that occur. These data include blood pressure. List five additional data. (Ref. 266)

    _____

    _____

    _____

    _____

Appendix 11-B

• •

Competency Checklist: Anesthesia

Under "Observer's Initials," enter initials upon successful achievement of competency.
Enter N/A if competency is not appropriate for institution.

NAME _____

	OBSERVER'S INITIALS	DATE

Preoperative assessment

1. Assesses patient/chart for anesthetic considerations (as applicable):

   a. coexisting disease

   b. NPO status

   c. allergies to medications, contrast dyes, tape, latex

   d. current medications, including herbal and nutritional supplements

   e. previous surgeries

   f. patient/family history of anesthesia complications

   g. substance abuse

   h. pregnancy

   i. diagnostic testing

   j. response to preoperative medications

   k. anxiety level

   l. knowledge level

   m. previous anesthesia—complications

2. Verifies that patient is in compliance with preoperative instructions.

3. Communicates assessment data to surgical team as appropriate.

4. Provides emotional support (answers patient concerns, provides reassuring touch, etc.) to patient/family.

5. Provides information as needed to patient/family.

6. Reinforces preoperative teaching with patient/family.

General Anesthesia

7. In preparation for induction:

   a. checks suction and places for easy access to patient's mouth

   b. applies monitoring equipment (ECG leads, blood-pressure cuff)

   c. places IV line

    d. applies safety strap   _____ _____

    e. limits patient exposure   _____ _____

    f. maintains quiet atmosphere   _____ _____

    g. remains at patient's side at head of table, provides reassurance   _____ _____

8. At induction, assists in intubation as needed (provides endotracheal tube, applies cricoid pressure, suctions, inflates cuff, etc.).   _____ _____

9. Following induction:

    a. checks position and pressure points and provides protective devices as needed   _____ _____

    b. applies warming devices as appropriate (lengthy procedure, large/deep incision, etc.)   _____ _____

10. Monitors fluid output and replacement and irrigating fluid.   _____ _____

11. During emergence and extubation:

    a. checks suction and places for easy access to patient's mouth   _____ _____

    b. remains at head of OR table by patient   _____ _____

    c. assists anesthesia care provider as needed (suction, ambu, O_2, etc.)   _____ _____

12. Provides report to postanesthesia care unit (e.g., patient name and age, surgical procedure, surgeon and anesthesiologist, anesthesia technique, estimated blood loss, fluid and blood administration, urine output, response to surgery/anesthesia, lab results, chronic and acute health history, drug allergies, expected problems/suggested interventions, discharge plan).   _____ _____

Regional Anesthesia

13. Implements procedures to alert others that patient is awake.   _____ _____

14. Assists in positioning patient for administration of regional anesthetic (e.g., provides stool for feet, instructs patient).   _____ _____

15. Provides safe environment for patient during positioning for administration of regional anesthetic (e.g., remains with patient).   _____ _____

16. Limits patient exposure limited during preparation for and administration of anesthesia.   _____ _____

17. Monitors and reports amount of local anesthetic agent administered.   _____ _____

Monitoring

18. Demonstrates ability to apply and use monitoring device and interpret data for:

    a. blood pressure   _____ _____

    b. cardiac rate and rhythm   _____ _____

    c. respiratory rate   _____ _____

    d. oxygen saturation   _____ _____

    e. mental status/level of consciousness   _____ _____

19. Demonstrates airway management, including use of oxygen delivery devices and equipment. _____ _____

20. Demonstrates ability to use resuscitative equipment. _____ _____

Emergency Preparations

21. Retrieves malignant hyperthermia supplies without hesitation. _____ _____

22. Explains protocol for malignant hyperthermia crisis. _____ _____

23. Ensures immediate availability of resuscitative equipment (IV, conscious sedation, and local procedures). _____ _____

24. Reports changes in patient condition and implements appropriate interventions. _____ _____

Documentation

25. Documents data as required by institutional policy. _____ _____

Anesthesia Machine

26. Identifies anesthesia machine components, oxygen flush button, monitors for ECG, blood pressure, pulse, respirations, breathing bag, carbon dioxide absorber canister, ventilator, flowmeters, scavenging system. _____ _____

OBSERVER'S SIGNATURE   INITIALS   DATE

_____

ORIENTEE'S SIGNATURE

_____

Chapter 11—Section Question Answers

Q1.   a, b, c, e
Q2.   False
Q3.   a, c, d, e
Q4.   Normothermia, unimpeded air exchange, adequate ventilation, maintenance of cardiac output and fluid volume, correct electrolyte and fluid balance, absence of allergic reaction, unimpaired thought process
Q5.   Aldrete
Q6.   True
Q7.   a, b, c, d, e, f
Q8.   Procedure, anesthesia provider, anesthetic agents and techniques, intraoperative medications, estimated blood loss, fluid and blood administration, urine output, response to surgery/anesthesia, lab results, chronic and acute health history, drug allergies, expected problems and suggested interventions, discharge plan
Q9.   False
Q10. False
Q11. a, b, c, d, e, f
Q12. a, b, c, d, e, f
Q13. True
Q14. True
Q15. b, c
Q16. False
Q17. True
Q18. a
Q19. Reduction of anxiety, sedation, analgesia, amnesia, prevention of nausea and vomiting, reduction of gastric volume and acidity, facilitation of induction, reduction in risk of allergic reaction, decreased secretions
Q20. True
Q21. True
Q22. True
Q23. Monitors cardiac rate, rhythm, and breath sounds
Q24. a, c, d, f
Q25. Dilation of blood vessels related to effect of anesthetic agents, inhibition of temperature regulating mechanism in the hypothalamus, exposure, cool irrigating fluids
Q26. Stockinette to make a head covering and Webril to wrap the limbs
Q27. True
Q28. True
Q29. a, e
Q30. Green, blue
Q31. Anesthetic gases are a health hazard
Q32. True
Q33. True

(continues)

Chapter 11—Section Question Answers (*continued*)

Q34. b, d, e, f

Q35. Hallucination

Q36. True

Q37. Narcotics are respiratory depressants

Q38. b

Q39. a, c, d

Q40. a, b, d

Q41. Limit exposure, close doors, keep unnecessary personnel from the room

Q42. a, b, c

Q43. True

Q44. False

Q45. a, b

Q46. a, b, c

Q47. False

Q48. Succinylcholine

Q49. Dantrolene sodium, 2.5

Q50. Cool irrigation, cool IV fluids, surface cooling with ice, cooling blanket, cool gastric/rectal lavage

Q51. Prepare OR table with cooling blanket, prophylactic administration of dantrolene sodium, bring malignant hyperthermia supplies or cart into the room

Q52. False

Q53. False

Q54. Nystagmus, slurred speech, unarousable sleep, hypotension, agitation, combativeness, respiratory depression, airway obstruction, apnea

Q55. True

Q56. True

Q57. a, c

Q58. Respiratory muscles are paralyzed, patient in respiratory distress and cannot breathe

Q59. False

Q60. True

Q61. b, c, d

Q62. a

Q63. True

Q64. b

Q65. True

Q66. False

Q67. a, b

Q68. Extremely slurred speech, not easily being aroused, inability to maintain patent airway, unresponsiveness to verbal commands

Chapter 11—Post Test Answers

1. Compromised perfusion, altered hypothalamic thermoregulation, ineffective airway, electrolyte imbalance, alteration in thought processes
2. True
3. False
4. May identify potential adverse reactions such as malignant hyperthermia
5. True
6. Age, medical history, physical status, procedure, patient preference, surgeon preference, anesthesia provider preference and expertise, whether surgery is elective or emergent, considerations for postoperative pain management, patient's previous anesthesia experience/recovery
7. False
8. False
9. b, a, c, d
10. a, b, c, d
11. True
12. True
13. b, c
14. Ventilation, liver, kidneys
15. bc, a, b, b, abc, c, abc, c
16. True
17. Succinylcholine
18. a, c, e
19. Provide suction (suction should always be functioning and immediately available and nurse should be prepared to assist the anesthesia provider), turn patient's head to the side, put patient into Trendelenberg, assist anesthesia provider
20. True
21. True
22. Tachycardia, tachypnea, unstable blood pressure, increased end-tidal CO_2, fever, sweating, cyanotic mottling of the skin, dark, unoxygenated blood in the field
23. b
24. Dantrolene sodium, 2.5
25. True
26. False
27. True
28. Full stomach and emergency procedure, patient with metabolic, renal, or hepatic disease and who cannot metabolize anesthetic agents
29. Spreads vertebrae and exposes desired interspaces to facilitate correct needle placement
30. True
31. Sensory pathways are blocked and pressure cannot be felt
32. True
33. a
34. Reaction—central nervous system toxicity, cardiovascular depression; Intervention—establish and maintain airway, assist or control ventilation with oxygen, administer sedation
35. Cardiac rate, cardiac rhythm, respirations, O_2 saturation, skin condition, mental status

12

Workplace Safety

LEARNER OBJECTIVES

After reading and completing "Workplace Safety," the learner will:

- identify chemical and physical hazards present in the operating room environment
- list the government organizations that publish regulations for healthcare worker safety
- define a *sentinel event*
- discuss the most common causes of operating room fires
- identify the ECRI recommendations to decrease the chance of a fire in the operating room
- define the acronyms *RACE* and *PASS*
- describe the components of a fire safety plan
- define the purpose of the Line Isolation Monitoring (LIM) system
- state the guidelines for healthcare workers to follow when working in a room where radiation is present
- discuss possible causes of low back pain in healthcare workers and the recommendations for injury prevention
- describe the precautions to use when working with methyl methacrylate
- identify the difference between localized and systemic latex allergy reactions

. . . .
Lesson Outline

I.   REGULATIONS
II. STANDARDS AND RECOMMENDATIONS
III. JOB SAFETY ANALYSIS
IV. PHYSICAL HAZARDS
  A. Fire
  B. Electricity
  C. Radiation
  D. Lifting and Moving
  E. Slips, Trips, and Falls
V.   CHEMICAL HAZARDS
  A. Formaldehyde
  B. Methyl Methacrylate
  C. Waste Anesthetic Gases
  D. Latex Considerations

This chapter addresses aspects of workplace safety that perioperative nurses most often cite as cause for concern. It does not cover all aspects of workplace safety or patient safety. Exposure to bloodborne pathogens is covered in Chapter 5, and patient safety is addressed throughout the text.

REGULATIONS

1. Trained safety personnel can be a valuable resource when designing and developing a safety program for the operating room. All staff should learn the basic safety requirements for the perioperative environment.

2. Building, electrical, and fire codes developed for each state and city are part of the creation of a safe environment for patients and healthcare workers. In addition to state and city regulations, organizations such as the Centers for Disease Control and Prevention (CDC), the National Institute of Occupational Safety and Health (NIOSH), the Occupational Safety and Health Administration (OSHA), the Joint Commission on Accreditation of Healthcare Organizations (JCAHO), the National Fire Protection Association (NFPA), and the Environmental Protection Agency (EPA) create regulations and recommendations for healthcare facilities that impact the workplace environment and perioperative nursing practice.

STANDARDS AND RECOMMENDATIONS

3. Occupational Safety and Health Administration (OSHA)—OSHA has the primary responsibility for publishing and enforcing workplace safety and health standards. Established in 1970, OSHA creates legal standards that must be economically feasible. OSHA can also assess the workplace for hazards and mandate changes to correct unsafe conditions. OSHA regulations carry the weight of the law, and healthcare facilities are generally vigilant in ensuring compliance.

Under OSHA's General Duty Clause, each employer must furnish each employee with a place of employment free from recognized hazards that are capable of causing or likely to cause death or serious physical harm to employees. Employers must create and implement an effective process that provides management support, involves employees in the plan, identifies problems, implements corrective actions, addresses employee and patient injury reports, provides periodic employee training, and evaluates ergonomics efforts (Gruendemann and Fernsebner, 1995, p. 268).

4. National Institute for Occupational Safety and Health (NIOSH)—NIOSH, also created in 1970, recommends standards based on public health considerations. Categories of standards include biological hazards such as bloodborne pathogens and tuberculosis; chemical hazards including ethylene oxide, glutaraldehyde, latex, and laser smoke control; and the physical hazards of ergonomics and musculoskeletal disorders and violence in the workplace.

Voluntary organizations, such as the Joint Commission on Accreditation of Healthcare Organizations (JCAHO) and the National Fire Prevention Association (NFPA), have developed standards and recommendations that are equally as important as those developed by OSHA and NIOSH, and require strict adherence.

5. JCAHO—JCAHO Standard EC.1.10 states in "Elements of Performance": "The hospital conducts proactive risk assessments that evaluate the potential adverse impact of buildings, grounds, equipment, occupants and internal physical systems on the safety and health of patients, staff and other people coming to the hospital's facilities . . . (JCAHO, 2004b, p. 3) and the hospital uses the risks identified to select and implement procedures and controls to achieve the lowest potential for adverse impact on the safety and health of patients, staff and other people coming to the hospital's facilities."

JCAHO Standard EC.9.10, "Elements of Performance," states: "The hospital monitors conditions in the environment, including injuries to patients or others coming to the hospital's facilities as well as incidents of property damage and occupational illnesses and injuries." (JCAHO, 2004, p. 24)

JOB SAFETY ANALYSIS

6. Job safety analysis can be applied to many work situations, including the OR, to analyze hazards and identify ways to overcome or eliminate them. Safety analysis methodology includes:

- identification of the various tasks in the work site
- breakdown of each task into the steps required to accomplish the task
- identification of any potential hazards
- suggestion of ways to reduce or eliminate the hazards
- development of standards for accomplishing the tasks
- periodic review of conditions in the work area

Safety standards are developed by the individual hospital department in conjunction with the facility infection control and employee health personnel. Following identification of the appropriate protective attire and work methodology, training and education of all employees is conducted to ensure that everyone understands the plan in order to avoid hazardous situations.

Ongoing monitoring is necessary to ensure that all personnel are familiar with the standards and are conducting their activities within the standard protocols. Monitoring results should be shared with personnel. Repeat training activities should be scheduled regularly to ensure that all personnel continue to comply with the standards, and any deviations should be addressed.

. . . .

SECTION QUESTIONS

Q1. Organizations with responsibility for regulating healthcare worker safety include OSHA, NIOSH, JCAHO and FDA. (Ref. 2)

True   False

Q2. Activities that employers must undertake to protect employees from hazards in the workplace include these three (Ref. 3):

_____

_____

_____

Q3. As part of the orientation process, each employee should receive safety training that is monitored at periodic intervals. (Ref. 6)

True   False

Q4. List 4 components of the job safety analysis (Ref. 6):

_____

_____

_____

_____

PHYSICAL HAZARDS

7. Some of the most important physical hazards for healthcare workers to maintain awareness of include fire, electricity, radiation, lifting and moving, and slips, trips, and falls.

Fire

8. Reports indicate that between 100 to 200 fires occur in the operating room each year. ECRI (formerly known as the Emergency Care Research Institute) reports that 10% to 20% result in serious patient injury. One or two fires are fatal, usually tracheal tube fires. Seventy-five percent of the fires occur in the oxygen-enriched area surrounding the patient's face. Frequent ignition sources include electrocautery (68%), lasers (18%), and light sources. Airway fires comprise 34% of the total, with 28% occurring on the face, head, neck, and chest of the patient (Bruley, 2003, p. 17). A small fire in an oxygen-enriched operating room can change to a large, life-threatening fire in seconds. Flames can reach a temperature of approximately 170°F (926°C) (ECRI 1992, p. 21). Smoke can make visibility difficult or impossible, and toxic fumes from burning synthetic materials can cause eye irritation or death if inhaled.

9. In January 2003, the JCAHO adopted the National Fire Protection Association's (NFPA) 2000 Life Safety Code for hospitals, ambulatory care centers, and other facilities. The Life Safety Code defines the requirements for facilities and procedures for safety from fire (Stewart, 2003, p. 26).

   In June 2003, the JCAHO issued a "Sentinel Event Alert on Preventing Surgical Fires" (JCAHO, 2003c, p. 1). A *sentinel event* is defined as an "unexpected occurrence involving death or serious physical or psychological injury, or risk thereof" (JCAHO, 2004a, p. 1). A healthcare or-

ganization that is accredited by the JCAHO is required to report any sentinel events that occur. A root-cause analysis focused on systems and processes and an action plan identifying process improvements to reduce the chances of another similar event must be submitted (Gruendemann, 1995, p. 27). Healthcare workers must:

- be trained in use of fire-fighting equipment
- be knowledgeable of rescue and escape methods
- be aware of hospital alarm systems and their use
- know how to contact the local fire department
- know the location of the medical gas shutoff valves (Koch, 2004, p. 48)

10. The fire triangle consists of ignition, fuel, and oxygen. All elements must be present for a fire to occur. The fuel source is anything that can burn. Examples of ignition sources include electrosurgery, laser, and fiberoptic cords.

11. Flammable anesthetics have been eliminated from operating rooms, but other hazards remain. Some potential sources of surgical fires include: an oxygen-enriched environment; electrical equipment; alcohol-based prepping and hand washing solutions; flammable chemicals; cylinders of compressed gas; draping materials; lasers; fiberoptic light sources and cables; patient care supplies; and trash.

12. Electrosurgical devices have been identified by ECRI as the most common cause of OR fires. The scrub person should know the location of the active electrode (ESU pencil) at all times. The ESU pencil should be kept in a location away from the patient and maintained in a protective holder with the holder secured so it will not be dislodged by personnel movements during the surgical procedure. The ESU pencil cord should not be wrapped around a metal surgical

instrument to secure it to the drapes. The active electrode should be cleaned periodically to remove buildup of eschar that can trap heat.

13. Fiberoptic cords and connectors become heated during use and should never be placed on the patient drapes because they have the potential to burn the patient and/or the draping materials. Headlights with fiberoptic cords should be removed when not in use or attached to the light source. Once detached, the fiberoptic cord should not be allowed to hang loose on the surgeon's back, where it has a potential to ignite the gown.

14. Oxygen supports combustion and, when used in close proximity to electrical equipment, requires constant vigilance. Surgery on or near the oxygen source, for example, surgery on the face, creates increased risk of fire. Often, surgical drapes used in conjunction with facial surgery create a tent effect where oxygen delivered via nasal cannula or endotracheal tube can become concentrated, creating a highly enriched oxygen environment. A spark in this environment can be disastrous. Draping should be done in a manner to prevent pockets where oxygen can concentrate.

15. Some materials that can contribute to the potential for combustion include patient hair, gases in the GI tract, skin degreasers, aerosol adhesives, ointments, breathing circuits, suction tubing, endotracheal tubes, and alcohol-based products. (Exhibit 12-1)

16. To reduce the risk of fires, alcohol-based hand washing products and patient prep solutions must be allowed to dry thoroughly or to evaporate following application. Prep solutions should not be allowed to saturate the drapes or pool in the patient's hair or on the linens or pillow.

17. ECRI recommendations that the perioperative nurse may implement include but are not limited to the following:

- questioning the need for 100% oxygen during facial surgery and replacing it with a lower concentration.
- ensuring that all flammable preps are thoroughly dry prior to placing drapes on the patient
- keeping sponges, gauze, and pledgets moist during surgery
- placing the electrosurgical pencil in a holster or a location off the patient when not in use
- disconnecting and removing contaminated ESU pencils
- checking the ESU alarm before use

- removing unnecessary foot pedals from area around surgeon's feet
- placing the laser on standby when it is not being used, placing wet towels around the laser incision site, and using nonreflective instrumentation
- keeping activated fiberoptic light sources from contacting surgical drapes or gowns (ECRI, as cited in Smith, 2004, p. 30)
- storing alcohol-based hand rubs in an area away from ignition and heat sources

18. Prevention is the best way to combat operating room fires.

19. In the event of a fire in the operating room, healthcare workers must be concerned about protecting both the patient and themselves. The acronym *RACE* is used to define personnel roles and responsibilities during a fire:

R - Rescue people from flaming materials.

A - Alert others by announcing "Code Red" and the location of the fire 3 times.

C - Confine or contain fire and smoke. Close the doors and shut off medical gas valves when leaving the room or when going from the fire area to a safe zone.

E - Extinguish the fire, if possible, using fire extinguishers. If the fire is immediately extinguished, call "Code Red all clear" and notify the Fire Department.

or

E - Evacuate to a safe place beyond the smoke or fire barrier doors, or outside. Activate the fire pull station when exiting the area. Remain with the patients and others in the safe area (Stewart, 2003, p. 27).

20. Fire safety training should include instruction in the use of fire extinguishers. When using an extinguisher, the acronym *PASS* identifies the steps of the process:

P - Pull the pin
A - Aim the nozzle
S - Squeeze the handle
S - Sweep at the base of the fire

21. Fire extinguishers are classified according to the National Fire Protection Association as follows:

- Class A—suitable for wood, cloth, paper, most plastics
- Class B—suitable for flammable liquids or grease
- Class C—suitable for electrical equipment

Exhibit 12-1   Fire Hazards and Appropriate Responses

Department/Services	Fire Hazard(s)/Fire Response Consideration(s)
Laboratory	Flammable materials such as Xylene, Methanol and other solvents with low flashpoints.
	Large volumes of formaldehyde solutions could present toxic environments for emergency responders in a fire situation.
Central Supply/Sterile Processing	Cartridges of 100% Ethylene Oxide (EtO) are flammable. EtO in any mixture (e.g., 90/10) could present toxic environments for emergency responders in a fire situation.
Surgical Suites	Surgical Suites are considered to have oxygen-enriched atmosphere (OEAs) due to the fact that oxygen concentration can exceed 23.5% by volume. Heat is present in overhead surgical lights, defibrilators, electrosurgical units, electrocautery units, and other sources. Fuels include prepping agents, open bottles or basins of volatile solutions, and most textiles (e.g. surgical drapes and gowns). Therefore, all the necessary ingredients are available in ample quantities to create a fire and thus put a patient and staff at risk.
Kitchens/Food Service	Grease fires represent a common fire hazard for those who prepare food.
Respiratory Therapy	Generally responsible for the storage and maintenance of large quantities of portable oxygen cylinders. Storage areas for bulk storage of these cylinders should be approved by the AHJ.
Hyperbaric Facilities	These areas are considered OEAs. Design and protocols should be conducted in accordance with NFPA 99 standards.
Magnetic Resonance Imaging (MRI)	MRI facilities represent evacuation issues for the patients being treated, and response issues for emergency responders. The magnet poses a potential risk for fire fighters responding to a room. In addition, emergency responders may have to purge the oxygen within the room to execute emergency response, which then creates an oxygen deficient atmosphere.
Engineering/Building and Grounds	Flammable materials such as gasoline and other fuels, oil based paints, and paint thinners are all present in large quantities.
Critical Care/General Nursing Areas	Areas such as the Intensive Care Unit, Neo-Natal Intensive Unit, Maternity, Labor and Delivery and Hemodialysis Units may have OEAs and also may represent significant challenges from an evacuation standpoint due to the fact that these patients are connected to hospital equipment or may out number staff by large quantities. Evacuation plans should be developed and approved by the AHJ.
Print Shops	Flammable solvents with large quantities of combustible material may be present.
Psychiatric Units	Evacuation may be an issue due to the fact that the Unit may be secured in accordance with the facilities Security Management Plan. Consult with the AHJ.
Linen and Laundry	Dryers and other heat sources are present. Ensure combustible material such as lint is adequately controlled.

22. The best fire extinguisher for the operating room is a halon extinguisher. It is usually marked for class B and C fires but is also effective against class A fires. It is lightweight and easy to handle.

23. A carbon dioxide extinguisher can be used for Class A, B, and C fires. It is heavier than a halon extinguisher and because of its size is usually wall mounted.

24. A pressurized water extinguisher, typically found in older operating room departments, is most suitable for class A fires. However, the fire hose sprays about 50 gallons a minute and is difficult to operate, and the force of the hose itself can cause injury.

25. Actual training sessions in a controlled area outside the building under the supervision of the local fire department can help employees to gain expertise and confidence when using fire extinguishers.

26. The education of staff begins at new-employee orientation and continues annually, including information about fire prevention, use of fire extinguishers, emergency response activities, and prevention of fire in the operating room.

27. Everyone on the surgical team must know the location of fire extinguishers, fire alarms, fire exits, and emergency shutoff gas valves. The locations of the alarms, extinguishers, and hoses must be posted in several sites. Fire blankets should not be kept in the operating room, as these will burn in the intense heat of a fire. They should be stored outside the OR and may be used in an area that is not oxygen enriched. Evacuation routes from all areas of the perioperative suite should be defined and posted in the hallways, OR lounge, and operating rooms. Hallways should be free of clutter that could hinder an evacuation. The perioperative nurse should be able to verbalize the evacuation route.

28. Each healthcare facility must:

    • have a fire safety plan
    • schedule safety education programs
    • conduct periodic fire drills

29. Each facility should develop a fire safety plan, involving representatives from OR nursing, clinical education, anesthesia, security, and the local fire and police departments. The chain of command should be decided upon and disseminated to all departments.

30. The fire safety plan should include:

    • a clear definition of responsibilities
    • methods for training staff members
    • scenarios for fire drills
    • instruction in the use of fire extinguishers
    • a plan for implementation of the code requirements
    • documents for life safety surveillance
    • an interim life safety plan for use in the event of construction
    • equipment, packaging materials, and supplies that must be retained for the fire investigation following any OR fire

31. Once the plan is finalized, education sessions for all departments involved should be scheduled to familiarize the entire staff with the plan and their roles. A safety officer should be appointed to be responsible for surveillance, conducting the fire drills, oversight of the required documentation, and an annual plan review.

32. The perioperative nurse must have a clear understanding of his or her responsibilities. Responsibilities may include but are not limited to the following:

    • identify the evacuation route
    • stay with the patient during evacuation
    • extinguish small fires with extinguisher
    • remove burning material from the patient and smother fire
    • turn off emergency shutoff valves
    • complete appropriate documentation

33. Fire drills should be conducted periodically to ensure that healthcare workers know their roles, whether they are at the location of the fire or away from the area. All employees should be familiar with the evacuation plans, proper methods of rescue and escape, location of the medical gases shutoff valves, fire alarm systems, how to contact the fire department, and the use of fire extinguishers.

34. Practice fire drills using different scenarios are invaluable in identifying portions of the plan needing revision or updating. A critique session following each fire drill can identify the need for changes or further education.

35. Life safety surveillance information should be collected and evaluated in a systematic way. In addition to fire safety, other topics may include facility and personnel security, hazardous substances, radiation safety, emergency preparedness, utilities, and infection control.

• •

SECTION QUESTIONS

Q5. The most common location for fires near the surgical patient is the _____, caused most often by _____. (Ref. 8)

    a. neck, electrocautery

    b. airway, laser

    c. face, laser

    d. airway, electrocautery

Q6. Define a *sentinel event*. (Ref. 9)

_____

_____

Q7. List 3 measures to ensure the security of the ESU pencil. (Ref. 12)

_____

_____

_____

Q8. Recommendations by ECRI to decrease the incidence of fires include using a lower concentration of oxygen during facial surgery, ensuring that all flammable preps are thoroughly dry prior to placing drapes on the patient, and keeping sponges, gauze, and pledgets moist during the surgical procedure. (Ref. 17)

True   False

Q9. Define the acronym *RACE*. (Ref. 19)

    R _____

    A _____

    C _____

    E _____

Q10. Either a halon or a carbon dioxide fire extinguisher can be used for most OR fires. (Ref. 22, 23, 24)

True   False

Q11. Development of the OR fire safety plan should include input from members of the following departments (Ref. 29):

    a. nursing, anesthesia, dietary

    b. security, clinical education, critical care

    c. local fire department, OR nursing, anesthesia

    d. OR nursing, housekeeping, clinical education

Q12. The role of the perioperative nurse during a fire does not include (Ref. 32):

    a. staying with the patient during evacuation

    b. notifying the patient's family

    c. removing burning material from the patient and smothering the fire

    d. completing the appropriate documentation

Q13. Other topics included in life safety surveillance may include hazardous substances, infection control, personnel security, and emergency preparedness. (Ref. 35)

    True   False

• •

Electricity

36. Electricity is one of the primary causes of hospital fires, increased by the use of inappropriate extension cords and/or equipment with frayed or faulty electrical cords. Additional hazards of using electrical equipment that is not functioning properly include shock, explosion, and burns.

37. The use of extension cords should be avoided, and many fire safety regulations prohibit their use. Equipment manufacturers must supply cords of sufficient length to allow equipment to be placed in the area of use. Each piece of equipment that is used in the operating room should be checked for function and electrical safety. Before use, the electrical outlets, switch plates, plugs, and power cords should be inspected for defects or damage.

38. Any new equipment should be inspected by the hospital biomedical engineering department prior to use. Labels or stickers should be placed on all equipment, denoting the date of inspection and the assigned hospital or department inventory number. The biomedical department is also responsible for documentation of regular inspections and preventive maintenance of all pieces of electrical/mechanical equipment. Every piece of electrical equipment should have a sticker showing the date of inspection and when the next inspection is due. If the inspection sticker is missing, or if the inspection has expired, the equipment should not be used.

39. Operating rooms are also equipped with a Line Isolation Monitoring (LIM) system. The LIM system continuously monitors ungrounded power systems that are isolated from the power supplied by the utility company. Ungrounded power systems may allow leakage to flow from the power system to ground. If the current passes through a person's body, it presents the potential for an electrical shock.

40. The LIM system measures the amount of current leakage and sounds an alarm if it exceeds the threshold for safety. The LIM system reduces the potential for electrical shock, cardiac fibrillation, or burns produced by excess electrical current flowing through the patient's body to ground.

41. In the event of an alarm, the perioperative nurse should immediately unplug the piece of equipment most recently plugged in and continue this process until the alarm ceases. The equipment responsible for the alarm should be removed from service until it can be ascertained that it is functioning properly.

Radiation

42. Surgical procedures performed under fluoroscopy or entailing intraoperative X-rays are the primary sources of potential exposure to radiation for operating room staff. Radiation safety training should be conducted as part of orientation and periodically thereafter.

43. The principles of time, distance, and shielding assist perioperative personnel to minimize their exposure to X-rays. When radiation is emitted at a constant rate, the dose received is dependent upon the amount of exposure time. The amount of time spent near the patient while radiation is being emitted should be as short as possible. During fluoroscopy or other procedures involving radiation, all personnel should remain at least 6 feet away from the X-ray tube.

44. Lead aprons and thyroid shields, along with leaded gloves and leaded eye protection in instances of lengthy exposure, are worn by perioperative personnel who must remain with the

patient while radiation is being used. A portable lead screen is another device that may be used for protection from radiation. Personnel should face the source of radiation while the radiation is being emitted.

45. Lead shielding devices should be checked at regular intervals by the X-ray department to ensure their integrity, and those with cracks discarded and replaced. If lead aprons are not handled properly, they can develop cracks that can permit radiation exposure to the healthcare worker wearing the apron. Aprons should be hung on a mobile or fixed rack designed for this purpose. They should not be folded.

46. Mobile lead shields may be placed in the room for nonscrubbed personnel to stand behind during the radiation emission time.

47. Personnel frequently assigned to procedures in which radiation is used should be monitored for exposure. A radiation monitoring badge, consisting of a strip of X-ray film encased in a plastic holder, should be worn on the neck area of the scrub attire above the lead apron. If two badges are worn, one should be worn at the neck above the lead apron and the other inside the apron (AORN, 2004a, p. 353). The amount of radiation absorbed by each badge should be measured monthly. They serve to monitor the amount of radiation experienced by each individual on the surgical team.

48. Any healthcare facility that uses therapeutic radionuclides for patient care should identify a ra-

diation safety officer to supervise the operation of the radiation safety program. Radionuclides are absorbed by the body, so personnel caring for the patients receiving them must take radiation safety precautions, in addition to standard precautions, with any bodily secretions from these patients.

49. The radiation safety officer will assist perioperative personnel in complying with government safety regulations and standards. Protective measures for perioperative personnel who are caring for a patient who has or is receiving therapeutic radionuclides include:

- using the principles of shielding, time, and distance to limit proximity to the radionuclides
- instituting contamination control measures
- notifying personnel caring for the patient postoperatively about the type and location of the radiation
- observing radiation precautions when transporting the patient
- keeping radioactive materials in a lead-lined container
- handling radioactive needles and capsules with forceps
- posting radiation warning signs on the doors to the operating room where the patient is located
- documenting all protective measures on the perioperative record

• •

SECTION QUESTIONS

Q14. New or loaner equipment may be used in the operating room immediately after it has been delivered. (Ref. 38)

True   False

Q15. What is the LIM system? (Ref. 39, 40)

_____

_____

Q16. The principles that assist perioperative personnel in limiting their exposure to radiation are (Ref. 43):

a. time, radiation level, and distance

b. distance, shielding, and radiation level

c. time, distance, and shielding

d. time alone

Q17. Name the personal protective equipment that should be worn when surgical procedures are performed under fluoroscopy. (Ref. 44)

_____

_____

_____

Q18. What type of monitoring device is available for healthcare workers who are present when intraoperative X-rays are being taken? (Ref. 47)

_____

Q19. If the patient is receiving radionuclides, no precautions or documentation is needed in addition to those used with X-ray or fluoroscopy. (Ref. 49)

True   False

● ●

Lifting and Moving

50. Work-related musculoskeletal disorders account for 1/3 of all occupational injuries and illnesses that are reported to the Bureau of Labor Statistics each year. Employers pay over $30 billion in worker compensation costs for musculoskeletal disorders each year. The average claim cost is $24,000, which increases to $40,000 if surgery is involved (Premier, September 28, 2004).

51. Indirect costs are estimated to be 4 to 7 times higher than direct costs, and can range from $147,000 to $300,000 (AORN, 2004b, p. 169). Indirect costs includes overtime, decreased morale, use of replacement workers, continual hiring and training cycles, and increased worker compensation and employee healthcare costs.

52. Back injuries are listed as the second most common reason for absenteeism in the workforce, following the common cold. Direct costs associated with occupational back injuries of healthcare providers average $37,000 (AORN, 2004b, p. 169). Healthcare workers experience 4½ more overexertion injuries than any other classification of workers (Premier, September 28, 2004).

53. Low back pain occurs more frequently in nurses than in the general population (Premier, September 28, 2004). Most back injuries last a short time and workers are able to return to work. However, for a small percentage of healthcare workers, the pain is long-term. Twelve percent of nurses leave the profession annually as the result of back injury (Sandel Medical Industries, Jan. 2004, p. 3). Factors that influence the number of back injuries include the aging workforce, staffing shortages, obesity of both patients and staff, and sicker, less mobile patients.

54. Most work-related injuries occur from cumulative injuries. Although the injury appears to be caused by a single incident, the underlying cause may be the previous years of repetitive trauma to the area. Lifting and moving heavy pieces of equipment and patients can cause injury when the healthcare worker exceeds his or her capacity to lift safely and puts excess force on the spine.

55. Lifting and moving surgical equipment, instrument sets, and patients causes many workplace injuries. Instrument sets often contain multiple, heavy, stainless-steel instruments that must be transported from place to place at different levels. Injuries include sprains and strains, acute or chronic lower back pain, and shoulder and neck injuries from lifting heavy instrument sets.

56. Factors that contribute to lifting injuries are height from which the item is lifted, the location and size of the item, and the gender, age, and training of the person doing the lifting. OR staff sometimes lift heavy articles and twist to the

side when moving them from place to place. In an effort to save time, staff may attempt to lift items, such as instrument sets, that are stored above shoulder level rather than use a ladder.

57. Using proper body mechanics when lifting heavy instrument sets can reduce the incidence of neck, shoulder, and back injuries. Safe lifting requires engineering designs to ensure that the physical conditions are safe for lifting; employee training in the correct lifting mechanics; and review of injury reports to identify common causes that need work redesign.

58. The following recommendations for lifting may prevent injury:

    • keep back straight
    • bend knees
    • clasp load close to the body
    • lift using leg muscles
    • do not turn or twist to pick up something
    • avoid lifting above shoulder level, lift objects that are chest high, use stool if necessary
    • when lifting, place feet apart to create a wide base of support

59. Preventing serious back injury when moving patients entails the use of adequate staff and lifting devices. An adequate number of staff members need to be present when moving patients postoperatively; 4 is the minimum number for anesthetized patients. A careful assessment of the patient will determine if additional personnel are needed. Safety devices used in the perioperative setting include slides, roller devices, and hoists.

60. Bariatric patients present special concerns. An estimated 30% of the general population is obese (Weise, 2004, p. 1). When the Body Mass Index (BMI) of the patient is greater than 38, special bariatric equipment will be needed. Lateral transfer devices should be used to move these patients. An air-driven mattress or friction-reducing sheet are useful.

61. Long periods of standing in one spot coupled with poor posture can cause back pain. When scrubbed, it is important to maintain good posture, stand with one foot on a standing stool, and change positions often.

62. Research demonstrates that specific interventions can reduce the reported rate of musculoskeletal disorders for workers who perform high-risk tasks. Support from top management is essential for a successful program. Both OSHA and JCAHO have identified safety as a top priority for healthcare institutions. Reduction of injuries and lost work time saves money in worker compensation costs and can lower the insurance premium for the facility. Promotion of a back injury prevention program requires a careful look at the extent and cost of injuries in the institution, a realistic and measurable goal, and a plan of action.

63. OSHA has identified the elements for a program to prevent back injuries (OSHA, Nov. 23, 1999):

    • wheels and other devices to move heavy equipment
    • mechanical devices for patient lifting
    • adequate staffing to prevent staff from lifting patients alone
    • training for new and experienced staff, addressing avoidance of back injuries
    • supervision of newly trained employees to validate learning
    • evaluation of workers prior to employment to identify preexisting back disorders

64. The action plan should review the current policies and procedures and identify needed changes to promote safety, determine the criteria for needing lifting assistance, assess the need for purchase and/or use of lifting equipment, and review the training needs for healthcare personnel.

    • The healthcare facility should first assess the current inventory of patient transfer equipment based on the patient population. It must decide what types of equipment will be needed and determine how frequently the equipment will be used. Thus the facility can ensure that adequate numbers of devices are available.

    • Policies and procedures focused on lifting protocols must become an important part of the program. Healthcare workers need definite criteria for making the decision on lifting assistance to ensure accountability for their actions.

    • Training programs should be provided for all levels of personnel, with the goal of training for management being focused on supporting the safe use of lifting equipment. Patient-care personnel should receive training to feel comfortable using the equipment and to ensure that they understand the benefits. Maintenance personnel should gain an appreciation for the preventive maintenance tasks they perform.

    • The program requires ongoing monitoring and evaluation in order to be successful (OSHA, Nov. 23, 1999).

Slips, Trips, and Falls

65. Workplace occupational hazards have been identified as a major contributor to nurses leaving the profession. Injuries to operating room personnel can easily occur if they are not aware of the physical hazards in the environment. Overexertion, repetitive stress injuries, and falls cost in excess of $6 billion in lost wages, healthcare expenses, legal costs, and worker compensation (Sandel Medical Industries, 2004b, p. 3).

66. The most common kinds of work accidents are slip and trip injuries. Slips and trips rose from 33% to 37% between 2000 and 2002. Falls take 715 lives per year and cause over 313,000 injuries that involve absence from work. Same-level falls account for 65% of all fall-related injuries. Average claim costs for a fall injury are almost $12,000 (Sandel Medical Industries, 2004b, p. 3).

67. Action can be taken by each person in the operating room to decrease the incidence of slips, trips, and falls:

- Placement of equipment, OR furniture, and supplies should allow for safe passage between them while carrying out patient care tasks.

- The multiple cords and hoses of electrical and mechanical equipment used in surgery present a tripping hazard and should be positioned out of the traffic pattern or safeguarded.

- Wet floors in the scrub sink area and in the operating rooms can cause slips and falls. Solutions spilled on the floor should be wiped up promptly.

- Nonskid protective footwear and support hosiery should be worn to safeguard the employee.

• •

SECTION QUESTIONS

Q20. Back injuries are the _____ most common reason for healthcare workers to be absent from work. (Ref. 52)

Q21. Factors contributing to the number of back injuries are (Ref. 53):

_____

_____

_____

Q22. Lifting and moving instrument sets can be accomplished easily and quickly because storage conditions promote safe transfer. (Ref. 55, 56)

True   False

Q23. List the principles for safe lifting. (Ref. 58)

_____

_____

_____

Q24. At least how many healthcare workers should be present when lifting a postoperative patient? (Ref. 59)

a. 2

b. 3

c. 4

d. 6

Q25. Name 4 elements of the OSHA back injury prevention program. (Ref. 63)

_____

_____

_____

_____

Q26. Ongoing monitoring and evaluation are needed to have a successful back injury prevention program. (Ref. 64)

True   False

Q27. Slips, trips, and falls have been identified as major factors in nurses leaving the healthcare setting. (Ref. 65)

True   False

Q28. Prevention of hazards leading to slips, trips, and falls are the responsibility of the healthcare facility. (Ref. 67)

True   False

• •

CHEMICAL HAZARDS

68. Each employee must be informed of the potential hazards of all chemicals used in the work setting, including information about disinfectants, skin prep agents, tissue preservatives, bone cement, chemotherapy agents, and any other chemicals used in the department. The Material Safety Data Sheet (MSDS) for each chemical must be readily available.

69. Manufacturers of chemical products must provide an MSDS for each chemical contained in the product. The MSDS describes hazards associated with the chemicals and describes first-aid measures in the event of exposure. Staff should know the location of MSDS sheets and be familiar with hazards and first-aid measures for the chemicals with which they work.

70. All employees must use the appropriate personal protective equipment and/or precautions when working with chemicals. Label instructions provided on the container must always be followed.

Formaldehyde

71. A 37% aqueous solution of formaldehyde is used in the operating room for preservation of surgical specimens. Formaldehyde can also be combined with water and methanol to make formalin.

72. Formaldehyde is a carcinogen (National Cancer Institute, July 30, 2004) that affects the nose and upper respiratory tract. It has a strong pungent odor that can cause watery eyes and respiratory irritation. When using formaldehyde, healthcare workers should wear gloves and ensure that there is adequate ventilation in the work area.

Methyl Methacrylate

73. Methyl methacrylate is an acrylic cement-type compound that polymerizes to form a strong plastic. Its uses include securing orthopedic prostheses and neurosurgical reconstruction of cranial bone.

74. Methyl methacrylate is supplied in separate containers of a liquid and a powder that are mixed just prior to being used. The combination forms polymethyl methacrylate, or PMMA. The liquid should always be poured into the powder to decrease the chance of aerosolization. The liquid component of PMMA is flammable.

75. Precautions must be taken when using methyl methacrylate, as it can cause skin rashes, itching and watering of the eyes, headache, and respiratory tract irritation. Personal protective equipment, including a face shield, should always be worn while mixing cement. Adequate ventilation using an exhaust hood or a suction evacuation bowl is necessary during the mixing process.

76. Double gloving is recommended when mixing the liquid and powder. The outside pair of gloves should be discarded once the cement has been mixed. Double gloving should be used by any staff who will be handling the cement to avoid penetration of the surgical gloves by the cement fumes.

77. Contact lenses should not be worn when working with methyl methacrylate because permeable lenses can be penetrated by the vapors, causing damage to the lens of the eye.

78. The use of electronic equipment should be deferred until the cement has set and all mixing equipment and supplies have been discarded.

Waste Anesthetic Gases

79. Anesthetic gases such as nitrous oxide and halothane are frequently used in the operating room. Exposure to waste gases may lead to neurologic problems or blood abnormalities.

80. NIOSH has set the recommended permissible exposure level for nitrous oxide of 25 ppm. Personal dosimeters are available to measure the levels of nitrous oxide present in the room. Each operating room is required to have a scavenger system in place so waste gases do not escape into the room atmosphere. Routine leak testing should be performed to ensure that the scavenger system is functioning properly.

Latex Considerations

81. Localized allergic reactions and skin irritation following contact with natural rubber latex have been recognized for many years, with the first reported case of hypersensitivity in 1979. Awareness of the potential for life-threatening systemic reactions has been increased with the advent of a sudden increase in systemic reactions.

82. Latex allergic reactions have been studied by clinicians, manufacturers, and regulatory agencies. The FDA issued a manufacturer's alert advising manufacturers how to reduce latex proteins in their products (FDA, Jan. 13, 1999). NIOSH issued a medical alert to healthcare professionals, advising them how to identify and treat reactions to latex (NIOSH, June, 1997).

83. Skin irritation reactions range from acute, with an immediate burning sensation and redness, to cumulative, with irritation that occurs after several weeks of exposure.

84. Latex allergy is different from irritant contact dermatitis. A true latex allergy may either be a type IV sensitivity or a type I hypersensitivity. Exhibit 12-2 illustrates the difference. (Exhibit 12-2)

85. Alternatives for operating room personnel include selection of nonlatex gloves, wearing glove liners, or changing brands of gloves, and monitoring for continuation of the allergic symptoms.

86. Localized allergic reactions can occur one to two days following contact with latex. Symptoms include redness followed by a rash and vesicles, with the skin becoming darker in color over time. Patch testing can assist with identification of the chemical causing the reaction. Once the chemical is identified, alternatives can be pursued. In severe cases, a temporary or permanent change of work area may be necessary.

87. Systemic allergic reactions to latex are less common but are the most hazardous. The reaction may occur immediately on exposure of the skin and mucous membranes to the allergen or after several incidences of contact with rubber latex. Usually caused by the proteins in latex, systemic reactions can occur on any contact with products made of rubber. Symptoms range from mild urticaria to anyphylaxis, and must be treated immediately.

88. Staff members diagnosed with a type I hypersensitivity to latex must avoid latex altogether and cannot work in an operating room environment. Many healthcare facilities have created latex-free protocols and often reserve specific operating rooms for patients who are allergic to latex. Staff members are provided with alternative latex-free products. The Safe Medical Devices Act requires all incidents of serious injury or death related to use of a medical device to be reported, including events involving latex allergy.

Exhibit 12-2   Reactions to Latex

Irritation	Delayed Hypersensitivity (also known as Type IV allergic reaction)	Immediate Type 1 Hypersensitivity
Non-allergic condition Dry skin Crusted skin lesions Papules Localized to contact area	Chemical allergy that activates the cellular immune system Symptoms appear 6 to 48 hours following contact. 　Dry crusted skin 　Eczema 　Hives 　Itching 　Redness 　Possible blisters Symptoms are localized but with repeated exposure may spread.	Allergic reaction mediated by IgE antibodies. It is a systemic reaction. Immediate onset 　Itchy eyes 　Rhinitis 　Hives 　Eczema 　Wheezing 　Swollen lips and tongue 　Asthma In rare instances may lead to shock and death.
Caused by friction or chemicals used in glove manufacturing.	Caused by reaction to chemicals used during manufacturing process or by manufacturing deficiency.	Caused by the proteins in latex.
Symptoms resolve when contact discontinued.	Symptoms resolve when contact discontinued. May not have reaction with change to another glove product.	Must avoid contact with all items containing latex

SECTION QUESTIONS

Q29. Manufacturers of chemical products must provide a document describing hazards associated with the chemicals and appropriate first aid measures in the event of exposure. This document is referred to as a(n). (Ref. 68, 69)

_____

Q30. What is the purpose of having formaldehyde in the operating room? (Ref. 71)

_____

Q31. What personal precautions must be taken when working with methyl methacrylate? (Ref. 75, 76, 77)

_____

_____

Q32. The FDA has issued a manufacturers alert advising latex manufacturers how to decrease the latex proteins in their products. (Ref. 82)

True   False

Q33. What alternatives do operating room personnel have if they suspect a latex allergy (other than a type 1 hypersensitivity)? (Ref. 85)

_____

_____

Q34. Define the symptoms of the following allergic reactions to latex (Ref. 86, 87):

Localized reaction _____

Systemic reaction _____

Q35. Allergic reactions to latex do not have to be reported, per the Safe Medical Devices Act. (Ref. 88)

True   False

● ●

● ● ● References

Association of periOperative Registered Nurses (AORN). (2004a). Recommended practices for reducing radiological exposure in the practice setting. In: *Standards, recommended practices and guidelines* (pp. 351–255). Denver, CO: Author.

AORN. (2004b). AORN position statement on workplace safety. In: *Standards, recommended practices, and guidelines* (pp. 169–171). Denver, CO: Author.

Bruley, M. (2003). Frequent questions on OR fire safety. *OR Manager, 19*(12), 17–18.

ECRI. (1992). The patient is on fire! A surgical fires primer. *ECRI, 21*(1), 19–24.

Food and Drug Administration (FDA). (1999). Premarket notification [510k] submission for testing for skin sensitization to chemicals in natural rubber products. Retrieved October 31, 2004, from www.fda.gov/cdrh/ode/944.pdf

Gruendemann, B., & Fernsebner, B. (1995). *Comprehensive Perioperative Nursing*, pp. 17–40, 267–288. Boston: Jones and Bartlet.

Koch, F. (2004). Fire safety in the OR. *Infection Control Today, 8*(8), 47–48.

National Cancer Institute. (2004). *Cancer facts.* Retrieved August 1, 2004, from http://cs.nci.nih.gov/fact/3_8.htm

National Institute for Occupational Safety and Health (NIOSH). (1997). Preventing allergic reactions to natural, rubber latex in the workplace. Publication No. 97-135. Retrieved Nov. 1, 2004 from www.cdc.gov/niosh/latexalt.html

Occupational Safety and Health Administration. (OSHA). (1999). Ergonomics program. retrieved October 31, 2004, from www.osha.gov/pls/oshaweb/owadisp.show_document?p_table=Federal_Register&p_id=16305

Premier. (2004). *Preventing back injuries in patient care.* Retrieved April 17, 2004, from http://www.premierinc.com

Sandel Medical Industries. (Jan. 2004). No. 2. Employee slips, trips and falls. [Brochure]. Author.

Sandel Medical Industries. (Jan. 2004). No. 5. On the job back injuries. [Brochure]. Author.

Smith, C. (2004). Home study program: Surgical fires—Learn not to burn. *AORN, 80*(1) 24–36.

Stewart, D. (2003). Fire and life safety for surgical services. *Surgical Services Management, 9*(2), 26–31.

Weise, E. (2004, July 16). Medicare redefines obesity as medical. *USA Today*, p. 1.

• • • Suggested Reading

Achmetov, T., & Gray, M. (2004). Adverse reactions to latex in the clinical setting: A urologic perspective. *Infection Control Resource, 2*(2), 1, 4–6.

Association of periOperative Registered Nurses (AORN). (2003a). Clinical issues. *AORN Journal, 77*(5), 1012.

AORN. (Sept. 2003b). Preventing surgical fires. *AORN Connections, 1*(9), p 12.

AORN. (Jan. 2004c). Survey identifies workplace safety issues of greatest concern. *AORN Connections, 2*(1), pp. 1, 4–5.

Bryant, K., Pearce, J., & Stover, B. (2002). Flash fire associated with the use of alcohol-based anti-septic agent. *American Journal of Infection Control, 30*(4), 256–257.

Flowers, J. (2004). Code red in the OR—Implementing an OR fire drill. *AORN Journal, 79*(4), 797–805.

International Occupational Safety and Health Information Centre (CIS). *International Hazard Datasheets on Occupation: Nurse, operating room.* Retrieved February, 2004, from http://www.ilo.org/public/english/protection/safework/cis

McCarthy, P., & Gaucher, K. (2004). Fire in the OR — Developing a fire safety plan. *AORN Journal, 79*(3), 588–600.

Van Milligan, G. (2003). Fire safety in the OR. *Advance for Nurses,* November 24, pp. 32–33.

Appendix 12-A

....

Chapter 12 Post Test

Instructions: Fill in the blank(s), mark the correct answer(s), or answer the question as appropriate.

1. Approximately 10 OR fires occur each year. (Ref. 8)

   True   False

2. The most common cause of fire in the OR is related to electrosurgery. (Ref. 8)

   True   False

3. The following items are potential sources for fire in the OR (Ref. 11, 12, 13, 15, 17):

   a. the ESU pencil

   b. fiberoptic cords

   c. hand cleaning solutions

   d. fire blankets

4. The acronym RACE stands for (Ref. 19):

   R _____ A _____ C _____ E _____

5. The best type of fire extinguisher for the OR is a _____ extinguisher. (Ref. 22)

6. Emergency shutoff valves should be turned off by fire department personnel only. (Ref. 32)

   True   False

7. Lead aprons should be hung on a rack when not in use. The reason is _____ . (Ref. 45)

8. Four factors that contribute to lifting injuries include (Ref. 56):

   _____

   _____

   _____

   _____

9. When scrubbed, techniques to prevent back pain resulting from long periods of standing in one place are maintaining good posture, _____, and _____. (Ref. 61)

10. The most common kinds of work injuries are trips and slips. (Ref. 66)

    True   False

Appendix 12-B

. . . .

Competence Checklist: Workplace Safety

Under "Observer's Initials," enter initials upon successful achievement of competency.
Enter N/A if competency is not appropriate for institution.

NAME _____

	OBSERVER'S INITIALS	DATE
1. Maintains active electrode in holster.	_____	_____
2. Does not wrap ESU cord around metal instrument.	_____	_____
3. Periodically cleans ESU active electrode tip of eschar.	_____	_____
4. Moistens gauze, sponges, etc., during surgery.	_____	_____
5. Prevents contact of activated fiberoptic cord with drapes and gowns.	_____	_____
6. Can state meaning of acronyms *RACE* and *PASS*.	_____	_____
7. Checks electrical cords before plugging in.	_____	_____
8. Identifies location of O_2 shutoff valves, LIM, fire extinguisher, evacuation route.	_____	_____
9. Can describe action to take if LIM alarms.	_____	_____
10. Wears lead apron and thyroid collar when potential for radiation exposure exists.	_____	_____
11. Hangs X-ray gowns on rack when not in use. (Does not fold.)	_____	_____
12. Uses correct body mechanics when lifting items and moving patients.	_____	_____
13. Places cords and equipment out of traffic pattern to prevent tripping injury.	_____	_____
14. Wears nonskid shoes.	_____	_____
15. Can locate MSDS sheets.	_____	_____
16. Uses suction bowl (exhaust hood) when mixing methyl methacrylate and wears double gloves.	_____	_____

OBSERVER'S SIGNATURE   INITIALS   DATE

_____

ORIENTEE'S SIGNATURE

_____

Chapter 12—Section Question Answers

Q1. False

Q2. Provide management support, involve employees in the plan, identify problems, implement corrective actions, address employee and patient injury reports, provide periodic employee training, evaluate ergonomics efforts

Q3. True

Q4. Identification of the various tasks in the work site, breakdown of each task into the steps required to accomplish the task, identification of any potential hazards, suggestion of ways to reduce or eliminate the hazards, development of standards for accomplishing the tasks, periodic review of conditions in the work area

Q5. d

Q6. An unexpected occurrence involving death or serious physical or psychological injury, or risk thereof

Q7. The scrub person should know the location of the active electrode (ESU pencil) at all times. The ESU pencil should be kept in a location away from the patient, maintained in a protective holder with the holder secured so it will not be dislodged by personnel movements during the surgical procedure. The ESU pencil cord should not be wrapped around a surgical instrument to secure it to the drapes.

Q8. True

Q9. R   Rescue people from flaming materials.

A   Alert others by announcing "Code Red" and the location of the fire 3 times.

C   Confine fire and smoke. Close the doors and shut off medical gas valves when leaving the room or when going from the fire area to a safe zone.

E   Extinguish the fire, if possible, using fire extinguishers. If the fire is immediately extinguished, call "Code Red all clear" and notify the Fire Department.

or

E   Evacuate to a safe place beyond the smoke or fire barrier doors, or outside. Activate the fire pull station when exiting the area. Remain with the patients and others in the safe area.

Q10. True

Q11. c

Q12. b

Q13. True

Q14. False

Q15. The LIM system measures the amount of current leakage and sounds an alarm if the current exceeds the threshold for safety

Q16. c

Q17. Lead aprons, thyroid shields, lead-lined gloves, eye protection

Q18. Radiation monitoring badge

Q19. False

Q20. Second

Q21. Aging workforce, staffing shortages, obesity of both patients and staff, sicker, less mobile patients

(continues)

Chapter 12—Section Question Answers (*continued*)

Q22. False

Q23. Keep back straight, bend knees, clasp load close to the body, lift using leg muscles, do not turn or twist to pick up something, avoid lifting above shoulder level, lift objects that are chest high, use stool if necessary, when lifting place feet apart to create a wide base of support

Q24. c

Q25. Wheels and other devices to move heavy equipment, mechanical devices for patient lifting, adequate staffing to prevent staff from lifting patients alone, training for new and experienced staff addressing avoidance of back injuries, supervision of newly trained employees to validate learning, evaluation of workers prior to employment to identify preexisting back disorders

Q26. True

Q27. True

Q28. False

Q29. Material Safety Data Sheet (MSDS)

Q30. Preservation of surgical specimens

Q31. Personal protective equipment, including a face shield, should always be worn while mixing cement; adequate ventilation; double gloving; contact lenses should not be worn

Q32. True

Q33. Selection of nonlatex gloves, wearing glove liners, changing brands of gloves, monitoring for continuation of the allergic symptoms

Q34. Localized reaction—redness followed by a rash and vesicles, with the skin becoming darker in color over time
Systemic reaction—mild urticaria to anyphylaxis; must be treated immediately

Q35. False

Chapter 12—Post Test Answers

1. False
2. True
3. a, b, c
4. R rescue, A alarm/alert, C confine/contain, E extinguish or evacuate
5. Halon
6. False
7. To prevent cracks
8. Age, gender, height from which item is lifted, training of person lifting, location and size of object/instrument set
9. Standing with one foot on stool, changing positions often
10. True

Active electrode: An accessory used in electrosurgery to deliver current from an electrosurgical generator to a patient for the purpose of hemostasis and/or cutting of tissue during surgery.

Aeration (ethylene oxide aeration): A process utilizing warm air circulating in an enclosed cabinet to remove residual ethylene oxide from sterilized items. The length of the process is determined by the composition of the sterilized items and the amount of residual ethylene oxide. The process generally takes from 8 to 12 hours.

Alcohol-based hand rub: A product containing alcohol intended for application to the hands for the purpose of reducing the number of microorganisms on the hands. Product is available as a rinse, gel, or foam. It is usually formulated to contain between 60% to 95% alcohol and contains emollients.

Aldrete postanesthesia scoring system: A scoring system used to evaluate the recovery of patients who have received general anesthesia. It evaluates patient activity, respiration, circulation, and oxygen saturation.

Anatomical timed scrub: A scrub procedure using a sponge/brush and an antimicrobial surgical scrub agent whereby a specified amount of time is allocated for scrubbing each surface of the fingers, hands, and portion of the arms with an antimicrobial agent.

Anesthesia standby: See moderate sedation/analgesia.

Antiseptic: A germicidal agent used on skin and tissue to destroy and prevent growth of microorganisms.

Asepsis: Absence of pathogenic microorganisms.

Aseptic practice/technique: The practices by which contamination from microorganisms is prevented.

Atraumatic suture: Suture that is attached to the needle during manufacture. The needle and suture are a continuous unit in which needle diameter and suture diameter are matched as closely as possible, thereby creating minimal trauma as the needle and strand are pulled through tissue.

Autoclave: A steam sterilizer.

Back table: Also referred to as an instrument table. A stainless-steel table covered with a sterile drape on which sterile surgical instruments are arranged for use during surgery.

Barrier (sterile): Material, such as a sterile drape or wrapper, that is used to protect sterility of items by preventing the entry or migration of microorganisms from an unsterile surface or area. Gowns, drapes, and package wrappers are examples of sterile barriers.

Bier block (intravenous block): A technique in which a local anesthetic agent is injected into a tourniquet-occluded extremity for purposes of analgesia.

Bioburden: A population of viable microorganisms on an item.

Biofilm: A collection of microscopic organisms that exist in a polysaccharide matrix and that adhere to a surface and prevent antimicrobial agents from reaching the cells.

Biological monitor (biological indicator): A sterilization monitor consisting of a known population of spores resistant to measurable and controlled parameters of a sterilization process.

Bonewax: Wax made from beeswax, used to stop bleeding from bone. It is used most often in neurosurgery and orthopedic surgery.

Bovie: Dr. Bovie was instrumental in developing the first spark-gap vacuum tube generator that produced cutting with hemostasis. Modern electrosurgical units are still often referred to as a "Bovies." The more accurate term is *electrosurgical unit.*

Bowie-Dick test: A test designed to test the steam sterilizer's ability to remove air and noncondensable gases from the chamber.

Capacitive coupling: The transfer of electrical current from the active electrode through the coupling of stray current into other conductive surgical equipment. Capacitive coupling can cause a burn injury, such as bowel perforation, during laparoscopic surgery that may go unnoticed and lead to peritonitis.

Capillarity: A process that allows tissue fluid to be soaked or absorbed into suture material and carried along the strand.

Certified registered nurse anesthetist (CRNA): A registered nurse with at least 2 years of anesthesia training after basic nursing school and acute care training.

Capnography: The measurement of the percentage of carbon dioxide exhaled during mechanical ventilation.

Chemical indicator: A device used to monitor one or more process parameters in the sterilization cycle. The device responds with a chemical or physical change (usually a color change) to conditions within the sterilization chamber. It is usually supplied as a paper strip, tape, or label that changes color or as a pellet that melts when the parameter has been met. A chemical indicator does not guarantee sterility.

Class 1—(process indicator) An indicator intended to demonstrate that an item has been exposed to the sterilization process. Usually a tape or paper strip that changes color to indicate exposure to the process. May be internal or external.

Class 2—Bowie-Dick test.

Class 3—(single parameter indicator) Indicator designed to react to one of the critical parameters of the sterilization cycle at a stated value of the chosen parameter.

Class 4—(multiparameter indicator) Indicator designed to react to two or more of the critical parameters of the sterilization cycle at stated values of the chosen parameters.

Class 5—(integrating indicator) Indicator designed to react to all critical parameters over a specified range of sterilization cycles and whose performance of the stated organism has been correlated to the performance of the stated test organism under the labeled conditions (AAMI, 2002, p. 2).

Circulating nurse: A perioperative nurse who is present during a surgical procedure, is not scrubbed, and is responsible for managing the nursing care of the patient and for coordinating and monitoring other activities during the procedure.

Clean wound (Class I): A wound in which the gastrointestinal (GI), genitourinary, or respiratory tract is not entered. No inflammation is encountered, and there is no break in aseptic technique. Examples of clean surgical procedures include her-

nia repair, carpal tunnel repair, and total joint replacement.

Clean contaminated wound (Class II): A wound in which the GI, genitourinary, or respiratory tract is entered under planned, controlled means. No spillage occurs, and no infection is present. Examples of clean contaminated procedures include cholecystectomy, cystoscopy, and colon resection.

Closed gloving: A method of donning sterile gloves in which the arms are inserted into the gown up to the point where the fingers reach the proximal edge of the gown cuff. Gloving is accomplished without the fingers or hands extending beyond the proximal edge of the gown. Only after the glove is donned are the fingers extended beyond the gown edge and inserted into the finger slots.

Contaminated: Soiled or potentially soiled with microorganisms. All items opened for surgery, whether or not they were used, are considered to be contaminated.

Contaminated wound (Class III): A wound in which gross contamination is present but obvious infection is not. Included in this category are incisions in which nonpurulent inflammation, gross spillage from the GI tract, a traumatic wound, or a major break in aseptic technique is encountered. Examples of contaminated procedures include gunshot wound, rectal procedures, colon resection with GI spillage, and inflamed but not ruptured appendix.

Cottonoid pattie: A small sponge made of compressed cotton. Often used in neurosurgery. There are a variety of sizes ranging from $1/4 \times 1/4$ inch to 1×6 inch.

Counted stroke scrub: A scrub procedure using a sponge/brush and an antimicrobial surgical scrub agent whereby a prescribed number of strokes is specified for scrubbing each surface of the fingers, hands, and arms.

Critical item: An item that is introduced beneath a mucous membrane or into a vascular space. Critical items *must* be sterile.

Decontamination: A process of cleaning, disinfecting, or sterilizing that renders items safe for handling by personnel not wearing personal protective equipment whereby they are no longer capable of transmitting infectious particles. Decontaminated items are NOT considered sterile.

Desiccation: An electrosurgical method of coagulation whereby an active electrode is in direct contact with tissue.

Dirty wound (Class IV): A wound in which an old traumatic wound with dead tissue exists or an infectious process is present. Examples of dirty or infected procedures include colon resection for ruptured diverticulitis and amputation of a gangrenous appendage.

Disinfectant: An antimicrobial agent used on inanimate surfaces to destroy microorganisms. The composition and concentration of the disinfectant and the amount of time an item is exposed to it determines the number and types of organisms that will be killed.

High-level disinfectants kill all bacteria, viruses, fungi, and some spores. High-level disinfectants are used only on instruments and medical devices.

Intermediate-level disinfectants kill vegetative bacteria, mycobacteria, viruses, and fungi. Intermediate-level disinfectants are used on environmental surfaces.

Low-level disinfectants kill vegetative forms of bacteria, lipid viruses, and some fungi. Low-level disinfectants are used on environmental surfaces.

Disinfection: Process that kills many or all living microorganisms with the exception of high numbers of spores.

Dispersive electrode: An accessory used in electrosurgery that is in contact with the patient and returns electrosurgical current from the patient to the generator.

Electrosurgery: A method of hemostasis that is provided when radio-frequency electrical current is passed through the patient's body. The energy is supplied from an electrosurgical generator, delivered to the patient from an active electrode, and returned to the generator via a dispersive electrode. Electrosurgery is used for purposes of cutting tissue or coagulating bleeding points.

Endogenous source of infection: A source of infection that arises from within the body.

Esmarch: Long piece of rolled latex used to drain the blood from an extremity. The extremity is elevated and Esmarch applied.

Ethylene oxide sterilization: A method of sterilization that utilizes ethylene oxide gas as the sterilant. It is used primarily for items that cannot tolerate the heat and moisture of steam sterilization.

Exogenous source of infection: A source of infection from outside the body.

Fasciculation: Skeletal muscle contractions that occur when groups of muscles that are innervated by the same neuron contract simultaneously. The contractions appear as twitching. Fasciculation following administration of depolarizing muscle relaxants progresses in a cephalocaudal sequence.

Flash sterilization: A steam sterilization process for sterilizing items that are needed immediately. Flash sterilization is utilized when there is insufficient time to process an item in the prepackaged method. Items that are flash sterilized are unwrapped and/or cannot be stored in a sterile state for future use.

Fluid proof: Prevents the penetration of fluids through an intact barrier.

Fluid resistant: Resistant to the penetration of fluids. Over time, fluids will penetrate.

Fulguration: An electrosurgical method of coagulation whereby sparking is used to coagulate large bleeders. The active electrode does not contact tissue. Sparks contact the tissue, causing superficial coagulation followed by deep necrosis. The purpose is to destroy tissue.

Gelatin sponge (Gelfoam): A sponge, resembling Styrofoam, made from purified gelatin solution and used for hemostasis.

Hemoclip: *See* ligating clip.

Indicator: *See* chemical indicator.

Induction: The period from the beginning of anesthesia through loss of consciousness.

Integrator: A device used to monitor more than one process parameter of the sterilization cycle. One example is a wicking paper that melts and progresses along the paper over time when the desired parameters have been achieved. The results are displayed in a window along the strip that indicates that the process is acceptable if the wicking reaches the target area on the strip.

Intraoperative: The period beginning when the patient is transferred to the operating room bed and ending with transfer to the recovery area.

Intravenous block: *See* Bier block.

Iodophor: A complex of free iodine combined with detergent that is used to kill microorganisms.

IV conscious sedation: *See* moderate sedation/analgesia.

Kitner: A small roll of heavy cotton tape that is usually clamped to a forcep and used for dissection or absorption.

Laminar air flow: A high-powered unidirectional air flow of about 100 ft/min; the air passes through a HEPA filter that removes all particles equal to or greater then 0.3 mu, with an efficiency of 99.7%. The intended purpose is to reduce airborne contamination.

Lap pad (tape): A square or rectangular gauze pad used for absorption where moderate or large amounts of blood or fluid are encountered.

Ligating clip: A stainless steel, titanium, or tantalum clip used to permanently clamp a vessel.

Local anesthesia: A form of regional anesthesia in which only a small, localized area is infiltrated with an anesthetic agent.

Local standby: *See* moderate sedation/analgesia.

Malignant hyperthermia: An emergency complication of general anesthesia that is characterized by a rapid rise in temperature (temperatures as high as 109.4°F [43°C] have been reported), extraordinary oxygen consumption, rapid uncontrolled muscle metabolism, and production of heat and carbon dioxide. Malignant hyperthermia is a crisis, and the patient will most likely die if not treated.

Mayo stand: A stand on top of which fits a removable stainless-steel tray. The legs of the stand slide under the operating room table and the tray extends over the patient. Instruments that are frequently used are placed on the Mayo stand. The scrub person hands instruments from the Mayo stand to the surgeon during the procedure.

Memory: A characteristic that causes a material to return to the state in which it was originally folded or placed.

Microfibrillar collagen (Avitene): A fluffy, white, absorbable material made from purified bovine dermis and used to provide hemostasis. Its application is topical. It is used for oozing or friable tissue.

Moderate sedation/analgesia (also referred to as IV conscious sedation, monitored anesthesia care [MAC], anesthesia standby, or local standby): A minimally depressed level of consciousness that allows a surgical patient to retain the ability to independently and continuously maintain a patent airway and respond appropriately to verbal commands and physical stimulation (AORN, 2004, p. 216). Medications are administered intravenously to provide sedation, systemic analgesia, and depression of the autonomic nervous system. This anesthesia technique may not require the presence of an anesthesia care provider. In the absence of an anesthesia care provider, the patient is monitored by the perioperative nurse with demonstrated competency in monitoring patients receiving moderate sedation/analgesia.

Monitored anesthesia care (MAC): *See* moderate sedation/analgesia.

Open gloving: Technique for donning sterile gloves. In this procedure, the fingers of the scrubbed person are extended beyond the cuff on the gown sleeve prior to gloving. Scrubbed hands touch only the inside of the gloves.

Oxidized cellulose: Oxidized cellulose (Oxycel, Surgicel, and Surgicel Nu-Knit) is a specially treated gauze or cotton that is applied directly to an oozing surface to control bleeding.

Passivation: A process used in making surgical instruments. The instrument is immersed in a nitric-acid bath solution that removes carbon steel particles and promotes the formation of a chromium oxide coating on the surface.

Peanut: A very small sponge approximately the size of a peanut that is commonly used for blotting blood. It is also used for dissection.

Peel pack: A see-through pouch made of plastic and paper, or plastic and Tyvek®, that is used to contain items during sterilization and to maintain them in a sterile state during storage.

Perfusionist: A member of the surgical team who is a highly skilled technician and who is responsible for operating the cardiac bypass equipment during open-heart surgery.

Perioperative: Encompasses the three phases of the surgical experience: preoperative, intraoperative, and postoperative. Perioperative nursing activities are activities that occur in any or all of the three phases.

Plasma (sterilization): Hydrogen peroxide gas plasma sterilizers use a unique technology consisting of hydrogen peroxide vapor and low-temperature gas plasma to rapidly sterilize most medical devices without leaving toxic residues. Plasma is a state of matter produced through the action of a strong electric or magnetic field. In hydrogen peroxide gas plasma sterilization, a plasma state is created by the action of electrical energy upon hydrogen peroxide vapor.

Pledget: Small piece of felt used as a support under friable tissues.

Plume: Smoke that results from cauterizing tissue—most often from application of electrosurgery.

Pneumatic sequential compression device: A device used to prevent formation of a thrombus. Device consists of a sleeve wrapped around the leg. The sleeve automatically inflates and deflates in sequential progression.

Postoperative: The period beginning when the patient is transferred to the recovery room and ending with resolution of surgical sequelae.

Preoperative: The period beginning when the decision to have surgery is made and ending when the patient is transferred to the operating room bed.

Prion: An infectious proteinaceous particle. Responsible for causing Creutzfelt Jakob disease and other spongiform encephalopathies.

Prep: *See* surgical prep.

Rapid readout biological monitor: An enzyme-based biological indicator that is used to monitor the sterilization process. Enzyme activity correlates to the inactivation of spores. Enzyme activity provides a reading that may be obtained soon after sterilization. A biological monitor is included within the product and may be incubated for an additional reading.

Raytex: Gauze sponge used where a small amount of blood or fluid is encountered. Supplied in 4 × 4 or 4 × 8-inch size.

Regional anesthesia: Regional anesthesia blocks the conduction of pain impulses from a specific region of the body. The patient is awake but does not feel pain during surgery.

Restricted area: An area within the operating room department where surgical procedures are performed and where sterile supplies are unwrapped. Surgical attire and hats are required apparel in this area. The Association of periOperative Registered Nurses (AORN) also recommends masks in this area.

Saturated steam: Steam that contains the greatest amount of water vapor possible.

Scrub: *See* surgical hand antisepsis.

Scrub person: A person who performs a surgical scrub on arms and hands, dons sterile attire, stands within the sterile field, and provides sterile instruments and other items to the surgical team during surgery. The scrub person is a member of the sterile team and is either a nurse or surgical technician/technologist.

Sellick maneuver: Manual compression of the esophagus between the cricoid cartilage and the vertebral column done for the purpose of visualizing the tracheal lumen and preventing regurgitation and aspiration during intubation.

Semicritical item: An item that makes contact with an intact mucous membrane but is not introduced below the membrane. Semicritical items may be sterilized but *must* be high-level disinfected when used on patients.

Semirestricted area: An area within the operating room department where surgical attire and hats are required. It includes peripheral support areas where clean and sterile supplies are stored. Traffic is limited to authorized personnel in surgical attire and to patients.

Sequential compression device: *See* pneumatic sequential compression device.

Shelf life: The amount of time an item may be assumed to be sterile. Shelf life is related to events and not to actual time. The longer an item remains on a shelf, the greater the possibility that an event will occur to cause contamination of the item. If no contamination occurs, the item is considered sterile for an indefinite amount of time.

Single-use device: A device manufactured for a one-time use. Not intended to be reused. Also referred to as a *disposable*.

Skin prep: *See* surgical prep.

Spore: An inactive, or dormant but viable, state of a microorganism that is difficult to kill. Sterilization methods are monitored by their ability to kill known populations of highly resistant spores.

Standard Precautions: Precautions designed to prevent the transmission of bloodborne and other pathogenic microorganisms. Under Standard Precautions blood, all body fluids, secretions, and excretions except sweat, whether or not they contain visible blood, nonintact skin, and mucous membranes are considered potentially infectious. Personal protective equipment, e.g., gown, gloves, mask, and eyewear, is appropriate when there is the potential for exposure to these patient fluids.

Steam sterilization: Process of sterilization that uses steam to kill all forms of microbial life.

Sterile: Free of all viable microorganisms, including spores.

Sterile field: The area immediately surrounding the patient into which only sterile items may be entered. A sterile field is created by placing sterile barriers over nonsterile items. The sterile field includes the area around the site of the incision and may include furniture covered with sterile drapes and personnel attired in sterile gowns and gloves.

Sterility assurance level (SAL): The probability of a viable microorganism, being present on an item after sterilization. The SAL for medical devices is 10^{-6}, or equal to or less than one chance in a million that there is a viable microorganism present on a device after sterilization.

Sterilization: A process that kills all living microorganisms, including spores.

Sterilizer (steam):
  Gravity displacement: A type of steam sterilizer in which steam displaces air through an outlet port by means of gravity.

Prevacuum: A type of steam sterilizer in which a vacuum is created to remove air at the beginning of the cycle and prior to steam entry into the chamber.

Pulse pressure: A type of steam sterilizer in which a series of steam flushes and pressure pulses at above-atmospheric pressure removes air from the chamber.

Strike-through: An event that occurs when liquids soak through a barrier from a sterile to an unsterile area or from an unsterile area to a sterile area. Strike-through renders items contained within the barrier unsterile.

Styptic: An agent used to cause blood vessel constriction. An example is epinephrine.

Superheating: Occurs when fabrics that are dehydrated are subject to steam sterilization. The temperature of the fabric exceeds the temperature of the steam. Superheating destroys cloth fibers.

Surgical conscience: An inner commitment to strictly adhere to aseptic practice, to report any break in aseptic technique, and to correct any violation, whether or not anyone else is present or observes the violation. A surgical conscience mandates a commitment to aseptic practice *at all times*.

Surgical counts: The counting of sponges, sharps such as blades and needles, and instruments that are opened and delivered to the field for use during surgery. Counts are performed prior to incision and before closing. Counts before incision and prior to closing should match. Counting is a safety mechanism to decrease the risk of items that are used during the surgery from being retained in the patient.

Surgical hand antisepsis: Antiseptic hand wash or antiseptic hand rub performed prior to surgery by surgical personnel to eliminate transient microorganisms and reduce resident hand flora. Done in preparation for gowning and gloving.

Surgical hand antiseptic: An antimicrobial product formulated to significantly reduce the number of microorganisms on skin. Products are broad spectrum and should exhibit both persistence and cumulative effect that prevents or inhibits proliferation or survival of microorganisms. Products used in preparation for gowning and gloving for surgery must be cleared by the FDA for use as a surgical hand antiseptic.

Surgical prep: Preparation of the patient's skin at the incision site. The patient's skin is cleansed with an antimicrobial agent to reduce the number of microorganisms at the incision site to as low a level as possible and to prevent rebound growth for as long as possible. The prep may or may not include hair removal at the incision site.

Surgical scrub: See counted stroke scrub, anatomical timed scrub, and surgical hand antisepsis. A process of cleansing the hands and arms for the purpose of removing as many microorganisms as possible from the hands and portion of the arms prior to donning a sterile gown and gloves.

Surgical site infection:

Superficial incisional: Infection involving only the skin or subcutaneous tissue.

Deep incisional: Infection involving deep soft tissue, e.g., fascia or muscle.

Organ/Space: Infection involving the visceral cavity or anatomic structures not opened during the surgery.

Suture: (**noun**) A strand of material used to tie a blood vessel so as to occlude the lumen or sew tissue together. (**verb**) To sew tissue using suture material.

Suture ligature: A tie with an attached needle that is used to anchor the tie through the vessel for purposes of hemostasis.

Tape: *See* lap pad.

Telfa®: Nonadherent wound dressing.

Tensile strength: The amount of tension or pull that a suture will withstand when knotted before it breaks. The tension or pull is expressed in pounds. Tensile strength determines the amount of wound support that the suture provides during the healing process.

Terminal sterilization: Sterilization of a wrapped package. Terminal sterilization permits storage of the sterilized item.

Thrombin: An enzyme made from dried beef blood that is used to control capillary bleeding. It is supplied as a white powder and may be mixed with water or saline to form a thrombin solution.

Tie: A strand of material that is tied around a vessel to occlude the lumen for purposes of hemostasis.

Tonsil sponge: Cotton-filled gauze in the shape of a ball with a long attached tape. It is used in the mouth or throat for absorption of blood. The tape extends outside the mouth to permit easy retrieval.

Transmission-Based Precautions: Transmission-Based Precautions are applicable for patients known or suspected to be infected or colonized with highly transmissible or epidemiologically important pathogens for which additional precautions are needed to prevent transmission. There are three types of transmission-based precautions:

Airborne, Droplet, and Contact. These are used in addition to Standard Precautions.

Airborne Precautions: Appropriate for protection against pathogens that are transmitted by the airborne route. Includes use of respiratory protection and special air handling and ventilation.

Droplet Precautions: Appropriate for protection against pathogens transmitted through droplets. Includes wearing a mask within 3 feet of an infected patient and positioning other patients at least 3 feet from infected patients.

Contact Precautions: Appropriate for protection against pathogens that are transmitted by direct or indirect contact. Includes wearing gown and gloves and cleaning and disinfecting patient equipment.

Tyvck®: Material made from high-density polyethylene fibers.

Universal Precautions: A method of infection control that requires that the blood and body fluid of all humans (patients and personnel) be considered infectious and that the same safety precautions be taken whether or not the patient is known to have a bloodborne infectious disease. The practice of universal precautions is a method of infection control that protects patients and operating room personnel. Universal Precautions have been incorporated into Standard Precautions.

Unrestricted area: An area within the operating room department where street clothes are permitted. Includes a control point where communication between the semirestricted and restricted areas is coordinated.

Washer-decontaminator: An automated processing unit that washes instruments for the purpose of decontamination. Includes washing, rinsing and a chemical or thermal process.

Washer-sterilizer: An automated processing unit that washes instruments for the purpose of decontamination. Includes washing, rinsing and sterilization. Instruments processed in a washer-sterilizer are not ready for patient use and must be subject to an additional sterilization process in a sterilizer.

Wound dehiscence: A partial or complete separation of the wound edges after wound closure as a result of failure of the wound to heal or failure of the suture material to secure the wound during healing.

Wound evisceration: The protrusion of the abdominal viscera through the incision as a result of failure of the wound to heal or failure of suture to secure the wound during healing.

Wound healing:

Primary intention: Wound healing occurs by primary union. Wounds heal by primary intention when minimal tissue damage occurs, aseptic technique is maintained, tissue is handled gently, and all layers of the wound are approximated. Wounds that heal by primary intention heal quickly and result in minimal scarring.

Secondary intention: Wound healing that occurs by wound contraction. Wound edges are not approximated. The wound is left open and healing occurs from the bottom upward. Granulation tissue forms in the wound and gradually fills in the defect.

Third (tertiary) intention: Wound healing that occurs when the wound is sutured several days after surgery. Wound suturing is delayed for several days to permit granulation to occur in an area where gross infection or extensive tissue was removed. Wound is only closed if there is no sign of infection.

• • • References

Association for the Advancement of Medical Instrumentation (AAMI). (2002). *Steam sterilization and sterility assurance in health care facilities.* (ANSI/AAMI ST46: 2002). Arlington, VA: Author.

Association of periOperative Registered Nurses (AORN). (2004). Recommended practices for moderate sedation/analgesia. In S*tandards, recommended practices and guidelines* (pp. 211–217). Denver, CO: Author.

Centers for Disease Control and Prevention, (CDC) Hospital Infection Control Practices Advisory Committee. (1997). *Part II: Recommendations for isolation practices in hospitals.* Retrieved July 3, 2004, from www.cdc.gov/ncidod/hip/isolat/isopart2.htm

Index

A

AAMI (Association for Advancement of Medical Instrumentation), 90
abdomen prep, 91
absorbable gelatin, 185
absorbable sutures, 240–241
accidents. *See* occupational hazards; patient injury
acid. *See* liquid peracetic acid sterilization
Active Electrode Monitoring (AEM), 195
active electrodes, 191–192
adhesives, skin, 248–249
advanced practice roles, 5
advocacy for patients, 3, 14. *See also* anxiety and fear, patient
anesthesia-related, 262, 292
dignity and comfort, 92, 133, 139, 281, 292
surgical positioning considerations, 141–142
transportation, 142
preoperative preparation, 6, 12
safety, 18, 65
AEM (Active Electrode Monitoring), 195
aeration cycles, 41
age of patients
educational considerations, 19
elderly, 19, 86, 139–140
pediatric patients
anesthesia for, 86, 268, 271, 276, 281
suture material considerations, 242
transportation of, 142
as preoperative assessment factor, 14
air filtration, 115
air pressure, 115
air removal tests, 29, 38, 47
airborne contaminants, 87–88, 114, 118
alcohol-based hand rubs, 97, 99–100, 311
alcohol-based prepping agents, 94

Aldrete postanesthesia scoring system, 261–262
allergies, 265
latex, 14, 101, 116, 321–322
medications, 14
tape, 141
American College of Surgeons guidelines, 18
American Society of Anesthesiologists guidelines, 265–266, 269
amnesia, resulting from anesthesia, 267. *See also* general anesthesia
analgesia, 267, 287–289. *See also* general anesthesia
anatomical timed scrub, 97
anesthesia, 259–305
anesthesiologist, role of, 6
anxiety reduced by, 267, 286
equipment, cleaning, 117
general anesthesia, 267, 273–287
malignant hyperthermia, 284–287
monitoring, 269–271
role and responsibilities of nurses, 281–284
moderate sedation (analgesia), 267, 287–289
monitoring during, 268–273
positioning patients, 132–133, 139–141, 289–290
postanesthesia. *See* postoperative period
preanesthesia and premedications, 265–268
previous complications with, 14
regional anesthesia, 267, 289–294
standby. *See* moderate sedation/analgesia
waste anesthetic gases, 321
antibiotic administration, preoperative, 12, 14, 268
antiembolectomy stockings, 142
antiseptic (antimicrobial) agents, 50, 91, 97, 99. *See also* sterilization and disinfection
anxiety and fear, patient
assessment for, 14–15
intraoperative, 292

as obstacle to patient education, 20
preanesthesia, 261–263, 265–267, 285. *See also* anesthesia
preoperative, 12, 17
reduction by anesthesia, 267, 286
AORN (Association of Perioperative Nurses)
anesthesia-related recommendations, 269
Official Position Statement on RN First Assistants, 5
Outcome Standards, 4, 12, 187
Perioperative Patient Focused Model, 2–3
Recommended Practice for Sponge, Sharp and Instrument Counts, 168
sterilization-related guidelines, 90, 108–112
tourniquet-related recommendations, 189
aperture drapes, 108
apnea. *See* general anesthesia
aprons, liquid-resistant, 97
argon beam-enhanced electrosurgery, 199
arms, patient, 134. *See also* positioning patients for surgery
arms, personnel. *See* scrubs and scrubbing
artificial nails as sources of infection, 87, 97
ASA (American Society of Anesthesiologists), 265–266, 269
aseptic practices, 83–130
antibiotics prior to surgery, 12, 14, 268
environmental sources of infections, 114–118
hand hygiene and prep, 87–88, 93, 97–100, 311
hypothermia, 143
prevention of infection, 12. *See also* sterilization and disinfection
Standard and Transmission-Based Precautions, 87–88
aspiration (pneumonitis), 266, 268, 283

assessment and interventions, 3, 6, 12–17
  age considerations, 19, 86, 139–140
  by anesthesiologist, 141
  communication of patient data, 20
  of patient knowledge, 17
  positioning patients for surgery, 139–140
  preanesthesia, 261–263, 265–267, 285. *See also* anesthesia
  preoperative preparation, 13–14
  wrong site surgery as result of inadequate assessment, 18
Association for Advancement of Medical Instrumentation (AAMI), 90
Association of Perioperative Nurses. *See* AORN
assurance. *See* advocacy for patients
atmosphere of operating room, 281, 292
attire, patient. *See* dignity, patient
attire, personnel
  gloves, 88, 97, 100–106
  gowns, 97, 100–106
  protective, 66, 87–88, 96, 315–316, 319
  scrubs and scrubbing, 5–6, 96–106, 112
    hand hygiene and prep, 87–88, 93, 97–100, 311
  surgical, 96–97
autoclaves, 29, 34–35, 46–49
automated systems. *See* mechanical cleaning
automatic blood pressure cuffs, malfunctioning, 134

B
babies as patients, 86, 271. *See also* pediatric patients
Bacillus atrophaeus spores, 48–49
back injuries, personnel, 317–320
"back" tables, draping of, 106
bacteria. *See* pathogenic microorganisms; spores; sterilization and disinfection
bagging the patient, 282
bandages for surgical positioning, 142
barbiturate induction agents, 276
bariatric patients, 140, 318
barriers and packaging materials, 69–72
basins, sterilizing, 73
beanbags for surgical positioning, 141

bedding, injuries caused by, 135
benzodiazepines, 277
BI (biological) monitors, 48–49
Bier blocks, 290–291
bioburden, 29
biofilms, 64, 66
biological hazards. *See* occupational hazards
biological monitors (BI), 48–49
bipolar electrosurgery, 190–192
blades, 216–219, 227
  counts, 172
  OSHA regulations, 88
blankets for surgical positioning, 141
bleeding. *See* hemostasis; tourniquets
blood flow restrictions, 135
blood pressure monitoring, 269–270
bloodborne pathogens, 88, 217
blunt dissectors, 218
body fluids safety precautions, 88
body temperature
  hypothermia, 143, 270–271, 283
  malignant hyperthermia, 271, 284–287
  monitoring, 270–271
bonewax, 186
Bovie machines, 190–192
Bowie-Dick Tests, 29, 38, 47
bowls, sterilizing, 73
box-lock joints, 216, 227
brachial plexus injuries related to surgical position, 134
breast prep, 94
breathing. *See* respiratory systems
bruises (pressure ulcers), 135
brushes. *See* scrubs and scrubbing
buccal bunch injuries related to surgical position, 134
burns. *See also* fire, risks of
  chemical, 188
  electrical, 143, 191, 194–196, 283

C
capacitive coupling, 195
capnography, 271
caps, 96
carbon dioxide, 271, 313
cardiac rate and rhythm monitoring, 269–270
cardiopulmonary resuscitation (CPR) certification, 292
care of surgical instruments, 215, 225–227. *See also* sterilization and disinfection
care planning, 3, 6, 12, 140. *See also* assessment and interventions

catheters during patient transfer, 143
caudal anesthesia, 290
cautery blades. *See* sharps
CDC (Centers for Disease Control), 30, 88, 236–237
cellulose-based wrappers, 70–71
Centers for Disease Control (CDC), 30, 88, 236–237
certification, CPR (cardiopulmonary resuscitation), 292
certified registered nurse anesthetist (CRNA), 6, 261
chart review, 14, 18–19. *See also* assessment and interventions
chemical burns, 188
chemical hazards, 41, 51, 188, 320–323
chemical hemostasis, 185–186
chemical indicators, 29, 47–48, 70, 74
chemical sterilization, 33, 42–43, 46–47
children as patients
  anesthesia for, 86, 268, 271, 276, 281
  educational considerations, 19
  suture material considerations, 242
  transportation of, 142
circulating nurse, role of, 6
circulation, monitoring of, 269
circulatory system compromise, 133
clamps, 218–219, 226–227
Class 1, 3, 4, and 5 indicators, 74
"claw hands", 134
clean wound classifications, 236–237
cleaning equipment, 39, 65–69. *See also* preparation of equipment; sterilization and disinfection
cleanup of operating room, 115–117
Clinical Nurse Specialists, 5
clips, ligating, 186
closed gloving, 101–102, 104
closure of wounds and counts, 171, 238–250
clothing. *See* attire, personnel
coagulation, 185
collagen formation, 238
combination packaging, 71
comfort of patient, 133, 269. *See also* dignity, patient
communicating with patient, 17–18. *See also* education, patient-family
communication of patient data, 6, 12, 14, 20, 262–263
communication, personnel. *See* talking in sterile fields
communication with patient, 17–18
compartment syndrome, 147

complications. *See* hemostasis; injuries, patient; malignant hyperthermia; occupational hazards; patient risk

concern. *See* advocacy for patients

conscience, surgical, 90

conscious sedation. *See* moderate sedation/analgesia

consciousness, monitoring of, 269

consent verification, 17

Contact Precautions, 87–88

contaminated wound classifications, 236–237

contamination, 64–66, 87–88, 104, 114, 118. *See also* sterilization and disinfection

contents. *See* labeling packages

control of infection. *See* infection injury

control, quality, 45–49, 52, 187–188

conversation in sterile fields, 112, 281, 292

coordinators, scheduling, 7

coping. *See* advocacy for patients

"correct count", 168–169

cotton as packaging, 70

cottonoid patties, 170

counted stroke scrub, 97

counts in surgery, 167–182

coupling, capacitive and direct, 195, 198

CPR certification, 292

creating a sterile field, 106–108

CRNA (certified registered nurse anesthetist), 6, 261

cross infection. *See* infection injury

cultural beliefs of patient, 17

cups, sterilizing, 73

curettes, 218

currents. *See* electrical hazards; electrosurgery and equipment

cutting and dissecting instruments, 216–219. *See also* electrosurgery and equipment; ultrasonic energy devices

D

Daily Air Removal Test, 38

damage. *See* injuries, patient; occupational hazards

danger stage of anesthesia, 281

dantrolene sodium, 285–286

data. *See* assessment and interventions; documentation

decontamination, defined, 64. *See also* cleaning equipment; sterilization and disinfection

deep vein thrombosis (DVT), 142

dehiscence, wound. *See* wound management

delayed primary closure, 237

delivery of equipment, 66, 110–112, 114–115

dentures, presence of, 14

desflurane, 274–275

desiccation, 193

detergents. *See* cleaning equipment

devices. *See* equipment

diagnosis, nursing, 3, 6, 12, 17–18. *See also* assessment and interventions; patient outcomes

diagnostic testing, preoperative, 265

dignity, patient, 92, 133, 139, 281, 292

surgical positioning considerations, 141–142

transportation, 142

direct coupling, 195, 198

dirty wound classifications, 237

discharge procedures, 17, 19, 261, 288–289

disinfection. *See* sterilization and disinfection

dispersive electrodes, 190, 192

disposal of equipment, 170–172

dissecting and cutting instruments, 216–219

dissociative induction agents, 276

documentation, 6

counts, 168–169, 172–176

disinfection, 52

electrosurgery, 198

inadequate review and risk for wrong site surgery, 18

package information and identification, 74

positioning patients for surgery, 154

quality control, 45–49

reusable textiles, 73, 107

skin prep and infection control, 94–95

"time out" final verification, 19

tourniquets, 189

donuts for surgical positioning, 141

Doppler ultrasound, 148

dorsal recumbent position. *See* supine position

double gloving, 104

drains, 249

draping, 106–109

dressings, surgical, 249–250

Droplet Precautions, 87–88

drugs. *See* anesthesia; medications

dry heat sterilization, 33

dust covers, 75

DVT (deep vein thrombosis), 142

dynamic air removal sterilizers, 35, 37–38

E

ECG (electrocardiograms), 270

education, nurse, 5

education, patient-family, 6, 12–20, 263, 266

elastic bandages for surgical positioning, 142

elbow injury, 134

elderly patients
    educational considerations, 19
    infection, increased risk for, 86
    positioning, 139–140

electrical hazards, 143, 191, 194–195, 283, 310–311, 315

electrocardiograms (ECG), 270

electrodes, active, 191–192

electrosurgery and equipment, 190–201
    dispersive electrodes, 190, 192
    ESU (electrosurgical unit), 190, 310–311
    fire hazards, 310–311

elevators (dissectors), 218

embarrassment, patient. *See* dignity, patient

emergency procedures, 14
    anesthetic classification, 266
    counts, 169
    for malignant hyperthermia, 271, 284–287
    wrong site surgery risks, 18

emotional support. *See* advocacy for patients

endogenous sources of infection, 86–87

endoscopic surgery, 197–198, 222–223, 227

endotracheal tubes, 143, 282–283

enflurane, 274

environment as source of infection, 87, 114–118

Environmental Protection Agency (EPA) registered products, 115–117

enzyme-based indicators, 47–49

EO (ethylene oxide gas) sterilization, 32–33, 40–41, 48, 73–74

EPA-registered products, 115–117

epidural anesthesia, 267, 290

equipment. *See also* attire, personnel; occupational hazards; sterilization and disinfection
    care and handling, 215, 225–227

(equipment *cont'd*)
classification of, 30
cutting and dissecting instruments, 216–219
disposal of, 170–172
draping, 108
electrosurgical, 190–201, 310–311
inspection of, 65, 68, 226–227, 315
instrument tables, 106, 141–142. *See also* positioning patients for surgery
manufacturing of, 215–216
needles, 88, 169, 172, 227, 245
packaging, 47, 69–75, 110, 244–245. *See also* preparation of equipment
positioning, 141–142
retractors, 219–221
as sources of infection, 87
suction, 221–222
unusual and wrong site surgery risk, 18
errors (wrong site surgery), 18–19. *See also* injuries, patient
Esmarch bandages, 187
esophageal or precordial stethoscopes, 269–270
ESU (electrosurgical unit), 190, 310–311
ethnicity, patient, 17
ethylene oxide (EO) sterilization, 32–33, 40–41, 48, 73–74
evaluation of recovery, 3, 6. *See also* patient outcomes
evidence of infection, 85
evisceration, wound. *See* wound management
excitement stage of anesthesia, 280
exogenous sources of infection, 87
expectations of patient. *See* patient outcomes
expiration dates of equipment, 74–75
exposure, patient, 92, 141, 292. *See also* dignity, patient
extinguishers, fire, 311–313
extraneous objects. *See* counts in surgery
extremities. *See* positioning patients for surgery
extubation, 283–284
eye pads, 141
eyewear, protective, 88, 96

F
fabric packaging, 70
face shields, 88, 96
facial nerve injuries related to surgical position, 134

facilities. *See* operating room
falls, personnel, 319
family-patient teaching, 6, 12–20, 263–266
fasciculation. *See* anesthesia
FDA regulations, 75, 97–98
fear and anxiety, patient
intraoperative, 292
as obstacle to patient education, 20
preoperative, 12, 14–15, 17, 268, 281
reduction by anesthesia, 267, 286
feelings, patient. *See* fear and anxiety, patient
femoral obturator injuries, 135
fenestrated drapes, 108
fever. *See* malignant hyperthermia
fiberoptic cords and connectors as fire hazards, 311
fibrin, 185
filtration, air, 115
fingernails, 97. *See also* hand hygiene and prep
fire, risks of, 195–196, 310–311, 315, 321. *See also* burns
flammable agents, 196, 310
flash sterilization, 29, 38–39, 65
fluid-proof and resistant gowns, 100
fluoroscopy and radiation hazards, 315–316
Food and Drug Administration regulations, 75, 97–98
food restrictions, patient, 266
foot injuries, personnel, 135
footwear, personnel, 96–97, 319
forceps, grasping, 218–219, 226
foreign body injury. *See* counts in surgery
forgetfulness, from anesthesia, 267. *See also* general anesthesia
formaldehyde, 320
forms. *See* documentation
frequent hand washing. *See* hand hygiene and prep
friction injuries, 135
fuel sources as fire hazards, 310
fulguration, 193

G
gas, methane, 196
gas sterilization
ethylene oxide (EO), 32–33, 40–41, 48, 73–74
low-temperature hydrogen peroxide gas plasma, 41–43
packaging methods, 73
gauges. *See* mechanical process indicators

gauze sponges, 170
gelatin, absorbable, 185
Gelfoam, 185
general anesthesia, 267, 273–287
malignant hyperthermia, 284–287
monitoring, 269–271
role and responsibilities of nurses, 281–284
generators, 190–191
Geobacillus stearothermophilus spores, 48–49
geriatric patients
educational considerations, 19
infection, increased risk for, 86
positioning, 139–140
gloves and gloving procedures, 88, 97, 100–106
glutaraldehyde, 51
gowns and gowning procedures, 97, 100–106
granulation tissue, 238
graphs. *See* mechanical process indicators
grasping clamps, 218–219
grasping forceps, 219, 226
gravity displacement sterilizers, 35
grieving, anticipatory, 17
grounding pads, 192
Guedel, Arthur, 280

H
hair as source of infection
removal of (patient), 90–91
surgical attire to contain, 96
halothane, 273–274
hand hygiene and prep, 87–88, 93, 97–100, 311
handling of surgical instruments, 215, 225–227. *See also* sterilization and disinfection
harm. *See* injuries, patient; occupational hazards
hats, 96
hazards. *See* occupational hazards; patient risk
HBV (hepatitis B), 88
heads and necks. *See also* positioning patients for surgery
injuries related to positioning, 134
prepping, 93
healing, 237–238. *See also* wound management
healthcare workers. *See* personnel
hearing aids, presence of, 14
height and weight, patient, 14, 140
hemorrhaging. *See* hemostasis; tourniquets
hemostasis, 184–187

argon beam-enhanced electro-surgery, 199
electrical (electrosurgery), 190–201
ultrasonic energy devices, 198–199
hemostatic clamps, 186, 218
hepatitis B (HBV), 88, 116–118
high-filtration masks. *See* masks
high vacuum sterilizers, 35
hinges, 227
hip prep, 92
HIV (human immunodeficiency), 88, 116–118
holding clamps, 218–219
home laundering of scrubs, 96
hoods, 96
hosiery, 319
housekeeping, 115–117
human immunodeficiency (HIV), 88, 116–118
humidity, 115
hydrogen peroxide gas plasma sterilization, 32–33, 41–42
packaging methods, 73–74
hyperextension injury related to surgical positioning, 133–134
hypnosis. *See* general anesthesia
hypodermic needles. *See* needles
hypothermia, 143, 270–271, 283
hypoventilation, risk of. *See* respiratory systems
hypoxemia, 270

I

ICDs (internal cardioverter defibrillators), 198
identification of equipment, 74
improper packaging, 47
in-house sterilization. *See* sterilization and disinfection
inactive electrodes, 192
incisions. *See* surgical site infections (SSI); wound management
incorrect counts. *See* counts in surgery
indicators. *See* quality control
induction phase, 281
infants as patients, 86, 271. *See also* pediatric patients
infected wound classifications, 237
infection injury. *See also* preparation of equipment
control of sources, 86–87, 90–118
evidence of, 85
prevention of infection, 12, 83–130. *See also* sterilization and disinfection
antibiotics prior to surgery, 12, 14, 268

environmental sources of infections, 114–118
hand hygiene and prep, 87–88, 93, 97–100, 311
hypothermia, 143
Standard and Transmission-Based Precautions, 87–88
risk of, 18
surgical site infections (SSI), 85, 237
infectious waste, 88, 116, 171
inflammatory wound healing, 237–238
information. *See* documentation; family-patient teaching
inhalation agents, 273–276
inhalation risks, 195–196
injuries, patient, 18. *See also* positioning patients for surgery
burns, 143, 188, 191, 194–196, 283
counts, 167–182
hemostasis, tourniquets, and electrosurgery, 184–201, 218, 291
instrumentation-related, 65, 214
positioning-related, 133–139
shock, 191
wounds, 236
wrong site surgery, 18–19
injuries, personnel. *See* occupational hazards
inspection of equipment, 65, 68, 226–227, 315
Institute of Medicine, 18
instruction. *See* family-patient teaching
instrument counts, 172–173
instrument tables, 106, 141–142. *See also* positioning patients for surgery
instruments. *See* equipment
insulation, 195, 227
integrating indicators, 29, 47–48, 70–74
integumentary system injuries, 135, 140
internal cardioverter defibrillators (ICDs), 198
interventions and assessments, 3, 6, 12–17
age considerations, 19, 86, 139–140
by anesthesiologist, 141
communication of patient data, 20
of patient knowledge, 17
positioning patients for surgery, 139–140
preanesthesia, 261–263, 265–267, 285. *See also* anesthesia

preoperative preparation, 13–14
wrong site surgery as result of inadequate assessment, 18
interviews. *See* assessment and interventions
intraoperative period, 2. *See also* anesthesia; equipment
cleaning equipment during, 65–66
counts, 167–182
intravenous agents, 276–278
intravenous blocks, 290–291
intravenous lines during patient transfer, 143
intubation, 282–283, 288. *See also* anesthesia
ionizing radiation, 33
irritants. *See* allergies
ischemia, 135
isoflurane, 274–275
IV. *See entries at intravenous*

J

jackknife position, 149–150
JCAHO (Joint Commission on Accreditation of Healthcare Organizations)
National Patient Safety Goals (2004), 18
standards and recommendations, 308–309
Universal Protocol for preventing wrong site surgery (2003), 18–19
jewelry, personnel, 97
job safety. *See* occupational hazards
Joint Commission on Accreditation of Healthcare Organizations. *See* JCAHO
joint pain related to surgical positioning, 133–134
joints in instrumentation, 216, 227
just-in-time sterilization, 30, 33, 42–43, 46–47

K

kidney elevators and braces, 151
kitner dissectors, 170
knee injuries, 135
knives. *See* cutting and dissecting instruments
knowledge, patient. *See* family-patient teaching
Kraske's position, 149–150

L

labeling packages, 74
laminar air-flow systems, 115
laminectomy frames, 141, 149

language barriers with patient, 17
lap pads, 170
lap sponges, 65
laparoscopic surgery complications, 195
laparotomy draping procedure, 109
laryngeal mask airway (LMA), 282
laryngoscopes, 282
lateral position, 136, 150–151
latex allergies, 14, 101, 116, 321–322
laundry and laundering. *See also* cleaning equipment; linens
    contaminated, 88
    home laundering of scrubs, 96
    reusable drapes, 107
lawnchair position, 147–148
lead shields, 315–316
leak testing, 321. *See also* Bowie-Dick Tests
learning needs of patient. *See* family-patient teaching
legal accountability, counts-related, 168
legs, patient. *See also* positioning patients for surgery
    leggings (drapes), 108
    lower extremity nerve injuries, 134–135
    protective coverings for, 97, 142
length of surgeries and positioning considerations, 140
lenses (contacts), presence of, 14
lesions, 135
liability, counts-related, 168
lifting and moving hazards, 317–320
ligating clips, 186
Line Isolation Monitoring (LIM) systems, 315
linens
    injuries caused by, 135
    reusable, 116
    sterilizing, 73
liquid peracetic acid sterilization, 33, 42–43, 46–47
liquid-resistant aprons, 97
listening to patients, 17, 20. *See also* advocacy for patients
lithotomy position, 135, 146–147
litigation, counts-related, 168
LMA (laryngeal mask airway), 282
local infiltration (anesthesia), 267, 291
local standby anesthesia. *See* moderate sedation/analgesia
lot control numbers, 74
low-temperature hydrogen peroxide gas plasma sterilization, 41–42

lower-extremity nerve injuries, 134–135
lubrication, 67
lumened instruments, 73, 225–226
lungs. *See* respiratory systems

M
MAC. *See* moderate sedation/analgesia
maintaining sterile field, 108–114
malignant hyperthermia, 271, 284–287
malnourishment and positioning considerations, 140
malpractice litigation, counts-related, 168
managers, perioperative nurse, 6–7
manual cleaning, 66, 225
manufacture of surgical instruments, 215–216
marking surgical site, 18–19
marking systems. *See* documentation
masks, 88, 96–97
massage, 135
Material Safety Data Sheets (MSDS), 320
materials, packaging, 69–72
maturation wound healing, 237–238
Mayo scissors, 217, 227
Mayo stands, draping, 106–108
MEC (minimum effective concentration), 52
mechanical cleaning, 66, 98
mechanical hemostasis, 186
mechanical process indicators, 45–47
medications. *See also* anesthesia
    allergies to, 14
    preoperative protocols, 267–268
    taken independently of surgery, 14, 265
memory loss, resulting from anesthesia, 267. *See also* general anesthesia
mental capacity of patient, 17
methane gas, 196
methods of sterilization. *See* sterilization and disinfection
methyl methacrylate, 320–321
Metzenbaum scissors, 217, 227
microfibrillar collagen, 185–186
microorganisms, 86, 97–98. *See also* infection injury
minimally invasive surgery, risks of, 195
minimum effective concentration (MEC), 52

miscommunication-related errors, 18. *See also* entries at communication
mobility impairments, preoperative assessment of, 14
moderate sedation/analgesia, 267, 287–289
monitoring. *See also* quality control
    anesthesia, 268–273, 288–289, 292
    blood pressure, 269–270
    chemical indicators, 29, 47–48, 70, 74
    devices during patient transfer, 143
    job safety analysis, 309
    precordial or esophageal stethoscopes, 269–270
    temperature, patient, 270–271
monofilament and multifilament sutures, 240
monopolar electrosurgery, 190–192
motor injuries related to surgical position, 134
mouth. *See* motor injuries related to surgical position
moving and lifting hazards, 317–320
MSDS (Material Safety Data Sheets), 320
multi-parameter indicators, 47
multiple procedures and risk for wrong site surgery, 18
muscle relaxants, 277–278
musculoskeletal injury, 133–134

N
nails (finger), 97
NANDA (North American Nursing Diagnosis Association), 12
narcotics, 276–277
National Fire Prevention Association (NFPA), 308–309
National Institute for Occupational Safety and Health (NIOSH), 308
National Nosocomial Infections Surveillance report, 85
National Patient Safety Goals (JCAHO), 18
nausea, 268, 290
necks and heads. *See also* positioning patients for surgery
    injuries related to positioning, 134
    prepping, 93
necrosis, 135
needles, 245–248. *See also* sharps
    broken, 172
    contaminated, 88
    counts for, 169
    holders, 227

neonate patients, 86, 271

nerve blocks, 267, 291

nerve injuries related to surgical position, 133–134

nervousness. *See* anxiety and fear, patient

neuro sponges, 170

neuromuscular blockers, 277–278

NFPA (National Fire Prevention Association), 308–309

nitrous oxide, 273–274

noise in operating room, 281, 292

nonabsorbable sutures, 241–242

nonbarbiturate induction agents, 276

noncritical items, sterilization and disinfection of, 30

noncrushing vascular clamps, 218

nonsterile team members, 6, 96

nonverbal support, 281. *See also* anxiety and fear, patient

nonwoven wrappers, 70–71

North American Nursing Diagnosis Association (NANDA), 12

nosocomial infections. *See* surgical site infections (SSI)

nothing by mouth (NPO) status, 14, 266, 283

nurse responsibilities and roles, 4–5, 12, 85. *See also* assessment and interventions

  advocacy and support, 12, 14

  anesthesia-related, 262, 292

  preoperative preparation, 6, 12

  safety, 18, 65

  anesthesia-related, 261–263, 281–289, 292

  counts, 168–169

  equipment preparation, 65, 216

  fire safety, 311

  patient-family teaching, 6, 12–20, 263–266

  positioning patients for surgery, 139–140, 154

  safety, 18, 65, 311, 313

  wound management, 250

nurses. *See also* personnel

  managers, 6–7

  nurse practitioners, 5

nursing diagnosis, 12, 17–18. *See also* assessment and interventions

nutritional assessment, 14, 140

O

obese patients, 140, 318

observation, patient, 14. *See also* assessment and interventions

occluding clamps, 218

occupational hazards, 307–328. *See also* attire, personnel

  bloodborne pathogens, 88, 217

  chemical hazards, 41, 51, 188, 320–323

  cutting and dissecting instruments, 216–219

  fires, 195–196, 310–311, 315, 321

  housekeeping, 115

  OSHA regulations

    back injuries prevention, 318

    Bloodborne Pathogens Standard, 88, 217

    General Duty Clause, 308

    glutaraldehyde exposure, 51

    personal protective equipment, 96–97

    universal precaution standards, 88

  personal protective equipment, 66, 87–88, 96, 225, 315–316

  plume inhalation, 195–196

  sharps, 88, 169, 172, 227, 245–248

open-gloving, 102–104

open wounds. *See* wound management

operating. *See* intraoperative period

operating room. *See also* occupational hazards

  controlling infection, 87, 114–118

  location of, 114

  patient dignity within. *See* dignity, patient

operating tables, 106, 141–142. *See also* positioning patients for surgery

oral medications. *See* medications

orbital blocks, 267

Ortho-phthalaldehyde, 51–52

OSHA regulations

  back injuries prevention, 318

  Bloodborne Pathogens Standard, 88, 217

  General Duty Clause, 308

  glutaraldehyde exposure, 51

  personal protective equipment, 96–97

  universal precaution standards, 88

outcomes. *See* patient outcomes

outfits. *See* attire, surgical

overexertion, personnel, 319

oxidized cellulose, 185

oxygen

  fire hazards, 310–311

  oxygenation, monitoring of, 269–270

oxygen-carbon dioxide exchange. *See* respiratory systems

ozone sterilization, 43

P

pacemakers, 198

packaging of equipment, 47, 69–75, 110, 244–245. *See also* preparation of equipment

padding for surgical positioning, 141

pain relief. *See* anesthesia; medications

paper packaging, 71, 73

paralysis, 134. *See also* neuromuscular blockers

PASS (fire extinguisher procedures), 311

pathogenic microorganisms, 86. *See also* aseptic practices; infection injury

patient data. *See* documentation

patient injury, 18. *See also* positioning patients for surgery

  burns, 143, 188, 191, 194–196, 283

  counts, 167–182

  hemostasis, tourniquets, and electrosurgery, 184–201, 218, 291

  instrumentation-related, 65, 214

  positioning-related, 133–139

  shock, 191

  wounds, 236

  wrong site surgery, 18–19

patient outcomes, 3, 6, 12, 17

  anesthesia-related, 260–263

  AORN Outcome Standards, 4, 12

  counts-related, 168

  electrosurgery-related, 196

  positioning-related, 132–133

  prevention of infection, 29–30, 65

  surgical instrumentation, 214

  tourniquet injury–related, 187

  wound management, 236

patient risk, 18

  aspiration, 268

  burns, 143, 188, 191, 194–195, 283

  infection. *See* infection injury

  instrumentation-related, 65, 214

  positioning-related, 133–139

  prevention of injury

    counts, 167–182

    hemostasis, tourniquets and electrosurgery, 184–201, 218, 291

    wrong site surgery, 18–19

  shock, 191

  wounds, 236

  wrong site surgery, 18–19

patient temperature

  hypothermia, 143, 270–271, 283

  malignant hyperthermia, 271, 284–287

  monitoring, 270–271

patients
  advocacy and support, 3, 14.
    See also dignity, patient
  anesthesia-related, 262, 292
  preoperative preparation, 6, 12
  safety, 18, 65
anxiety and fear
  assessment for, 14–15
  intraoperative, 292
  as obstacle to patient education,
    20
  preanesthesia, 261–263,
    265–267, 285. *See also*
    anesthesia
  preoperative, 12, 17
  reduction by anesthesia, 267, 286
assessment and interventions, 3, 6,
    12–17, 139–140
  age considerations, 19, 86,
    139–140
  by anesthesiologist, 141
  communication of patient data,
    20
  of patient knowledge, 17
  positioning patients for surgery,
    139–140
  preanesthesia, 261–263,
    265–267, 285. *See also*
    anesthesia
  preoperative preparation, 13–14
  wrong site surgery as result of
    inadequate assessment, 18
children
  anesthesia for, 86, 268, 271,
    276, 281
  educational considerations, 19
  suture material considerations,
    242
  transportation of, 142
communicating with, 17–18
cultural beliefs and ethnicity, 17
dignity and comfort, 92, 133, 139,
    281, 292
  surgical positioning considera-
    tions, 141–142
  transportation of, 142
education of, 6, 12–20, 263, 266
elderly
  educational considerations, 19
  infection, increased risk for, 86
  positioning, 139–140
positioning. *See* positioning
  patients for surgery
preoperative preparation, 11–25
recovery. *See* postoperative period
  as source of infection, 86–87,
    90–95
transferring, 142–143, 154, 318

peanuts, 170
pediatric patients
  anesthesia for, 86, 268, 271, 276,
    281
  educational considerations, 19
  suture material considerations, 242
  transportation of, 142
peel packs, 71
peracetic acid sterilization, 33,
    42–43, 46–47
perineum prep, 92–94
Perioperative Patient Focused Model
    (AORN), 2–3
peroneal nerve injuries, 135
personal protective equipment
    (PPE), 66, 87–88, 96, 225,
    315–316
personnel, 2. *See also* attire
  anesthesiologist, role of, 6
  managers, 6–7
  movement of within operating
    rooms, 112, 114
  nonsterile team members, 6, 96
  nurse practitioners, 5
  nurse responsibilities and roles,
    4–5, 12, 85. *See also* advocacy
    for patients; assessment and
    interventions; dignity, patient
  anesthesia-related, 261–263,
    281–289, 292
  counts, 168–169
  equipment preparation, 65, 216
  fire safety, 311
  patient-family teaching, 6,
    12–20, 263–266
  positioning patients for surgery,
    139–140, 154
  safety, 18, 65, 311, 313
  wound management, 250
scrubbed personnel, 5–6, 96–106,
    112
  as sources of infection, 87,
    96–106, 112
surgeons, 6, 18
photodetectors, 270
physical deformities as risk for
  wrong site surgery, 18
physical hazards, 310–320
physiologic assessment, 14–17
pillows for positioning, 141
plan of care, 3, 6, 12, 140. *See also*
  assessment and interventions
plastic packaging, 71, 73
plated instruments, inspection of,
    227
platelet plugs, 185
pledgets, 170
plume inhalation risks, 195–196

pneumatic sequential compression
    devices, 142
pneumatic tourniquets, 187–190, 291
pneumonitis (aspiration), 266, 268,
    283
point-of-use sterilization, 43
polypropylene wrappers, 70–71
popliteal knee supports, 135
positioning patients for surgery,
    131–166
  anesthesia stage, 132–133,
    139–141, 283, 289–290
  basic positions, 144–151
  devices for, 141–142
  impact of, 133–139
  initial position techniques, 143
postanesthesia. *See* postoperative
  period
posterior tibial injuries, 135
postoperative period, 2
  anesthesia, recovery from, 261
  cleaning equipment, 66
  complications related to position-
    ing, 133–139
  discharge, 17, 19, 261, 288–289
  patient-family teaching, 19–20
  removing surgical attire, 104
  transfer of patient, 154
  wound management, 235–237
posture, personnel, 318
pouch packages, 71, 73
PPE (personal protective equip-
    ment), 66, 87–88, 96, 225,
    315–316
practice settings, 5
preadmission and patient-family
  teaching, 19
preanesthesia, 261–263, 265–267,
    285. *See also* anesthesia
precautions. *See* occupational hazards; prevention of infection;
  prevention of injury
precordial or esophageal stethoscopes, 269–270
preexisting conditions, 140
pregnancy and anesthesia, 265
premature infants, 86, 271
premedication and anesthesia,
    267–268
preoperative preparation, 2, 11–25.
    See also assessment and interven-
    tions; family-patient teaching;
    positioning patients for surgery
  anesthesia, 281. *See also* anesthesia
  diagnostic testing, 265
  hair removal, 90–91
  nursing diagnosis and intervention,
    12, 17–18

prevention of infection, 12, 83–130. *See also* sterilization and disinfection

antibiotics prior to surgery, 12, 14, 268

environmental sources of infections, 114–118

hand hygiene and prep, 87–88, 93, 97–100, 311

hypothermia, 143

Standard and Transmission-Based Precautions, 87–88

prevention of wrong site surgery, 18–19

skin prep and infection control, 5–6, 96–106, 112

prep solutions, 5–6, 90–106, 112

preparation for surgery. *See* preoperative preparation

preparation of equipment, 63–82. *See also* sterilization and disinfection

care and cleaning, 225–226

cleaning instruments, 39, 65–69

electrosurgical equipment, 197

inspection of equipment, 65, 68, 226–227, 315

packaging equipment, 69–75, 110, 244–245

storage of equipment, 43, 69–75

tourniquets, 188

preparing patients for surgery, 11–25. *See also* prevention of infection

antibiotic administration, 12, 14, 268

assessment and interventions, 13–14

communication of patient data, 20

draping, 106–109

nursing diagnosis, 12, 17–18

patient-family teaching, 19–20

prevention of wrong site surgery, 18–19

prepping agents, 94

pressure, air, 115

pressure (hemostasis), 186

pressure points, illustrated, 136–137

pressure ulcers, 135

pressures, time, 18

prevacuum sterilizers, 35, 37–38

prevention of accidents. *See* occupational hazards

prevention of infection, 12, 83–130. *See also* sterilization and disinfection

antibiotics prior to surgery, 12, 14, 268

environmental sources of infections, 114–118

hand hygiene and prep, 87–88, 93, 97–100, 311

hypothermia, 143

Standard and Transmission-Based Precautions, 87–88

prevention of injury. *See also* positioning patients for surgery

basic surgical instrumentation, 213–234

counts, 167–182

hemostasis, tourniquets and electrosurgery, 184–201, 218, 291

in workplace. *See* occupational hazards

wound management, 117, 235–237

wrong site surgery, 18–19

primary intention, 237

printout records. *See* mechanical process indicators

prion contamination, 66–67

procedure verification, 14, 17–19

procedures, multiple, 18

process indicators, 47

professional growth, 5

proliferation wound healing, 237–238

prone position, 136, 148–149

prophylactic antibiotics, 12, 14, 268

prosthetic devices, presence of, 14

protective attire and equipment, 66, 87–88, 96, 315–316, 319. *See also* occupational hazards

prothrombin, 185

psychological preparation of patient. *See* preoperative preparation

psychosocial preoperative assessment, 14–15

pulse oximetry, 270

Q

quality control

disinfection, 52

documentation, 49

sterilization and disinfection, 45–49

tourniquets, 187–188

questions. *See* family-patient teaching

R

RACE (fire procedures), 311

radial nerve injury, 134

radiation hazards, 315–316

radio-frequency electrical currents. *See* electrosurgery and equipment

radiopaque strips, 170

rapid readout biological monitors, 48–49

ratchets, 227

reassurance to patient. *See* advocacy for patients

Recommended Practice for Sponge, Sharp and Instrument Counts (AORN), 168

record keeping. *See* documentation

recovery. *See* postoperative period

regional anesthesia, 267, 289–294. *See also* anesthesia

Registered Nurse First Assistant (RNFA), 5

regulations. *See also* JCAHO

FDA regulations, 75, 97–98

infectious waste regulations, 171

OSHA regulations

back injuries prevention, 318

Bloodborne Pathogens Standard, 88, 217

General Duty Clause, 308

glutaraldehyde exposure, 51

personal protective equipment, 96–97

universal precaution standards, 88

relaxation stage of anesthesia, 280

religious beliefs of patient, 17

repetitive stress injuries, 319

reprocessing single use devices, 75

resident microorganisms, 97

respiratory systems, 133, 269–270

responsibilities of nurses. *See* role and responsibilities of nurses

restricted areas, 114

results. *See* documentation; patient outcomes

retained foreign bodies. *See* counts in surgery

retention sutures, 242–243

retractors, 219–221

return electrodes, 192

reusable textiles, sterilizing, 73

reuse of single use devices, 75

reverse Trendelenburg position, 146

rigid containers, 71–72

ring stands, 106

risks, occupational. *See* occupational hazards

risks, patient, 18

aspiration, 268

burns, 143, 188, 191, 194–195, 283

infection. *See* infection injury

instrumentation-related, 65, 214

positioning-related, 133–139

(risks *cont'd*)
prevention of injury
counts, 167–182
hemostasis, tourniquets and electrosurgery, 184–201, 218, 291
wrong site surgery, 18–19
shock, 191
wounds, 236
wrong site surgery, 18–19
RNFA (Registered Nurse First Assistant), 5
role and responsibilities of nurses, 4–5, 85. *See also* assessment and interventions
advocacy and support, 12, 14
anesthesia-related, 262, 292
dignity of patient, 92, 133, 139, 141–142, 281
preoperative preparation, 6, 12
safety, 18, 65
anesthesia-related, 261–263, 281–284, 286, 288–289, 292
counts, 168–169
equipment preparation, 65, 216
patient-family teaching, 6, 12–20, 263–266
positioning patients for surgery, 139–140, 154
safety, 18, 65, 311, 313
wound management, 250
role and responsibilities of surgical team, 5–7. *See also* anesthesia
role of surgeon, 6, 18
room temperatures, 115
rubber goods, sterilizing, 73
rubbing. *See* friction injuries

S
safety. *See* occupational hazards; patient risk; prevention of infection; prevention of injury
safety pins. *See* sharps
SAL (Sterility Assurance Level), 30
sandbags for surgical positioning, 141
sanitation, operating room, 115–117. *See also* sterilization and disinfection
scalpels. *See* cutting and dissecting instruments
scar tissue, 238
scheduling, 7, 117–118
sciatic nerve injuries, 135
scissors, 217, 226–227. *See also* cutting and dissecting instruments
scopes, 222–223, 227
screw joints, 216
scrubs and scrubbing, 5–6, 96–106, 112

hand hygiene and prep, 87–88, 93, 97–100, 311
sealing packages, 74
secondary intention, 237
securing patients. *See* positioning patients for surgery
sedation. *See* anesthesia
self-retaining retractors, 219–221
Sellick maneuver, 283
semi-fowlers position, 147–148
semi-sitting position, 147–148
semibox lock joints, 216
semicritical items, 30
semirestricted areas, 114
sensitivities. *See* allergies
sensory impairments, preoperative assessment of, 14
sensory loss related to surgical position, 134
serrated instruments. *See* surgical equipment
setup of operating room. *See* preoperative preparation
sevoflurane, 274–275
sharps
counts, 172
cutting and dissecting instruments, 216–219
disposal of, 116
needles, 88, 169, 172, 227, 245–248
OSHA regulations, 88
shearing injuries, 135
sheets for surgical positioning, 108, 141
shelf life of sterilized equipment, 74–75
shivering. *See* hypothermia
shock injury, 191
shoe covers, 96–97
shoulder braces, 134
shoulder prep, 92
signs of infection, 85
single parameter indicators, 47
single use devices, reuse of, 75
site verification, 14, 17–19, 142–143
sitting position, 137, 147–148
skeletal-muscle relaxation. *See* general anesthesia
skin. *See also* wound management
cutting and dissecting instruments, 216–219
infection risks, 86. *See also* infection injury
integumentary system injuries, 135, 140
intraoperative monitoring, 269

irritations and latex allergies, 14, 101, 116, 141, 321–322
preoperative assessment of, 14
prep (patient) and infection control, 90–95
prep (personnel) and infection control, 5–6, 96–106, 112
tapes and adhesives, 248–249
skin adhesives, 248–249
sleep. *See* general anesthesia
slips (falls), personnel, 319
smoking history, 265
sound in operating room, 281, 292
sources of infection. *See* prevention of infection
Spaulding classification of surgical devices, 30
spinal anesthesia, 267, 289–290
spiritual beliefs of patient, 17
splash guards, 96. *See also* masks
sponges. *See also* scrubs and scrubbing
counts, 170–172
lap, 65
spores, 29. *See also* sterilization and disinfection
SSI (surgical site infection), 85, 237
staff. *See* personnel
stainless steel instrumentation, 215
Standard Precautions, 87–88
standards and recommendations. *See* AORN; occupational hazards
standing positions, personnel, 318
stands. *See* Mayo stands, draping; ring stands
stapling devices, 248
steam sterilizers, 29, 33–35, 46–49, 66, 72–74
steam-flush-pressure-pulse sterilizers, 35, 38
sterile team members, 5–6, 97–106
sterilization and disinfection, 27–62. *See also* preparation of equipment
aseptic practices, 12, 83–130.
antibiotics prior to surgery, 12, 14, 268
environmental sources of infections, 114–118
hand hygiene and prep, 87–88, 93, 97–100, 311
hypothermia, 143
Standard and Transmission-Based Precautions, 87–88
Bowie-Dick Tests, 29
creating and maintaining sterile fields, 106–114

disinfection, 31
methods of sterilization, 32–35
  dry heat, 33
  ethylene oxide (EO), 32–33, 40–41, 48, 73–74
  flash sterilization, 29, 38–39, 65
  hydrogen peroxide gas plasma, 32–33, 41–43, 73–74
  ionizing radiation, 33
  just-in-time, 30, 33, 42–43, 46–47
  liquid peracetic acid, 33, 42–43, 46–47
  low-temperature hydrogen peroxide gas plasma, 41–42
  prevacuum sterilizers, 35, 37–38
  steam, 29, 33–35, 46–49, 66, 72–74
  steam-flush-pressure-pulse, 35, 38
  thermal, 33–34
  quality control, 45–49
  sterile storage, 43, 69–75
  Sterility Assurance Level (SAL), 29–30
stethoscopes, esophageal or precordial, 269–270
stirrups, 134–135, 148. *See also* lithotomy position
stockinette drapes, 108
stockings, antiembolectomy, 142
storage, sterile, 43. *See also* packaging of equipment
stretcher safety, 142–143
strike-through, 110
styptics, 186
substance abuse and preoperative assessment, 14
suction, 221–222
superheating, 73
supine position, 134, 136, 144–145
supplies. *See* equipment
support for patients. *See* advocacy for patients
support hosiery, 319
surgery. *See also* intraoperative period; postoperative period
  emergency, 14, 18
  location of. *See* operating room
  multiple surgeons, 18
  preparation for. *See* preoperative preparation
  role and responsibilities, 6, 18
  site verification, 14, 17–19, 142–143
surgical conscience, 90
surgical dressings, 249–250
surgical equipment. *See also* attire; occupational hazards; sterilization and disinfection
  care and handling, 215, 225–227

classification of, 30
cutting and dissecting instruments, 216–219
disposal of, 170–172
draping, 108
electrosurgical, 190–201, 310–311
inspection of, 65, 68, 226–227, 315
manufacturing of, 215–216
needles, 88, 169, 172, 227, 245–248
packaging, 47, 69–75, 110, 244–245
positioning, 141–142
retractors, 219–221
as sources of infection, 87
suction, 221–222
unusual and wrong site surgery risk, 18
surgical hand antisepsis, 97–100
surgical site infections (SSI), 85, 237. *See also* infection injury; sterilization and disinfection
surgical smoke risks, 195–196
surgical team, 5–7. *See also* personnel
surgical wounds. *See* wound management
suture materials, 238–245. *See also* needles
swaged needles, 245, 248
symptoms of counts, 168
symptoms of infection, 85

T
tables, operating, 106, 141–142. *See also* positioning patients for surgery
talking in sterile fields, 112, 281, 292
tapes, 141
  wound management, 248–249
teaching patients and families, 6, 12–20, 263–266
team members. *See* personnel
temperature, patient
  hypothermia, 143, 270–271, 283
  malignant hyperthermia, 271, 284–287
  monitoring, 270–271
temperatures, room, 115
temperatures, sterilizers. *See* sterilization and disinfection
tensile strength, 238
tertiary intention, 237
testing. *See* diagnostic testing, preoperative; quality control
textile packs, sterilizing, 73
thermal sterilization, 33–34

thermometers. *See* mechanical process indicators
thromboplastin, 185
"time out" final verification, 19
time pressures and wrong site surgery, 18
timed scrubs, 99
tissue. *See also* wound management
  cutting and dissecting instruments, 216–219
  infection risks, 86. *See also* infection injury
  integumentary system injuries, 135, 140
  intraoperative monitoring, 269
  irritations and latex allergies, 14, 101, 116, 141, 321–322
  preoperative assessment of, 14
  prep (patient) and infection control, 90–95
  tapes and adhesives, 248–249
titanium instrumentation, 216
tolerance to procedure, 269
tonsil sponges, 170
topical anesthesia, 291–292
tourniquets, 187–190, 291
towels as drapes, 108
toxic reactions, symptoms of, 291
tracking systems. *See* documentation
traffic patterns and sterile fields, 114–115
tranquilizers, 277
transfer of patient, 142–143, 154, 318
transient microorganisms, 98
Transmission-Based Precautions, 87–88
transmission of infection. *See* prevention of infection
transportation of equipment, 66, 110–112, 114–115
trauma. *See* injuries, patient
Trendelenburg position, 133, 145–146
trips (falls), personnel, 319
tubing, sterilizing, 73
Tyvek packaging, 71, 73

U
ulnar nerve injury, 134
ultrasonic cleaning, 67, 225
ultrasonic energy devices, 198–199
ultrasound, Doppler, 148
understanding, patient. *See* family-patient teaching
underweight patients, 140
uneasiness. *See* anxiety and fear, patient

United States Pharmacopeia suture standards, 240
universal precautions, 88
unrestricted areas, 114
unscrubbed personnel, 96
USP suture standards, 240

V
vacuum sterilizers, 35
vapor phase hydrogen peroxide sterilization, 43
vascular surgery, 140
venous thrombosis, 133
ventilation systems, 115, 142–143, 269
verification of patient identity and procedure, 14, 17–19, 142–143
violations, reporting, 90
vital signs, preoperative assessment, 14
vomiting, 268, 290. *See also* aspiration

W
warm-up jackets, 96

washer-sterilizer or washer-disinfectors/decontaminators, 64–66
waste, infectious, 88, 116, 171
waste anesthetic gases, 321
waveforms. *See* electrosurgery and equipment
weight and height, patient, 14, 140
Wilson frames, 149
wood, sterilizing, 73
workplace safety, 307–328. *See also* attire
    bloodborne pathogens, 88, 217
    chemical hazards, 41, 51, 188, 320–323
    cutting and dissecting instruments, 216–219
    fires, 195–196, 310–311, 315, 321
    housekeeping, 115
    job safety analysis, 309–310
    OSHA regulations
        back injuries prevention, 318
        Bloodborne Pathogens Standard, 88, 217
        General Duty Clause, 308

    glutaraldehyde exposure, 51
    personal protective equipment, 96–97
    universal precaution standards, 88
    personal protective equipment, 66, 87–88, 96, 225, 315–316
    physical hazards, 310–320
    plume inhalation, 195–196
    regulations, 308
    sharps, 88, 169, 172, 227, 245–248
    standards and recommendations, 308–309
wound management, 235–258
    classification of, 236–238
    closure, 238–250
    counts, 117
    delayed, 86
woven fabric packaging, 70
wrong site surgery, 18–19

X
X-rays
    count procedures and, 170–171
    radiation hazards from, 315–316